Short Notes for Dental PG Entrance Examinations

Including Review for Undergraduate Students

Volume III

- Operative Dentistry
- Pedodontics
- Oral Surgery
- Prosthodontics
  - Fixed Partial Dentures
  - Complete Dentures
  - Removable Partial Dentures
- Periodontics

This volume covers the following subjects

- ❖ Operative Dentistry
- ❖ Pedodontics
- ❖ Oral Surgery
- ❖ Prosthodontics
  - ❖ Fixed Partial Dentures
  - ❖ Complete Dentures
  - ❖ Removable Partial Dentures
- ❖ Periodontics

List of Contributors

1. **Dr Sandeep Goyal** MDS (Orthodontics)
   Associate Professor, Instt. of Dental Studies and Tech., Modinagar
2. **Dr Sonia Goyal** MDS (Oral & Maxillo-Facial Surgery)
   Sr. Lecturer, Instt. of Dental Studies and Tech., Modinagar
3. **Dr. Akshay Bhargava** MDS (Prosthodontics)
   Associate Professor, ITS Dental College, Murad Nagar.
4. **Dr. Nimit Garg** MDS (Periodontics)
   Sr. Lecturer, DJ Dental College, Modi Nagar.
5. **Dr. Bhavna Gupta** MDS (Pedodontics)
   Sr. Lecturer, MM Dental College, Mullana, Ambala.
6. **Dr. Ajay Bansal** MDS (Oral Pathology)
   Dr. R. Ahmad Dental College, Calcutta.

Short Notes for Dental PG Entrance Examinations

Including Review for Undergraduate Students

Volume III

SANDEEP GOYAL MDS (Orthodontics)
Associate Professor
Institute of Dental Studies and Technology
Modinagar, UP

Edited by

Sonia Goyal MDS (Oral and Maxillofacial Surgery)
Senior Lecturer, Institute of Dental Studies and Technology
Modinagar, UP

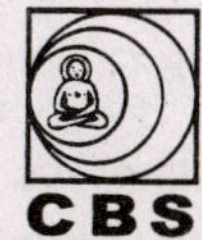

CBS PUBLISHERS & DISTRIBUTORS
NEW DELHI • BANGALORE

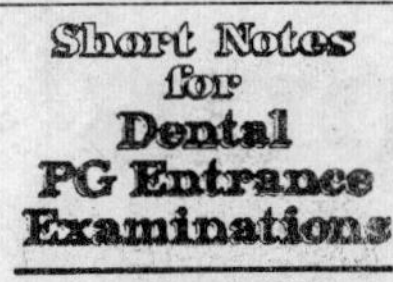

First Edition : 2006
Reprint : 2008

ISBN : 81-239-1233-1

Production Director : Vinod K. Jain

Published by :
Satish Kumar Jain for CBS Publishers & Distributors,
4596/1-A, 11 Darya Ganj, New Delhi - 110 002 (India)
E-mail : cbspubs@del3.vsnl.net.in
Website : http://www.cbspd.com

Branch Office :
Seema House, 2975, 17th Cross, K.R. Road,
Bansankari 2nd Stage, Bangalore - 560070
Fax : 080-6771680 • E-mail : cbsbng@vsnl.net

Typeset at CBS P&D Typesetting unit and printed at
Asia Printograph, Shahdara, Delhi - 110032 (India)

Dedicated

to

My Parents

and

My Family

Acknowledgment

I bow my head to God Almighty for all the grace He has bestowed upon me to bring out this book.

I am thankful to my parents for their unforgettable sacrifices and choicest blessings.

I affirm my deep gratitude towards my respected teachers: **Dr D N Kapoor**, Professor and Head, **Dr V P Sharma**, Professor, and **Dr Pradeep Tandon**, Professor, Department of Orthodontics and Dentofacial Orthopedics, Faculty of Dental Sciences, KGMC, Lucknow, for all their blessings, ideas and inspiration.

My sincere thanks to respected **Dr Sanjay Tiwari**, Professor and Head, Department of Endodontics, GDC, PGIMS, Rohtak, for all his support, appreciation and magnanimous help during my career.

I acknowledge my wife **Dr Sonia Goyal,** MDS (Oral & Maxillofacial Surgery), for her calm support, constant advice, contributions and editing of this project.

I acknowledge **Mr. Tarsem Garg**, Chairman, MM Education Trust, Mullana, Ambala, for his support and appreciation of the work.

I wish to thank **Dr Ragini**, Professor and Head, Department of Orthodontics, and Principal, ITS Dental College, Murad Nagar, for her support, blessings and advice.

I acknowledge **Mr S K Jain** and **Mr Y N Arjuna** and the team of CBS Publishers and Distributors for their best suggestions and help in getting this work published in the present form.

Last, but not the least, I acknowledge all my family members and friends for their best wishes to boost my morale.

Dr Sandeep Goyal

Preface

PG entrance examinations have seen a changed trend in recent times as the questions are mainly based on theoretical knowledge of the students, rather than totally on the available question-banks in the market. After receiving a good response for volume I from students and teachers, I have tried to improve upon the deficiencies in volume I and make modifications in volume II.

Volume III of *Short Notes for Dental PG Entrance Examinations* is the compilation of clinical subjects. It contains oral surgery, pedodontics, prosthodontics (fixed partial dentures and complete dentures), periodontics and conservative dentistry. Endodontics and orthodontics have already been covered in Volume I.

Again, emphasis has been given to compile the information in the tabulated form for easy reasoning and learning. Comparative evaluation has been done for many topics, especially in prosthodontics and oral surgery. We have tried our best to incorporate recent information also from the point of view of PG entrance examinations.

As I have emphasised in volumes I and II, I would mention here again that no compilation is complete in itself. It is the reader who can critically evaluate the book and contribute in its improvement. So I request all of you to send me your suggestions for improvement of volumes in their subsequent editions for the best advantage of the coming generations who strongly aspire to become dental specialists.

Again, I do not claim that this book will fulfil all the requirements of each student, therefor the aspirants are advised to refer the textbooks for detailed study of the topic of their interest.

I request the readers to evaluate the volumes critically and send me their invaluable suggestions for the improvement of the contents, because only criticism leads to progress and improvements. These suggestions will be solicited in future editions volumes of this book.

My e-mail addresses are: goyalsandeep2000@sify.com and goyalsandeep2000@rediffmail.com .

Lastly, I thank all of you for showing your faith in me and I wish all of you the success in your exams and fulfilling your dreams.

Dr Sandeep Goyal
Email: goyalsandeep2000@sify.com
goyalsandeep2000@rediffmail.com

Contents

1

Operative Dentistry

- **Operative** dentistry is defined as the diagnosis, prevention and Rx of defects of natural teeth. These defects can be dental decay, erosion, abrasion, attrition, hypoplasia, trauma, etc.
- **Diagnosis** is the statement of the nature of the disease or other conditions made after correlating the history of patient; signs and symptoms; clinical examination and the lab tests.
- **Prognosis** is an advanced indication or forecast of the course of the disease. It is the prediction of the duration, course and termination of a disease and patient's response to the Rx.
- **Signs** are the conditions related to the disease, which are observed by the doctor.
- **Symptoms** are those conditions related to the disease, which are observed by the patient and told to the doctor.
- **Treatment planning** is the blue print of the case management. It is a carefully sequenced series of events or services designed to eliminate or control the etiological factors, repair the existing defects and create a functional maintainable environment.
- **Dental emergencies** are those events in which, the patient is in dental related pain or in immediate threat of damage to the dentition or its supporting tissues, e.g. trauma.
- **Dental urgencies** are those incidents in which the patient is not experiencing pain nor is there immediate threat of sustaining damage to the dentition or supporting tissues. They do not require immediate attention.

- **Post-op. complications** are related to previously performed dental procedures, arising especially shortly after treatment. These are related to _____________.

RECENT RESTORATIVE TREATMENT

- **Chief complaint** is a symptom described related in the patients own words.
- **Cavity** = it is any defect in enamel/dentin due to pathologic process of dental caries.
- **Cavity preparation** = it is the performance of those dental surgical procedures required to expose the carious lesions, permit removal of affected tissues and so shape the remaining enamel and dentin as to contribute to a biologically and mechanically sound restoration.

Fundamental aims of operative dentistry are:

- Prevention
- Interception
- Preservation
- Restoration

Different systems of tooth designation:

1. **Universal system/American system** of tooth numbering (By ADA–CDA)

	(R)	(L)	
(1)	A B C D E	F G H I J	Primary teeth
	T S R Q P	O N M L K	
(2)	1 – 8	9 – 16	Permanent teeth
	32 – 25	24 – 17	

2. **Zsigmondy/Palmer system**–1861

- **Oldest system**, most widely used.
- Also known as angular/**grid** system/Chevron or set/square system.

8 – 1	1 – 8
8 – 1	1 – 8

E – A	A – E
E – A	A – E

3. 2-Digit system (FDI) system–1971

- First digit indicates quadrant.
- Second digit indicates tooth.
- Quadrants = 1–4 in permanent dentition.

  5–8 in primary dentition.
- Quadrants are allotted in clockwise sequence and start from upper right.
- Digits should be pronounced separately.

18 – 14 13 12 11	21 22 – 28
48 – 41	31 – 38

4. European system: for permanent teeth

8+ 7+6+5+4+3+2+1+ \\+1+2+3+4+5+6+7+8

8-7-6-5-4-3-2-1- \\-1-2-3-4-5-6-7-8

for primary teeth

05+04+03+02+01+ \\+01+02+03+04+05

05-04-03-02-01-\\-01-02-03-04-05

DIAGNOSIS OF DIFFERENT CONDITIONS

Vitality Tests (Refer to pedo/endo sections also.)

- Vitality tests indicate whether a viable nerve supply exists.
- Percussion verifies whether there is PDL inflammation.
- Electric pulp testing relies on direct electrical stimulation of sensory Ns of pulp.
- Lack reproducibility; depends on subjective nature of pain.

RADIOGRAPHY

VERTICAL ANGULATIONS

Teeth	Incisor	Canine	Premolar	Molar
Upper	+ 40 (50–60)	+ 45 (45–50)	+ 20 (35–40)	+ 10 (20–30)
Lower	– 15	– 20	– 10	– 5

- For incisors = the rays are through the nose to the extension of ala-tragus line.
- For canine = ala of nose along the interdental space between canine and first PM.
- Where the perpendicular from mid point of the infraorbital margin crosses the line of concentration/ala–tragal line or above the corner of mouth.
- Perpendicular 1 cm behind the outer canthus of eye crosses ala–tragus line.
- Anode film distance = 20 cm.
- Buccal object/SLOB/Clark's rule: it is also known as tube shift technique.

Entry point of rays

Teeth	Incisors	Canines	Premolars	Molars
Upper	Tip of nose	Ala tragus line	Zygomatic buttress	Zygomatic arch
Lower	Mid point of chin/symphysis 1 cm above the mandibular lower border	Corner of mouth	B/w para-symphysis and body of mandible	Angle of jaw

- For Mandible = Tragus–corner of mouth line should be parallel to floor.

- For Maxilla = ala-tragus line parallel to floor.
- Parallel cone technique = also known as 16″ technique.

Size of films

No.	Use	Size	
0	Pedofilm	22 × 35 mm	
1	Only 2 anteriors (less projection)	24 × 40 mm	
2	Adult film	32 × 41 mm	Mostly commonly used
3	Occlusal	57 × 76 mm	

Prevention from 2° radiations

1. 6 feet distance in a zone of 90°–135° from x-ray source.
2. 3 feet brick wall.
3. 1 feet concrete.
4. Gypsum boards on wall = 8–12 mm thick.
5. Lead point.
6. Lead shield.
7. Lead apron = 0.5–1.0 mm; mostly 1.0 mm.

   *Why lead? Due to its high atomic no. and compact crystal lattice, the x-rays cannot pass.

Types of lead aprons: Type 1, 2, 3 or heavy/medium/low; heavy is used for the patient, medium by operator.

- IOPA x-ray shooting requires time = 0.4 sec.
- Radiograph is C/I in pregnancy especially in 1st trimester and in untreated thyrotoxicosis/hyperthyroidism.
- **Inherent filter** = occurs due to glass tube and mineral oil; is approx 0.7 mm Al.
- Total filter = 2 mm Al.
- Mineral oil = to dissipate heat generated; so rest of the filter, i.e. 1.3 mm Al; by Al filter, etc.
- **Machine** = 70 kvp × 8 mA.

R/G

- Bite wing R/G help determine the proximal carious lesions.
- By the time, the proximal lesion can first be seen on enamel, the demineralization has often extended into dentin.
- Surface lesions without cavitation can get remineralised by fluorides.
- B/W, R/G are taken every 2 years because the carious progress is slow.
- Enamel, sclerotic dentin, primary dentin have descending order of radiopacity.
- 4 B/W R/G are required for the posterior segments of both arches.
- B/W R/G is exposed at 8° vertical angulation to minimize vertical overlapping.
- A devital posterior tooth usually requires a minimum of an MOD —protected cusp or only cast gold restorations because of susceptibility of fracture of tooth.
- Teeth of older patients require CUSP protection, because of increased friability with age.

Electric pulp tester: different types of responses are noted as follows.

No response	Either tooth is not vital or cusps are highly calcified; apical periodontitis
Moderately transient	Vital pulp
Painful transient	Hyperemia; reversible pulpitis
Painful lingering	Irreversible pulpitis

- The EPT and ultrasonic scaling are absolutely contraindicated in patients having pacemakers.
- If moderate transient response, it means the tooth is vital.
- A current of 5–20 mA is sufficient to modify the normal pacemaker function.
- False +ve readings = tooth is non-vital; it may be due to the factors, i.e. pulp tester touching the metallic restoration; improper

isolation; anxiety of the patient; liquefaction necrosis; coagulation; moist gangrenous pulp.

- Periapical lesions do not respond to pulp vitality tests except liquefaction necrosis and tooth having more than one root canals.
- False negative response = is due to heavily premedicated patients.
- In internal resorption = EPT is normal.
- Reversible pulpitis = sensitive to cold stimulus; relieved by hot stimulus.

ODONTALGIA is defined as pain in a tooth.

Referred pain = pain is often not well–localized within the oral region.

- Spontaneous pain and sensitivity to percussion are clinical s/s, which correlate with pulpal/PA response.
- Spontaneous pain is related to IRREVERSIBLE PULPITIS while sensitivity to percussion is related to PA inflammation.
- A single evoking stimulus of cold/sweets/biting pressure = implies reversible pulpitis.
- Spontaneous pain/prolonged sensitivity to heat, which is not relieved by cold–implies irreversible pulpitis.
- **Dentinal pain** = sharp, jabbing pain of short duration (< 1–3 min) upon removal of stimulus is a sign of reversible pulpitis.
- **Pulpal pain** = dull aching/throbbing pain of longer duration (> 5 min) indicates irreversible pulpitis.

DENTINAL PAIN (Also refer to section of endodontics in Vol. I.)

- Is a sharp lancinating pain.
- Easily localised.
- Immediately initiated by specific stimuli, e.g. heat/cold.
- Lasts for a few seconds to a few minutes after removal of stimulus.

PULPAL PAIN

- Dull, throbbing ache.
- Pulp does not contain proprioceptive nerve endings, so *pain is poorly localized*.

- Not associated with a stimulus.
- Slowly responds to heat.
- Reaction continues for a minute to hours.
- Sensitivity to heat checked by placing WARM impression compound for 5 sec.
- Ice/metal instrument chilled with ETHYLENE CHLORIDE spray is placed for 5 sec. to test sensitivity to COLD.
- Ability of pulp to recover from injury depends on its blood supply and not on the nerve supply.
- Pain of reversible pulpitis = subsides after removal of stimulus.
- Pain of irreversible pulpitis = lasts for several hours; pulsatile in nature; worse at night; cold helps in decreasing the pain; pain remains after removal of stimulus.

Erosion

- It is the loss of E/D from slow dissolution.
- Is a form of **chemical reduction** of hard tissues.
- Incisors have the greatest degree of erosion.
- It is generally seen in patients taking acidic drinks, having hyperacidity, etc.
- Lesion is of sharp V-shape.
- Lesion is most sensitive in initial stages, gradually becomes less sensitive as 2° dentin is deposited.

Abrasion is a **mechanical reduction** of hard tissues usually occurring over a long period of time.

Cervical abrasion occurs mainly from ***faulty total brushing***.

Attrition is loss of occlusal and incisal enamel, which occurs throughout life. Due to Aging/Stress. It is also a form of **mechanical reduction** of hard tissues.

Bruxism is diagnosed by the p.o. atypical wear facets on the teeth, which are generally outside the general range of masticatory functions.

Fractured cusps are most commonly the lingual cusps, mandibular molars and cusps of maxillary premolars.

Cracked tooth syndrome is due to incomplete fracture of tooth. There is sensitivity to cold.

- Sharp pain on RELEASE of pressure during mastication.
- Symptoms gradually intensify with time.
- Diagnosis by asking the patient to bite on a wooden stick.

Cracked tooth syndrome = diagnosis is done by asking the patient to bite gently on small rubber polishing wheels or an orange wood stick.

♦ Its best treatment is CAST RESTORATION.

REVERSIBLE PULPITIS

♦ Most common form of ODONTALGIA associated with reversible pulpitis is POSTOPERATIVE HYPERSENSITIVITY.

♦ Cavity preparation may lead to REVERSIBLE pulpitis, so should be made with adequate coolant, with sharp bur and with intermittent pressure.

♦ Gold has more thermal conductivity than amalgam and so gold castings have a potential for greater thermal sensitivity.

♦ Formation of reparative dentin and occlusion of dentin may result in decrease in sensitivity due to increased thickness of remaining dentin.

IRREVERSIBLE PULPITIS

♦ Electric pulp testing = NIL response.

♦ Tooth may feel elongated and sensitive to percussion.

♦ R/G = widened PDL.

Periapical pain = PDL has proprioceptors and so patient can localize the affected tooth.

♦ Acute periapical abscess = severe pain; tender tooth; drain pus and relieve the occlusion for its treatment.

MAXILLARY SINUSITIS

♦ Throbbing pain in all maxillary posterior teeth.

♦ May be result of common cold also.

- Is due to that the apices of teeth closely approximate the wall of sinus.

DISPLACED TEETH

- Intruded teeth usually re-erupt within 6 mos. in a young patient with no root fracture.
- EPT will normally give NO RESPONSE for at least 1 month after trauma.

Avulsed teeth: permanent anterior teeth of young adult = should be REPLANTED AS SOON AS POSSIBLE; tooth should be free in all excursive movements; RCT should be done within 2 weeks.

Root fracture: refer to section of pedo also

- **If in apical 3rd**—should be stabilized by splinting with adjacent teeth; successful in young teeth due to wide open apices.
- Prognosis is poorest if fracture is in gingival 3rd root.
- Most difficult to treatment = if fracture is in mid 3rd of root.
- **Union/healing**—refer to section on pedo also.

VERTICAL ROOT fracture—Poorest prognosis.

- **Attrition** is loss of surface tooth structure due to direct frictional forces between contacting teeth. It is a **physiological** process.
- **Abrasion** is a saucer shaped or wedge shaped lesion; loss of surface tooth structure due to a direct contact between teeth and external objects, e.g. tooth brush abrasion is most common; abrasives on powders, etc.; it is a **pathologic** process. It involves **only cementum**, as it is soft.
- **Erosion** is wedge-shaped lesion; loss of tooth structure due to chemico-mechanical means in the absence of specific bacteria; it is one of the most predominant oral **pathologic changes,** e.g. by excessive soft drinks; hyperacidity; recurrent vomiting tendency; excessive intake of citrus juices; it involves **enamel** only.

DISCOLORATION OF TEETH It is of 2 types (Refer to pedosection also).

- **Extrinsic** is due to surface staining.
- **Intrinsic** is internal and is due to changes in one or more tooth tissues.
- **Tetracycline** has 9 times more affinity for dentin than enamel; it forms chelates with calcium; can cross placenta; gets secreted in breast milk.
- **Fluorides**
- **Corrosion** products of amalgam enter in dentinal tubules; also the products of pulp necrosis, blood, etc.
- **Porphyria**

Bleaching

- 5 parts of 30% H_2O_2 + 1 part ethyl ether
  sodium perborate + 30% H_2O_2 to make paste
  heated at 110°–130°F for 1–3 min.

Indirect pulp capping

- Leaving some softened dentin at base of cavity to avoid pulp exposure.
- Softening of dentin precedes bacterial invasion.
- Pulpitis does not occur until bacteria are within 0.5–1.0 mm of pulp.
- $Ca(OH)_2$ with alkaline pH is bacteriostatic and helps formation of calcific bridge of secondary dentin and arrests the caries.

Materials required

ZOE	Sterilises the underlying dentin Decreases PG synthesis Aids remineralisation; hygroscopic
$Ca(OH)_2$	Alkaline pH Bacteriostatic Helps calcific barrier formation Zone of pulpal necrosis occurs, which gets mineralized with Ca^{++} ions from the pulp.

Materials required (*Contd.*)

Ledermix	Triamcinolone acetonide + dimethyl chlortetracycline mixture Antiinflammatory and bacteriostatic Also decreases pulp defenses.

CARIES (Also refer to section of oral pathology in Vol. I.)

Characteristics of caries

- **Caries** is the slowly progressing, irreversible decay of dental hard tissue, which is characterized by demineralization of inorganic part and disintegration of organic structure.
- Carious lesion tends to spread more rapidly in lateral direction along DEJ than along the dentinal tubules.
- **Bacteria responsible** for caries is *Strept. mutans.*
- Sugar responsible = sucrose.
- **First sign** of caries is opacity.
- **Difference between opacity of caries and hypoplasia/ hypocalcification** = incipient caries lesion becomes translucent after wetting and again becomes opaque after drying. But, the developmental defects are not affected by wetting process.

Facts about caries

- **Miller's chemoparasitic theory** = dissolution of inorganic salts, i.e. HA crystals of the tooth occurs by acids produced.
- *Strept. mutans* is main bacteria for initiation of caries, and **lactobacilli** is for P and F caries and **actenomyces** in root caries.
- **Main sugar** implicated in caries = **sucrose.**
- **Rampant caries** occurs on smooth facial surfaces of teeth; also seen in xerostomia after radiation therapy.
- **Initial caries** starts with *S. mutans*; then lactobacilli aciduric bacteria predominate in the larger lesions.
- SnF_2 is the most effective in decreasing *S. mutans*, levels in saliva, among the various Fluoride preparations available.

Caries disclosing dyes

- Used to find out the soundness of the dentin.
- **0.5% solution of basic fuchsin** in propylene glycol is used.
- Stained dentin has 1300 times more bacteria per mg of dentin than the unstained dentin.
- **Plaque disclosing agents** = 4% erythrosine.
- 5% Na–MFP is the abrasive in tooth powders.
- Saliva can be cultured on selective MSB medium to find out the count of *S. mutans*. MSB contain bacitracin and sucrose broth.
- High caries Risk = if *S. mutans* level is 10^6 CFU/ml (CFU = colony forming units).
- Best caries prevention is by = F + professional debridement + dietary counselling.
- Medium for lactobacilli uses pH = 5.
- If > 10^5 CFU/ml of lactobacilli = implies high caries.
- If < 10^4 CFU/ml of lactobacilli = low caries risk.
- **Xylitol is most effective sucrose substitute** in decreasing decay.
- 10^6 strept mutans bacteria/ml of saliva are required to start the caries.
- **Acidogenic theory** = acids produced from carbohydrates decalcifies inorganic part of teeth, and then the organic part is disintegrated creating cavities.
- **Proteolysis theory** = organic part of tooth is attacked first with certain lytic enzymes. This leaves the inorganic part without a matrix support, which gets washed away creating cavities.
- **Caries triad** = there must be 3 factors, i.e. host/tooth + parasite/bacteria + medium/carbohydrate. A fourth factor has been added to it as time (Keyes triad).
- Caries susceptibility of a tooth is inversely proportional to its F, Ca and Sn contents.
- Caries susceptibility of a tooth is inversely proportional to salivary phosphate content.
- Higher organic content of saliva indicates more plaque accumulations.

- Higher alkaline saliva predisposes to less decay.
- Serous saliva/low viscosity causes more self-cleansing action.
- Higher quantities of saliva flow lead to less caries.
- Plaque adheres to tooth surface with a sticking polysaccharide known as **dextran.**
- *Strept. mutans* is the main cariogenic bacteria.
- Sucrose is the main carbohydrate causing caries.
- Anti-caries bacteria = veillonella.
- Genetic modification to prevent caries.
- **Fluorides** = decrease caries activity by decreasing solubility of tooth structure, decreasing surface energy of tooth surface, decreases plaque adhesion interferes in carbohydrate metabolism by bacteria.
- Increasing phosphate content in diet = decreases the solubility of inorganic substance of the tooth.
- Vitamin K = is anti-cariogenic.
- ***First component of enamel to be involved in caries is the interprismatic substance.*** Caries spreads in the form of a cone; the base of cone is towards DEJ in P and F caries and away from DEJ in smooth/convex surfaces.

Caries progress: Also refer to the sections of oral pathology and pedodontics.

- In P and F, the caries spreads along the divergence of enamel rods in the form of a CONE, the base of the cone is at DEJ.
- Spread of caries along DEJ is more RAPID than through enamel.
- Caries through dentin spreads as CONE, the base is also at DEJ.
- P and F caries = is seen as a small external clinical lesion, but internally more spread.
- Smooth surface lesions = base of cone is at outer enamel surface. Starts below plaque and below the contact areas.

First component of dentin involved is ***protoplasmic extensions within the dentinal tubules***, which are wider at DEJ and narrower at pulp. So caries cone in dentin has its base at DEJ.

Classification of caries–by Black–

Class	Features
I	P and F cavities at occlusal surfaces of M, PM, and pits on buccal/lingual surfaces of I/PM/M.
II	Cavities on proximal surfaces of PM/M. **Smooth surface** lesion.
III	Proximal surface of incisors/cuspids, but not involving incisal edges. **Smooth surface** lesion.
IV	On proximal surfaces of I/C, involving incisal edges. **Smooth surface** lesion.
V	In gingival 3rd of any tooth; mostly seen in older age group due to gingival recession.
VI	MOD cavity; and incisal edges and cusp tips of teeth.

Black's classification of caries = is a **therapeutic classification**; as it is based on Rx and restoration designs.

Class	Features
I. on all teeth	Begin in structural defects, e.g. P and F and grooves, e.g. occlusal surfaces of M and PM; the occlusal 2/3rd of buccal and lingual surfaces of molars; and the lingual surfaces of anteriors.
II. on posterior teeth	On proximal surfaces of M and PM.
III. on anterior teeth	On proximal surfaces of anteriors without involving incisal edge and angle.
IV. on anterior teeth	On proximal surfaces of anteriors and involving incisal edge and angle.
V. on all teeth	At gingival 3rd of facial/lingual surfaces of anterior and posterior teeth.
VI. on all teeth	On incisal edges and cuspal tips or on any highly self-cleansable areas.

Types of cavities: Classification of decay

Type	Features
Incipient/initial/	Is ***the first attack*** on a tooth surface.
Recurrent/secondary primary caries	Is seen ***under or around the margins*** or surrounding wall of an existing restoration.
Acute or rampant caries	Is a ***rapidly invading*** process, which involves several teeth. Lesions are soft and light coloured and mostly with severe pulpal reactions.
Chronic caries	Are of variable depth, longer standing; and tend to be fewer in number; dentin is hard and dark in colour.
Pit and fissure caries	Originates in P and F of teeth, e.g. on lingual surface of maxillary incisors; and buccal, lingual and occlusal surfaces of posterior teeth.
Smooth surface caries	Originates on all surfaces without P and F and grooves.
Forward decay	i.e. when caries cone in enamel is larger than in dentin or of same size, it is known as forward decay, as seen ***in Pit caries***.
Backward decay	When caries process in dentin is much faster than enamel, the lateral spread of caries may occur, which undermines the enamel. It may attack the enamel from the dentinal side. It is seen in ***smooth surface lesions***.
Senile caries	Are associated with ageing and are present almost on root surfaces.

Types of cavities: Classification of decay *(Contd.)*

Type	Features
Residual caries	Is that which is not removed during a restorative process, either by accident, neglect or intention.
Simple caries	Which involves ***only one surface*** of the tooth.
Compound caries	Which involves ***two surfaces*** of the tooth.
Complex caries	Which involves ***more than two surfaces*** of the tooth.

Features of carious lesions

- Opacity adjacent to Pit/fissure as evidence of undermining/ demineralization.
- Loss of normal translucency of enamel showing undermining.
- **Decalcification of enamel is first stage** of caries process.
- Decalcified enamel is white and opaque.
- White spot seen due to **subsurface demineralization**; the area is soft.

Smooth surface carious lesions = seen on proximal surfaces just below the contact area; have broad area of initiation. It is diagnosed by:

- If MR (marginal ridge) is opaque due to undermining of enamel.
- R/G shows radiolucency due to break in surface continuity.
- Transillumination used for anterior teeth—loss of TRANSLUCENCY is seen.
- Bite wing R/G are taken for posterior teeth.

Differences between acute and chronic caries

Acute caries	Chronic caries
The acids dissolving the tooth structure precede the bacteria producing them in respect to pulp	The bacterial are preceding the acids produced by them or are at the same level pulpally.

Differences between acute and chronic caries

Acute caries	Chronic caries
Is of shorter duration	Longer duration
Soft and easily scooped out	Hard
Colour is straw yellow	Dark brown to black
Odourless	Foul smelling
In younger age	In older age
Little or no reparative reaction of pulp	+ve reaction
Deepest dentinal layer is considered sterile as it has only acids but no bacteria	Entire carious mass is infected

Number of line and point angles in different cavities

Cavity	Line angles	Point angles
I	8	4
II	11	6
III	6	3
IV	11	6
V	8	4
VI	14	8

Classification of prepared cavities: According to the depth of the cavity.

Class	Features
Class A depth	i.e. cavity with minimum depth. Remaining dentin is of maximum thickness possible.
B	Extends beyond the minimum depth required by mechanical and biological factors; a substantial thickness of dentins remains.
C	Extends into dentin such that only a thin, but intact wall of dentin remains.
D	Actual or subclinical exposure of pulp is observed.

Principles of cavity preparation: According to Black:

1. Outline form
2. Retention/resistance form
3. Convenience form
4. Removal of remaining carious dentin
5. Finishing of the enamel wall
6. Cleaning of cavity/toileting.

Steps in cavity preparation: From Marzouk:

- Outline form
- Resistance form
- Retention form
- Removal of carious dentin
- Convenience form
- Establishing the configuration and correlations of enamel walls
- Debridement
- Observing and practising the biologic forms

Outline form	Is the locations that the peripheries of cavity will occupy on tooth surface; for most intracoronal preparations: the depth of cavity should be to include DEJ and 0.5 mm in dentin. It is due to 3 reasons: • DEJ is very sensitive, where maximum interconnections of dentinal tubules exist. • To give bulk to the restorations. • To take advantage of elasticity of dentin during insertion and function.
Retention form	**Principal means of retention are:** • Frictional retention. • Elastic deformation of dentin. • Inverted truncated cones or undercuts. • Dovetail **Auxiliary means of retention:** • Grooves = cut in dentin. • Internal boxes = have definite walls and floors. • Posts = made from wrought/cast metals and placed in root canals. • Pins = made from cast/wrought metals. • Triangular area = placed in dentin. • Etching. • Cement/luting agents = **least effective** methods. • If occlusal loading helps to seat the restoration rather than displacing it, it is an ideal auxiliary retention form.
Removal of	**0.2–0.5% basic fuschin dye** stains the dentin irreparable decay areas.
Debridement	• H_2O_2 • Water–air jet • Cavity cleaners = e.g. citric acid; ascorbic acid; acetic acid in a conc of 1–10%. • Smear layer is only removed by 10% EDTA • Chisel, etc.

- **Outline form** = is the form of area of the tooth surface to be included within the outline or enamel margins of finished cavity.
- **External outline form** = the external boundary or perimeter of the prepared cavity.
- **Internal outline form** = is the inner dimension and detail of the prepared cavity.
- **Retention form** = prevents the restoration from being displaced.
- **Resistance form** = enables the restoration to withstand the stresses of mastication.
- **Convenience form**–provides ease for placing the restorative materials, i.e. for instrumentation, condensation, adaptation and finishing.
- Enamel walls must be parallel to the general direction of enamel rods and be supported by an intact DEJ.
    - Heavy flow of thin saliva—helps in bathing the teeth and decreases caries. It has anti-caries effect due to immunoglobulins and fluorides.
    - A gingival sulcus depth of 1–2 mm buccally and lingually, and 2–3 mm inter-proximally is normal.
    - Normal physiologic changes in colour of tooth is deepening of colour and increased opacity due to loss of enamel, and thickening and sclerosis of dentin.

OCCLUSION

Central parts of TMJ are avascular and without sensory nerves. They are capable of functional stress bearing without injury or pain.

Supporting Cusps

- Lingual cusps of maxillary and buccal cusps of mandibular posteriors and cusps tips/incisal edges of anteriors.
- They contact in the **centric stops** of opposing teeth.
- In normal angle's class I occlusion = the centric stops on mandibular teeth are fossae and marginal ridges.
- Centric stops play a significant role as the physical determinants of occlusal stability.

- TMJ has **no receptors** that monitor forces on joint but may depend on inputs from teeth and muscles for monitoring loading.
- CR = is a position, where almost wholly rotary (hinge-like) open and closing jaw movements can be made up to approx 25 mm.
- Average movement/slide from CR to CO is approx 1 mm; it is in anterior direction; it is known as **freedom-in-centric**. CO is 1 mm anterior to CR.
- Optimal condylar position for maximum intercuspation is slightly anterior to the midmost uppermost position, i.e. on the anterior slope of articular eminence.
- RCP: seldom seen as a functional position in natural dentition; helps in relating the mandible to maxilla in a patient.

Position	Features
Premature contacts	areas for PC in CR are mesial inclines of maxillary teeth and the distal inclined of mandibular teeth (MU-DL).
Balancing interferences	on maxillary molars are mesial/distal cusps ridge along with the buccal incline of the lingual cusps.
Working side interferences	lingual inclines of buccal cusps of maxillary posterior teeth and buccal inclines of lingual cusps of mandibular molars.
Protrusive interferences	on Md Post tooth = mesial inclines of marginal ridges; mesial inclines of triangular ridges.
Protrusive interferences	On Mx molars/PM = distal inclines of triangular ridges; distal inclines of marginal ridges.

PERIODONTAL ASPECTS (Refer to perio section also.)

- Most vulnerable part of periodontium is the junction between gingival epithelium and the tooth.

- Epithelium which joins directly and adheres to the tooth surface is known as junctional epithelium; while the attachment itself is known as epithelial attachment.
- Epithelial attachment is weak and is supported and maintained by tonus of the firm, free and circular gingival collagen fibers, which hold the gingiva close to the tooth.
- JE and EA have cell turn over time of approx. 7–10 days.
- After injury, the EA is reestablished by regenerating epithelial cells within a week and during this time, the bacteria are eliminated by PMN cells.
- PD disease is most often initiated and maintained by PLAQUE.
- Depth of normal gingival sulcus is 1–2 mm buccally, lingually and 2–3 mm proximally.
- Probe stops approx. 0.5 mm short of CT attachment to the tooth under normal pressure.
- After Rx and PD diseases, 4–6 weeks time is required for gingival health to return to normal.
- Less the gingival shrinkage after the surgery—the better are the esthetic and functional results.

ELECTRO SURGERY (Also refer to section of oral surgery.)

- Can be used safely only for gingivoplasty of free gingiva.
- Hyperplastic tissues may be removed with it, but should be done before the preparation of a restoration.
- Margins of restoration should be placed SUPRA-GINGIVALLY.
- Subgingival margins cause inflammation of tissues.
- It should not extend more than 0.5–1.0 mm under free marginal gingival.
- **Contour** = over contouring is more damaging than under contouring. It interferes with plaque removal. It interferes with ***sealing-cuff effect*** of gingiva against the tooth.
- Contact areas or I/d soldering joints should be placed as far occlusally as possible and should be convex and easy to clear.

TYPES OF PONTICS (Refer to prosthodontics section also.)

- **Sanitary pontics** = should be given in mandibular posterior area.

- **Ridge saddle pontics** = is in touch with the tissues—so makes plaque removal almost impossible.
- **Bullet pontics** = contact only at a point at the ridge.
- Antibiotics especially TETRACYCLINE may be required during maintenance plan for Rx of acute infection in a pocket.
- NaF and SnF_2 rinses help against sensitivity.
- APF should not be used for patients with porcelain crowns. It tends to stain the crowns.

SPLINTING (Also refer to perio for indications and details.)

- Used to maintain the PD support of teeth; it enhances the functional stability and esthetics. It also helps during healing phase.
- *Temporary/provisional splinting* = is required when continuous trauma interferes with comfortable function and to maintain teeth in favourable esthetic/functional position after ortho Rx.
- Ortho Rx can be done to intrude teeth with deep pockets.
- Intrusion does not eliminate the pocket, but makes them intra-bony due to new tooth position, which has better chance of reattachment after PD Rx.

PREVENTIVE MEASURES

- Acquired pellicle formation is the first stage of plaque formation due to absorption or precipitation of a protein layer on the tooth surface; it forms in less than 30 min, after through cleaning.
- Some cationic molecules about a nitrogen atom have preventive effect on plaque formation.
- Sucrose is the main sugar causing plaque and caries.
- Harmful effects of sucrose get increased by increasing thickness of plaque, because it then interferes with the ***buffer system of saliva*** and so low pH at tooth surface may lead to caries.
- Best prevention from caries and PD disease is by :
  - Regular professional tooth cleaning.
  - Fluoride application.
  - Tooth brushing instructions.

MECHANICAL MEANS OF PLAQUE CONTROL (Also refer to pedo and perio sections for details and table.)

- Multi-tufted soft bristles brushes with a bristle diameter 0.007–0.008 inch and with will finished rounded tips.
- **Bass method** = at 45°, bristles pushed into gingival crevice, but it does not remove plaque over the free gingiva.
- **Circular scrub method** = better than Bass method; light pressure used; brush moved in 2–4 mm diameter with circular movements; more effective near the interdental areas.
- 5–8 circular scrub movements are to be made for each brushing position with some overlap as the brush is moved around the dental arch.
  - ***Disclosing solution*** = Bismarck brown.
  - Most effective cleaning of exposed I/D surfaces is provided by = **Charter's method**.

Floss (Classification of floss)

- Multi-tufted floss spreads out in a tape like fashion.
- More effective plaque removal occurs with unwaxed floss.
- For tight i/d contents = waxed floss is easier than unwaxed floss.
- Concave i/d surfaces that cannot be cleansed with floss are cleaned with special inter-proximal brushes.
  - Gingival massage helps in reducing gingival inflammation by removing plaque and crevicular toxins, rather than by stimulation of circulation and metabolism.
  - **Forced irrigation** = it should be used with caution in patient with active periodontitis especially with H/O rheumatic fever or diabetes, as it may lead to bacteremia.

CHEMICAL MEANS OF PLAQUE CONTROL (Also refer to sections of pedo and oral pathology.)

- 0.2% **chlorhixidine gluconate,** but may cause taste change and staining of the teeth after prolonged use.
- Other cationic disinfections also have plaque inhibiting properties.
- Fluorides.

- SnF_2 and MFP decrease the incidence of caries.
- 2% NaF, 8% SnF_2, 1.23% APF can decrease decay by 40%.
- APF should not be used on ceramic crowns, as it tends to ERODE the surface of porcelain.
- NaF is easier to formulate than APF.
- Taste of SnF_2 is objectionable.
- 0.05% NaF = if used daily.
- 0.2% NaF = if used weekly.
- Maximum dose recommended in packs to be sold = **264 mg of NaF.**

P AND F SEALANTS (Also refer to sections of pedo and dental materials.)

Prophylactic odontotomy is conservative preparation of non-carious fissures and filling them with Ag; by Hyatt 1923.

Enameloplasty—by Bodecker; enlarging the P and F to form wide, non-retentive grooves to remove enamel faults.

Buonocore 1955—etching and bonding of resin helped 86% reduction of occlusal caries.

- Fluorides can decrease smooth surfaces caries but has little effect on P and F caries.
- A resin sealant coating is applied to enamel defect, which adheres to the demineralized ends of acid-etched enamel rods.
- Loss of this sealant can occur by abrasive wear, by bond failure or by premature contacts.
- So occlusal interferences should be removed especially if a fluid resin is used.
- P and F sealant should extend up the cuspal inclines adjacent to the fissures to a sufficient distance to attain an undetectable junction with enamel.
- Most common materials used as P and F sealants = BIS–GMA, MMA, urethane diacrylate resins.
- Sealants can be pure or can have 15–20% wt. fillers of silanated glass particles.

- Filled resins have more viscosity/less flow and permit better control during placement, improved wear resistance.
- Sealants are **most effective in decreasing caries in young children** when applied shortly after permanent tooth eruption.
- So **sealant Rx in children and young adults is indicated** for non-carious teeth.
- Sealants are **C/I on primary molars**, on carious P and F, on interproximal lesions.
- It is best to seal non-carious P and F; however the bacteria present in sealed carious fissures loose their viability and potential to produce demineralization; because they get cut off from saliva and carbohydrates.
- **Sucrose** or other lightly refined carbohydrates in plaque are essential for caries.
- Ortho Rx creates a favourable dental alignment and may intrude periodontally involved teeth for a better bone support.
- Teeth active in mastication collect less plaque than nonfunctional teeth.
- Most common cause of gingival recession is FAULTY TOOTH BRUSHING.
- Recession also occurs in teeth with extreme facial or lingual inclination with respect to the alveolar process.

INSTRUMENTS

Classification: Divided in 6 categories by black:

1. Cutting instruments: hand; rotatory
2. Condensing instruments
3. Plastic instruments
4. Finishing and polishing: hand; rotatory
5. Isolation instruments
6. Miscellaneous

INSTRUMENTS

- Hand cutting instruments
- Rotary cutting instruments
- Ultrasonic instruments

Hand cutting instruments

- Excavators = hatchet; hoe; spoon excavators; discoid and cleoids.
- Chisels = straight; monangle; binangle; triple angle.
- Special form of chisel = hatchets; GMT; angle formers; Wedelstaedt chisel; offset hatchet; triangular chisels; hoe chisel.

Rotary instruments

- A rotary tool should be large in diameter, when used with low speeds.
- In ultra high speed, the diameter of tool should be decreased.
- Maximum cutting efficiency of a cutting tool of uniform width ranges between 5000–6000 surface feet/min.
- Heat production is directly proportional to = pressure; RPM; area of tooth in contact with the tool.
- Pulp gets permanently damaged if a temperature of 130°F is reached.
- **Vibration** = a rotation of approx 6,000 rpm sets up a fundamental vibrational wave of approx 100 cycles/sec. This is most annoying to the patient and dentist. But vibrations above 1300 cps are imperceptible to patients, which occur at ultra high speed.

Finishing and polishing instruments

- Burs
- Paper carried abrasives
- Brushes
- Rubber
- Cloth
- Felt

Restoring instruments

- Mixing instruments
- Plastic instruments
- Condensing instruments
- Burnishing instruments
- Carvers
- Files
- Knives
- Finishing and polishing instruments

HAND CUTTING INSTRUMENTS: 3 parts:

1. Handle/Shaft.
2. Shank—connects the shaft to blade.
3. Blade/Nib—also known as point/head. It is the functional end of instrument, bears cutting edge, etc.

INSTRUMENT FORMULA

3-Unit formula

1. Width of blade = in tenths of a mm
2. Length of blade = in mm.
3. Angle of blade with axis of handle; in hundredths of a circle or centigrades.

4-Unit formula

- i.e. if cutting edge is at an angle other than 90° to blade length.
- It is placed at 2nd position in the formula.
- Describes the angle formed between cutting edge and central axis of the shaft; in centigrades.

Important points

- All hand-cutting instruments are excavators differing in the shape of cutting edge.

- According to Angle/Angles in shank-4 types.

Straight	No angle
Monangle	One angle
Binangle	Two angles
Triple angle	Three angles

Contra angle = i.e. angling of shank to bring the cutting edge or working point into close proximity to the central axis of instrument.

- **Single plane instrument** = instrument with 2 or more angles in the shank in a single plane; it could be laid on the table top, e.g. hatchet.
- **Double plane instrument** = e.g. GMT; has a curved blade; curved blade has lateral scraping ability. All double plane instrument are *lateral cutting instrument.*

TYPES OF HAND CUTTING INSTRUMENTS

Chisel
- One sided bevel.
- Cutting edge is ⊥ to plane of instrument.
- If cutting edge is distal to the shaft, it is known as CONTRA - BEVELED/REVERSE beveled chisel.
- Used with *push motion.*
- Monangle/Binangle chisels for MAXILLARY ARCH.

HOE
- Angle of blade is greater than 12.5°C
- Used with *pull motion.*

Hatchet
- CE/cutting edge is in the plane of instrument.
- R and L pair.
- Used for planning/cleaning Enamel and Dentin.
- May be bi-beveled placing the CE in the centre; used to refine line ∠ and point ∠.
- Generally used in MANDIBULAR ARCH.

Angle
- CE is at an ∠ to the BLADE.

Former
- ∠ of CE to the blade axis is 80–85°C.
- 4-unit formula = i.e. ∠ of CE to the shaft.
- Used to accentuate line and point ∠ in internal outline form in cavities.
- Used in *lateral scrapping motion.*
- Blade is beveled on sides and at ends to form 3 cutting edges.
- is a **modified chisel**.

Gingival margin trimmer—is a **modified hatchet**.
- ♦ CE is at an angle other than a right ∠ to the axis of blade (while in hatchet, CE is at 90° to blade axis).
- ♦ Blade of GMT is curved (while hatchet has straight blade).
- ♦ R and L pair.
- ♦ Used to bevel gingival cavosurface margin.
- ♦ Mesial GMT = 10–80–6–12.
- ♦ Distal GMT = 10–95–6–12 (Higher no. is always of Distal GMT).

Spoon excavators—modified hatchet; double plane.
- ♦ Rounded cutting edge.
- ♦ Action is *scooping/spooning nature.*
- ♦ Used for lateral scrapping.
- ♦ Paired.
- ♦ For removal of carious dentin.

Cleoid discoid instrument—modified double end chisel.
- ♦ Cutting edges = spoon shaped.
- ♦ Used for carving of amalgam and wax.

Abrasion
- ♦ Is the action of wearing away **by friction**.
- ♦ e.g. diamond, silicon carbide, aluminum oxide, silicon dioxide.

Airbrasive technique (By RB Black.)
- ♦ It is non-mechanical preparation of cavities.

- **30–50 micron aluminium oxide** particle under **110 psi pressure** of CO_2 stream are propelled at tooth surface and funneled through a tungsten carbide nozzle with a lumen of 0.018″.
- Precise, sharply defined cavities not possible with this technique.
- Used generally for smaller carious lesions.

Other important points

- Mimp function of rotary instruments = action of cutting and abrading.
- Cutting instruments consist of = a six-bladed bur.
- Tungsten carbide burs = harder than SS burs.
  - At higher speeds (70,000 rpm) = lighter force increases cutting efficiency of diamond points.

Ultrasonic method

- Frequency used—15000–30000 cycles/sec.
- **Al_2O_3 particles** in water slurry is used.
  - **Atraumatic Restorative Techniques** (ART): here, no rotary instruments are used; gross caries removal is done with the help of excavators; the defect is filled with GI cements; it is mostly used in backward/developing countries.

Bur designs

Parts	Features
Bur tooth	It ends up in the cutting edge or blade. It has 2 surfaces: 1. tooth face = which is the side of the tooth on the leading edge. 2. back . flank = which is the side of the tooth on the trailing edge.
Rake angle	Angle which the face of the bur tooth makes with the radial line from the centre of the bur to the blade.

Bur designs (*Contd.*)

Parts	Features
	1. negative = if face is beyond or leading the radial line. 2. zero = if radial line and tooth face coincide with each other; also known as radial rake angle. 3. positive = if radial line leads the face ST rake angle is on the inside of the radial line.
Land	Plane surface immediately following the cutting edge.
Clearance	Angle between the back of tooth and the work. If back surface of tooth is curved—it is known as radial clearance.
Tooth angle	Is between face and back.
Flute or chip space	i.e. the space between adjacent teeth of the bur.

Important points about burs

- More positive the rake angle, greater is the bur's cutting efficiency.
- Radial rake angle bur cut more effectively than with negative rake angle.
- With negative rake angle = the cut chips move directly away from the blade edge and often fracture in small bits/dust.
- With positive rake angle, the chips are larger and tend to clog the chip space. The size of bur tooth is decreased and its tooth angle is decreased, so the bulk is decreased, which can get fractured during cutting.
- Larger clearance angle results in less rapid dulling of the bur.
- No. of teeth in a bur = 6–8.
- If no. of teeth is decreased = thickness of chip removed by each flute increases.
- If no. of teeth is less = the clogging tendency is decreased, but, because they remove more material, the bur wears faster and rougher.

- Bur with straight flutes produces less temperature than with spiral flutes.
- Fewer the no. of teeth, the greater is the tendency of vibrations.
- Burs can be latch type and friction grip types; burs revolve clockwise.
- Round burs = ¼; ½; 1, 2, ——— 10.
- Wheel burs = 14, 15.
- Inverted cones = 33 ¼; 33 ½; 34; 35 ——— 39.
- Plain cylindrical fissure burs = 55 ——— 59.
- Cross cut cylindrical fissure bur = 555 ——— 560.
- Plain tapered fissure bur = 169 ——— 172.
- Cross cut tapered fissure bur = 699 ——— 703.
- Round nose fissure burs = all burs can be round ended. The number 1 will be added to previous numbering, i.e. 155; 1555; 1169, etc.
- Pear shaped = 229 ——— 333; mainly used in **pedodontics.**
- End cutting burs = 900 ——— 904.
- **Run out** is the eccentricity or maximum displacement of bur head from its axis of rotation. Average acceptable run out is 0.023 mm.
- **Load** is the force exerted by the dentist on the tool head. For low speed, 1000 gm, i.e. 2 lbs; for high speed 2–4 oz is used.
- **Finishing burs** should be at least 12 fluted.
- SS burs for amalgam.
- Tungsten carbide burs for composite resins.

Speeds used in dentistry

Ultra low speed	300–3000 rpm
Low speed	3000–6000 rpm
Medium high speed	20000–45,000 rpm
High speed	45,000–100,000 rpm
Ultra high speed	> 100,000 rpm

Speed classification

Speed	Frequency
Conventional/low speed	< 10,000 rpm
Increased/high speed	10,000–1,50,000 rpm
Ultra speed	> 1,50,000 rpm

Important points

- Pulp is larger than it appears on R/G.
- Cutting instruments should be sharp, concentric and of proper shape and dimension for removal of caries.
- Removal of deep, pulp encroaching caries should be done by low rotational speeds and bulk removal of enamel and dentin by high speeds.

Instrumentation

- Position of pulpal floor of cavity should ideally be placed in = 0.5 mm into the dentin.
- Unsupported enamel should be removed.
- With spoon excavator, the forces of removal of dentin are directed LATERALLY.
- Slow speed is used for removal of carious dentin; use light forces while removing it.

Steel bur has more number of flutes than the carbide bur and so gives a smoother cutting action.

- Air water coolant is used to dissipate heat.
- **Washed field technique** = i.e. high velocity evacuation of coolant.
- Fiber optic hand pieces = increases visualisation of the operative site.
- Ultra speed = is best for penetration through bulk of enamel and extensive removal of enamel.
- Low speeds = for caries removal and cavity refinements.

ROTARY PROCEDURES: For cavity preparation are:

1. **Penetration** = ultra speed; round bur is used.
2. **Extension** = ultra speed; straight/plain fissure bur.
3. **Excavation** = low speed; for caries removal; lighter touch; round bur used.
   - Round carbide bur is more sharp, with less cutting blades; more difficult to control in delicate procedures.
4. **Refinement** = with plain/non-cross cut fissure bur,
   - Excavation of caries lesion should be carried out at low rotational speeds, especially the deep caries encroaching the pulp.
   - Placement of retention areas and other refinements also require low speed. Should always be placed in the dentin without undermining the enamel.
   - Crosscut burs should not be = used with ultra speed; as they become more of an abrading instrument than a milling instrument.

Noise emission is air turbines

- More noisy.
- Vibration frequencies are > 5000 cps.
- Speech range = 250–3000 cps.
- Intensity of > 85 decibels can lead to hearing diseases.
- Dental ball bearing air turbine noise is = 75–100 db.
- Air bearing hand piece = 60–70 db.
- Effective insulation of walls can increase noise absorption.
- Operate intermittently to reduce fatigue.

At ultra speed

1. At 3–5 lac rpm, only 2–4 oz light force are enough for cutting.
2. Tactile discrimination for the amount of tissue removed is absent.
3. Use small dimension burs for good control.

Instrument grasp methods

1. Pen grasp.
2. Inverted pen grasp.
3. Palm and thumb grasp.
4. Modified palm and thumb grasp.

Instrument grasps

Pen grasp grasp	Very accurate control most effective and universally used grasp.
Inverted pen	Used in upper teeth 3rd/4th finger rests on adjacent tooth of the same jaw.
Palm and thumb	Used on maxillary teeth esp of right side. Thumb rests at some distance from the point of operation.
Modified palm and thumb grasp	Greater freedom of movement and delicacy of control. Prevents instrument slippage. Hand is only about half-closed. End of thumb is used for the rest.

- **Pen grasp** = most frequently used; esp in **mandibular arch**; 2-handed control of both hand and rotary instrument is recommended.
- **Inverted pen grasp** = palm and finger tips are directed towards the operator. Used in maxillary arch on both L/R side. Dentist stands behind the patient at 11 O'clock .
- **Palm and thumb grasp** = Tip of thumb is the rest or pivot. Mostly used in **maxillary arch**.

Sterilization (Refer to section on Microbiology Vol. II)

- Is complete destruction of all microbial life including spores.
- Cutting edges of instrument must be protected during autoclaving by an oil emulsion coating.
- Autoclaving is the most reliable method; done at 121 C × 15 psi × 10 min.

Disinfection: It is the destruction of most of the pathogens from inanimate surfaces; can be done by:

1. 100°C water × 30 min.
2. 2% alkaline glutraldelyde for 10 min (for 10 hrs if instruments have been used in a TB patient or spores forming infection).
3. 1% NaOCl × 10 min.
4. 2% formaldehyde and 20–30 min.
5. Quaternary Ammonium compounds are not effective *vs* spores/virus and should not be used for disinfections.

For scrubbing the **chair/handles,** etc.

1. Detergents = to remove dried blood
2. 90% isopropyl alcohol or 70% ethyl alcohol = remove dried blood/saliva.
3. 5% iodophor in 70% isopropyl alcohol.
4. Air-water syringe line should be flushed for 3 min to decrease **Pseudomonas aeruginosa.**
   - Corrosion of instruments made of SS and Tungsten carbide can be prevented by using 2% sodium nitrite solution coating.
   - Autoclaving is done at 121 C × 15 psi × 10 min, i.e. (249.8°F) or at 258°F × 35 psi × 5 min
   - Ethylene oxide gas × 3 hrs applications; (total 24 hrs with aeration also).

BIOLOGICAL CONSIDERATIONS

Mechanical properties of teeth

- Compressive strength of enamel supported by vital dentin is = 36000–42000 psi.
- Compressive strength of vital dentin = 40000–50000 psi.
- Modulus of elasticity of enamel supported by vital dentin under compression = 70 lac psi.
- MOE of vital dentin = 19 lac psi.
- Tensile strength of dentin is about 10% less than its compressive strength.

- Tensile strength and compressive strength of enamel is same.
  - Dentin is the secretory products of pulp.
  - Enamel is hardest substance in the body due to its high mineral content, approx 95% inorganic and 5% organic + water.
  - KHN of different dental tissues is

Enamel	–343
Dentin	– 68
Cemetum	– 40

  - Enamel is 5–20 × more resistant to abrasion than dentin.
  - Enamel rod = are made of many HA crystals, extend at right angles from dentin outward to the tooth surface.
  - Rod sheath contains more ORGANIC substance than the rod and so not as susceptible to demineralization by acids.
  - Fluoride prevents caries by decreasing the enamel dissolution by making fluorapatite crystals, which are more resistant to acids produced. Fluoride facilitates redeposition of mineral as apatite, when acid attack has subsided.
  - Walls of the cavity should be parallel to enamel rods direction leaving no unsupported enamel, which otherwise gets broken.
  - Cavity preparation with an inter-cuspal distance of 1/4 to 1/3 results in sound enamel. If width is 1/2 the ICD, the cavity walls require increasingly greater divergence (inlay taper) to be parallel to enamel rods.
  - For amalgam: the buccal/lingual/gingival walls of proximal box should be at right angles to the cavosurface for supported enamel rods.
  - For gold: Bevel is used for proper adaptation of gold to the margins of the cavity.
  - For class 5 cavity:
    1. Occlusal and gingival walls are diverging.
    2. Cavosurface angulation of occlusal walls must become more OBTUSE as the position of this margin approaches the occlusal surface of the tooth. It may be 120–130° to assure a sound enamel margin.
  - Cuspal protection = minimum restoration required is gold only.

Biologic aspects of dental materials: Pulp injury may occur due to:

- Heat and desiccation.
- Pressure generated during condensation of gold and silver
- Due to inherent irritational potential of materials, e.g. silicate cement; composite resin; so a protective base should be placed below them.
- Remaining dentin thickness is less.
- Presence or absence of reparative dentin below the cut dentin.

Acid etching

- Increases surface area by creating the micro-pores in the enamel surface **by 200 times** for bonding by creating micro-mechanical pores in the surface.
- 37–50% of buffered orthophosphoric acid for 1 minute. Latest researches say that etching time of 15–20 sec is enough.
- Rinse for at least 15 sec for washing; and air dry the surface for 60 sec. The air should be free of oil, etc.
- Etched Enamel surface appears as frosty/chalky white.
- Longer etching results in greater loss of enamel.
- A cavosurface bevel of enamel = gives more uniform etching.
- Etched pattern consists of 3 zones from surface inwards:

Pattern	Depth
Etched zone/enamel removed	10 micrometers
Qualitative porous zone	20 micrometers
Quantitative porous zone	20 micrometers

So composite resin tags can penetrate up to 50 microns into enamel to give retention.

- Provides higher surface energy to enhance WETTING.
- Demineralisation of rod ends occurs, in which resin flows to form RESIN TAGS.

- The bond is micro-mechanical/MECHANICAL.
- Salivary contamination deposits salivary mucoid material and remineralisation of etched enamel. So re-etching is to be done.
- Etched enamel returns to pre-etched state if exposed to oral atmosphere for 1 hrs.
- Complete remineralisation occurs within 45 days after etching.
- Acid etching of dentin = Removes smear layer, opens the dentinal tubules to the pulp, which act as pathway of micro-leakage to pulp.

Enamel

- 95% mineralized/inorganic component. Due to its uniformity, the pattern of acid etching is good; but the dentin contains both organic and inorganic components and so its etching pattern is not that good for good retention as of enamel. So dentin bonding agents are required.
- Demineralization—initially a **whitish lesion** with **decreased translucency**.
- Increased demineralization increases its OPACITY and friability, decreased hardness.

Dentin

- Carious dentin is soft and tends to be penetrated by explorer under light pressure.
- A clear **chatter sound** comes on normal dentin.
- KHN of sound/primary dentin = 61.
- KHN of reparative dentin = 40.
- **0.5% Basic Fuchsin** in propylene glycol for 10 sec = this stain affects that dentin, whose collagen fibers have been denatured irreversibly. Cross-linking of these fibers is reduced beyond Remineralisation.

Dentin: refer to section of dental histology for details

DIFFERENT TYPES OF DENTIN: From lowest to highest permeability are:

- Calcific barrier dentin.

- Sclerosed dentin.
- Primary dentin.
- Secondary dentin.
- Tertiary/reparative dentin.
- Globular dentin.
- Granular dentin.
- Dead tract dentin.
- Forms the greatest bulk of the tooth.
- 70% inorganic + 30% organic.
- Made of collagen fibers and ground substances of mucopolysaccharide.
- KHN = 68, (enamel = 343), i.e. enamel is 5 times harder than dentin.
- Dentinal tubules = are of S shape curve.
- 30000–70000 /mm^2 of dentin = number of tubules per square mm of dentin.
- Only 100–150 micron thickness of dentin from the pulp contains free nerve endings. That is why the pain is felt during cavity preparation at that point.
- Pain in dentin is due to **tactile stimuli** like pressure; **probing,** etc. It is due to **rapid inflow** of the dentinal fluids from the dentinal tubules to the pulp.
- **Pain due** to osmotic stimuli like **sweets** is due to **rapid outflow** of the fluid form the dentinal tubules.
- Pain due to thermal stimuli is also due to **rapid outflow (cold stimuli)**; or **inflow (hot stimuli)** of dentinal fluid.
- **Pain transmission** = is through **hydrodynamic theory** of dentin sensitivity. Fluid in dentinal tubules moves under stimuli and stimulates the free nerve endings in pulp/dentin. No pain killer is effective in such conditions.
- Sensitive dentin indicates that the underlying tubules are open to the pulp.
- Fluid pressure is higher in pulp than in oral cavity.

- Air drying of freshly cut dentin causes evaporation of dentinal fluid causing fluid movement and sensitivity due to stimulation of pulpal nerves and pain.
- Bases applied in the cavity compensate for the lost dentin tissue. Bases/Varnish/Liner also compensate for setting shrinkage of restorative materials.
- Varnish/Base materials plug the dentinal tubules and prevent fluid movement in dentin, and thus prevent the hypersensitivity.
- Potassium nitrate containing tooth pastes also help in reducing the sensitivity.
- **Dentin bonding agents** = bonding to dentin is difficult due to its high organic and water content and presence of smear layer. DBA help to overcome these problems esp in class V and II cavities extending on dentin or cementum. DBA removes the smear layer, exposes the collagen and opens the dentinal tubules. Then DBA is applied, which has difunctional ends, the hydrophilic end attaches to dentin and the hydrophobic end bonds to the composite resin.

Important points

- 1 mm square of cut dentin exposes 30000–45000 dentinal tubules.
- Carbide burs are more cool–cutting than steel burs.
- Rotary abrasive instrument stones are not used on vital dentin as it may increase the temperature. So abrasive action should be confined to enamel and superficial 1 mm of dentin.
- **Effective depth** = is the thickness of dentin bridge between floor of cavity and roof of pulp chamber.
- If pulp temperature increases by 11 F—it may cause destructive reaction in pulp.
- Most deleterious speed is 3,000–30,000 rpm.
- In making pin holes, the speed should not exceed 3,000 rpm.
- Instrumentation pressure should not be more than 4 oz, when using high speed and 12 oz with low speed.
- When RPMs are increased, the size of cutting head should be decreased.

- Desiccation of vital dentin results in the **aspiration of nuclei of odontoblasts** into the tubules and may increase the permeability of vital dentin to the irritants.
- Cementum is thinnest over the cervical portion of the root and becomes thick towards the apex. It is the softest of all the hard tissues of tooth.

Factors affecting health of pulp and dentin

- Irritation stimuli lead to pulpal inflammation and then reparative dentin formation.
- *High speed cutting* with *copious water coolant* and a *light force* = results in MINIMAL HISTOLOGIC alteration of pulp.
- Cavity depth = dentin having remaining **thickness of 2 mm** or more acts as a good barrier vs the trauma of instrumentation.
- Pulpal response is more in larger and deeper cavity.
- Reparative dentin acts as an INSULATOR.
- Compressed air = prolonged use of dry air on a prepared cavity causes a DELAYED HEALING RESPONSE.
- 30 sec compressed air drying can cause pulpal inflammation and displacement of odontoblasts cells in the dentinal tubules. In most cases, this damage is REVERSIBLE.

DENTIN PRETREATMENT

Smear Layer: Amorphous layer of organic film and debris deposited on DENTIN during cutting is called smear layer.

- Acts as a cavity liner by sealing the dentinal tubules.
- But inhibits effective ion exchange and bonding of GI to tooth surfaces. So dentin should be pretreated to remove it.
- Should be SELECTIVELY removed from dentin surface leaving the tubules filled.
- Open tubules may allow dentinal fluid to come on dentin surface, reducing proper bonding or/and irritant may go towards pulp.

Agents used

- Citric acid
  (a) Poly-acrylic acid = Best; leaves tubules partially occluded
  (b) EDTA
- Tannic acid
  - PAA/Poly-acrylic acid conditioning is done for 10–20 sec. But longer time can remove peritubular dentin and open the tubules.

Smear layer

- It is an uniform amorphous layer, which occludes the dentinal tubules.
- It prevents penetration of bacteria in the tubules, but does not prevent penetration of fluids through the dentin, e.g. bacterial products may cause pulpal inflammation.
- It greatly reduces dentin permeability and protects the dentin from hydrostatic forces.
- DILUTE EDTA is used to scrub the smear layer, but leaving the tubules blocked.
- **Potassium oxalate** can be used as a cavity liner. It removes smear layer and forms a calcium oxalate layer. It decreases dentin permeability and is resistant to ACID ATTACK.
- It can also provide ADEQUATE seal at the dentin interface and can be used to Rx dentin hypersensitivity.

Direct pulp capping (DPC)

- Its purpose is to preserve pulp vitality by using a medicament on exposure site, which provides an environment for the tooth to heal, e.g. $Ca(OH)_2$ is the best choice.
- A small, pin - point exposure **in young patient** has more chances of success due to VASCULARITY OF PULP AND SIZE OF exposure.
- Mechanically exposed teeth have greater chances of success than carious exposure, due to less pulpal inflammation and bacterial toxins.

Indirect pulp capping (IPC)

- Involves removal of all carious dentine except the deepest layer to prevent exposure.
- Placing calcium hydroxide dressing on some residual carious dentin, for the formation of reparative dentin.
- Helps in formation of reparative dentin by the pulp.
- It causes cell death of bacteria at high pH of 11–12, especially of those bacteria having pH optima below 7 as of most of aciduric organisms.
- It makes the remaining carious sterile of bacteria (with cannot withstand high pH).
- Best success in young patients due to large volume of pulpal tissues and good vascularity, which helps good healing.

BASIC Rx PROCEDURES

A. There are 4 **major zones of activity** around the operation field:

1. Operator's zone
2. Transfer zone
3. Assistant zone
4. Static zone.

B. Positions

- 12 O'clock = for U/L POSTERIOR segment.
    - Requires use of mouth mirror.
    - Requires severe bending of back and neck.
- 11 O'clock = most UNIVERSAL POSITION.

  Access to all areas except = most distal areas of mandibular right posterior teeth and cervical areas on right posterior teeth.
- 9 O'clock/7 O'clock = alternate position for mandibular right posterior teeth.

Transfer zone: Located near oral cavity, where instruments are transferred between operator and assistant. It is just in front of and slightly below the patient's mouth.

Assistant zone: At 3 O'clock position.

Static zone: Contains auxiliary equipments.

Operator's position

- Operator seated well back on stool.
- Feet flat on floor.
- Legs relaxed and relatively together.
- **Thighs parallel** to the floor.
- Back straight and supported by back-rest.
- **16–18 inches** is the optimal eye to work distance.
- Usual operating position is between 10 to 12 O'clock with respect to the patient.
- Lower leg making a 90 degree angle with upper leg
- Straight line unobstructed of area of operations.

Patient's position

- In semi-supine or supine position.
- Operative field/oral cavity should be over the **operator's lap** at the height of operator's elbow.
- Operators **forearm should be parallel** to the floor.
- Patient's **ankles and chin should be at the same level**. If legs are higher than head, it may cause POSTURAL HYPOTENSION.
- For LA = supine position. But patient should be more upright for inferior alveolar block.

Dentist and patient seating positions

Quadrant	Dentist	Patient
Lower right	7–9 O'clock	2–4 O'clock
Lower front	Same	Same
Lower left	10–11 O'clock	3 O'clock
Upper and lower front	Same	Same
Upper arch with mirror	11–12 O'clock	3–5 O'clock
Upper right facial and left	7–10 O'clock	

Assistant's position: His head/stool should be 4–6″ higher than the operator to improve the vision. It is usually placed between 2 or 3 O'clock position. Assistant seated at a higher position than dr. so that his knees are at the level of patient's head and his feet rest on the foot rest of his stool.

Light position

- Operatory light should be placed at an arms length from the operator.
- Higher light position is used for mandibular arch.
- Lower light position is used for maxillary arch.
- Lower light position is used for indirect vision.
- Higher light position is used for direct vision.

ISOLATION

Various methods of attaining the isolation are:

1. Anti-Sialogogue drugs, e.g. atropine; propantheline bromide.
2. An aesthetics.
3. Saliva ejectors and high vacuum evacuating devices.
4. Absorbents and cotton rolls.
5. Rubber dam.

Ideal isolation = by rubber dam.

An astringent retraction cord = decreases seepage from gingival crevice.

Adrenaline impregnated cord = **0.5 mg/inch adr**.

Rubber Dam: By SC Barnum (1860s).

♦ Parts of rubber dam:

Parts	Features
RD sheet	• rubber sheet of 5 × 5 or 6 × 6 inches size • 5 types = thin (0.006 inches); medium (0.008 inches); heavy (0.010 inches); extra heavy (0.012 inches); special duty (0.014 inches). • are of green or blue colour for colour contrast; • dull side of the sheet faces towards occlusal side to avoid light reflection.
RD holder	Mostly Young's holder is used.
RD clamp/	2 types = winged; wing less; smaller size retainers for premolars; larger size for molars; no. 212 clamp is used for retracting the RD sheet during class V restorations; its bow is placed towards distal side;
RD punch Clamp holding devices	

♦ Types = light, medium, heavy and extra heavy.

Hole punching

♦ 2 inches RD material peripheral to lower anteriors; lateral to U/L posteriors on each side.

♦ 1–1.5 inches peripheral to upper anteriors.

♦ Holes for anterior teeth follow a curve.

♦ Holes for premolars follow a straight line parallel to midline.

♦ Holes for molars follow a straight line, slightly inclined towards midline.

- For class V lesion, the hole is punched 2–3 mm away from normal arch line. And a clamp of 212 series is used.
- Isolation of anterior teeth = at least one tooth behind the one being operated to the opposite canine.
- Interseptal rubber should have 4–5 mm width. It helps in gingival retraction and prevents the seepage due to its snug fit.
- Single tooth isolation is used for RCT.
- In RCT, light or medium RD sheet is used.
- Removal = done by clipping the interseptal rubber.
    - Made of latex; indicated for **absolute dryness**.
    - **Dark coloured** = for good contrast; for decreasing light reflection.
    - 5″ wide = used with Young's frame.
    - 6″ wide = used with Enodon frame.
    - Mostly heavy weight is needed, as it also helps in **retraction of gingival** tissues.
    - RD clamp for securing on posterior tooth.
    - Enodon frame helps in formation of a RD pouch, in which water gets collected, which can be removed by saliva ejector.
    - Anti-sialogogues = atropine 5 mg given 1/2 hr before the appointment.

Factors/Important points

- Involve at least one tooth posterior to the being operated extending to some position beyond the MIDLINE into the adjacent quadrant.
- More teeth isolated, the better is the access and easier isolation.
- Dental floss should be tied to the RD clamps = it helps in retrieval of the clamp, if it becomes dislodged toward pharynx.
- RD clamp is first placed in LINGUAL CERVICAL position. A uniform **4-point contact** of the jaws of the clamp is ideal.
- Superior border of RD sheet should be JUST BELOW THE NARES, not obstructing BREATHING.

- Normal spacing from the border of one hole to the adjacent hole = 4 mm, except in Maxillary anterior region, where 5 mm space is required.
- While removing, the I/D rubber is cut for easy removal.

VARNISHES, BASES AND LINERS

Ideal requirements of a protective base:

- Well tolerated by the pulp (Biocompatible).
- Should promote reparative dentin formation.
- Should provide adequate pulp protection.
- Should have adequate physical properties to withstand forces.
- Antibacterial properties.
- Obtundent effect on pulp.
- Be compatible with restorative materials.
- Eg ZOE; $Ca(OH)_2$, glass-inomer, etc.

VARNISHES (Also refer to sections of pedo and dental materials.)

Varnishes are the film forming solutions.

- Made of natural gums, synthetic resins or rosins.
- e.g. copal resin dissolved is chloroform.
- These are the solution of resins in **volatile solvents.**
- Produce a resinous solute layer of a few micron thickness upon evaporation of organic solvent.
- Less soluble than cavity liners.
- Multiple layers (2–3) are better than single layer, it helps to seal the holes/defects due to formation of bubbles during evaporation of solvent.
- Should **not be used beneath composite resins,** because CR results in discontinuous varnish film.
- Provides no thermal insulation; but only helps to **prevent the microleakage.**
- Also helps to reduce the dentinal sensitivity.
- Decreases pulpal response.

- Decreases penetration of corrosion products in dentin and of acid from $ZnPO_4$ cement.
- Can be used even on CAVOSURFACE margins as it is **insoluble in the oral fluids.**
- Should be placed below ZnPO4 cement to prevent acidic attack on the pulp.
- Can be applied to enamel, dentin and cavosurface margins.
- MMA (BIS–GMA monomers destroy varnish layers and should not be used.)

Liners (Intermediary bases) (Also refer to sections of pedo and dental materials.)

- These are the liquids in which $Ca(OH)_2$/ZnO are suspended in natural/synthetic resins.
- Minimize/prevent micro leakage.
- Also change physiologic environment by their peculiar chemical characteristics.
- It provides a chemical barrier; very thin layer is applied.
- Thin membrane is formed; it is **soluble in oral fluids**; so should not be placed on Cavosurface margins, it provides very little thermal insulation due to its thinness.
- Liners-Prevent microleakage; have some therapeutic effect on pulp. Does not have proper strength; are soluble in oral fluids.
- Sound dentin is the best barrier between pulp and restoration.
- Liner contains resin and ZnO/$Ca(OH)_2$ dissolved in volatile liquids.
- Varnish does not contain ZnO/$Ca(OH)_2$.
- Both are used in liquid form.

Cavity Liner suspensions

- Made of $Ca(OH)_2$, ZnO in resinous solutions; are used esp with composite resins.
- They form thicker films.
- Should not be placed on cavosurface margins, because of high solubility and so microleakage can occur.

- If placed on enamel, the opacity mars the esthetics, so must be restricted to dentin.
- $Ca(OH)_2$ in methylcellulose can also be used, but it does not adhere to dentin as compared to resin-containing liners.
- Can be used for pulp capping if $Ca(OH)_2$ is present in it.

Intermediary base

- Acts as a protective barrier.
- It has therapeutic effects also, e.g. $Ca(OH)_2$ in Direct Pulp Capping/IPC.
- It has low compressive strength and Mod of Elasticity (MOE).
- Provides a chemical protective barrier; if bulky, then provides thermal insulation.
- Thicker layer used—so better thermal insulators.
- e.g. $Ca(OH)_2$; modified ZOE, they retard penetration of acid.
- Eugenol–has topical anesthetic property; obtundent effect, decrease discomfort associated with dental caries and instrumentation; used to cover deeper dentin in class C deep caries.
- Eugenol is C/I with resin materials, as it hampers with the polymerization of resins.

ZOE

- Excellent sealing qualities.
- Bacteriostatic.
- **ZOE beneath composite resins is C/I,** because eugenol retards the polymerization of resin and dissolves the liner.
- A set matrix consists of unreacted ZnO particles held in a ZINC-EUGENOLATE material.
- Acts as a competitive inhibitor of ***Enz. PG synthetase*** at 10^{-5} to 10^{-4} mol/L range. Aspirin acts as antiinflammatory effect by an irreversible inhibition of the same enzyme.
- It inhibits SENSORY N. ACTIVITY reversibly in 10^{-4} to 10^{-3} mol/L range.
- It is irreversibly NEUROTOXIC above 10^{-3} mol/L.

- A reversible VASODILATOR in 10^{-4} to 10^{-3} mol/L range.
- Reversibly inhibits RESPIRATION in mammalian cells in 10^{-4} to 10^{-3} mol/L range.
- Cells get killed by prolonged (12 hrs) exposure to 10^{-3} mol/L and by brief (minutes) to 10^{-2} mol/L. Cells survive prolonged exposure to 10^{-4} mol/L.
- Eugenol kills a range of intra oral organisms at 10^{-3} to 10^{-2} mol/L.

Mechanisms of ZOE (Also refer to sections of pedo and dental materials.)

- ZOE seals and excludes dietary substrate from bacteria, preventing decomposition.
- Kills microorganisms and halts spread of the lesion and bacterial toxins and so helps pulpal recovery.
- A conc. of 10^{-4} mol/L is there in the pulp adjacent. to intact dentin for at least 10 weeks—it decreases sensory nerve activity, increases blood flow and clearance of toxins; decreases PG synthesis and inflammation.
- Low thermal conductivity of ZOE and a good barrier to chemical diffusion will also decrease other insults to the pulp.

Calcium hydroxide (Also refer to sections of pedo and dental materials.)

- Used for direct and indirect pulp capping (DPC/IPC).
- Used for weeping canals in RCT.
- Used for Rx of internal resorption; apexification and apexogenesis; periapical resorption, etc.
- Is **acid etching resistant** liner beneath filled/unfilled CR.
- Helps in producing reparative dentin and so pulp to heal.
- BACTERICIDAL.
- May cause dystrophic calcification and obliteration of pulp chamber, which may be due to extensive and repeated irritation/ microleakage and reparative dentin formation only.
- ZOE should not be used on exposed pulp or under CR.

Mechanism of action of calcium hydroxide

- $Ca(OH)_2$ in contact with pulp immediately causes severe inflammatory response. $Ca(OH)_2$ causes following reactions adjacent to the tissue it is placed:
  - LOCALISED NEUROSIS of pulp.
  - Inflammatory cells collect here.
  - Undifferentiated mesenchymal cells proliferate to form odontoblasts.
  - Reparative dentin forms in approx 1 month after the capping.
  - Causes formation of reparative dentin.
  - It is basic with pH = 11.
  - It causes a **superficial zone of coagulation necrosis.** New odontoblasts then develop through differentiation of undifferentiated mesenchymal cells in pulp and cause reparative dentin formation.

Cement Bases, e.g. Zinc phosphate/GI/Zinc poly-carboxylate/ Reinforced ZOE (Also refer to sections of pedo and dental materials.)

- Its main function is to **replace the dentin thickness lost** due to caries and cavity preparation.
  - **It provides** chemical/thermal insulation .
  - Have low thermal conductivity; high compressive strength and stiffness.
  - Replaces the lost bulk of dentin
  - Bases with compressive strength up to 200 psi are capable of supporting amalgam condensation.
- Provides bulk and strength; thermal insulation.
- $Zn(PO)_4$ cement has thermal conductivity similar to dentin and a high compressive strength.
- GI = has ability to bond to dentine and high compressive strength; a good sealing capacity. It chemically adheres to the dentin or enamel. No microleakage (Chemical adhesion).

- Bases are not required below CR, because the conductivity of CR is same as dentin. But $Ca(OH)_2$/GI may be used as liners to act as barrier to the monomer of resin and to microleakage.
- e.g. $ZnPO_4$/Reinforced ZOE/GI/Zinc-poly carboxylate cements.
- GI/Zn-PC = form chemical bond and get adhesion to dental tissues.
- Grooves may be placed for retention of cement bases into dentin by burs-grooves are directed LATERALLY from the pulp to avoid pulp exposures.

Strength requirement for cement bases

- Strongest cement, e.g. $ZnPO_4$/GI should be used to minimize tensile stresses and to bear the occlusal stresses.

  $Ca(OH)_2$—used in 3 special circumstances.
- Direct pulp capping—as protective chemical barrier below the resins.
- Indirect pulp capping—as protective chemical barrier below the resins.
- For primary teeth esp if much loss of dentin is there.
- Thermal insulating property = can be used below silver-amalgam in class B depth cavities.
- Has no OBTUNDENT features.
- Compressive strength = 1500–4000 psi; not suitable under heavy occlusal pressure.
- Light cure $Ca(OH)_2$ material = has compressive strength = 12,000 psi.

$ZnPO_4$

- Varnish should be placed before $ZnPO_4$ to cover the dentin to prevent acid insult.

Reinforced ZOE

- Nonirritating to dentin.
- No cavity varnish required.

Zn–PC

- No liner required below it.
- Adhesive to tooth.

GI cement = ABC

A. Adhesion to enamel/dentin.
   - Good support to restorative materials.

B. Biocompatible.
   - Under CR = for S and with technique.

C. Fluoride = anti-caries.

Mixing

Reaction between $ZnPO_4$ powder and liquid is **exothermic**. So use cool slab and wide area for mixing.

- Cool slab permits INCORPORATION of more powder and hence more strength.
- 70° F temperature is required for cooling slab.
- 6 increments spatulated for 15 sec each and so 90 sec are required for proper mixing.

Glass–Ionomer cement

- Setting reaction is not exothermic.
- Reaction of PAA with aluminosilicate glass is fast = so cement must be placed, at proper time for proper adhesive bond.
- In water hardening cements = polyacid is dried, which is mixed with H_2O before mixing.
- Insertion of mix should be completed before the loss of gloss = to form a good adhesion to dentin.
- But in very deep cavity = the pulpal walls should be protected by using $Ca(OH)_2$.

Provisional restorations

- Maintains the position of the prepared tooth.
- ZOE acts as obtundent to the pulp.

- ZOE seals the cut dentin from oral fluids.
- After placing in the cavity = the hot water cotton pallet is wiped over the cement surface to HASTEN THE SETTING.

GI–CR laminate technique or scientist technique

It is used to fill the pits and fissures of a tooth to prevent the development of caries. Base of the fissures is sealed with GI cement as it is adhesive and releases the fluoride as anti-caries effect; the CR is placed on the GI after etching; as it is stronger and can withstand the heavy occlusal forces.

Gingival tissue M/M (Also refer to section on prosthodontics.)

A. **Mechanical method**
   - By extra heavy weight rubber dam = causes tissue retraction; prevent seepage of fluids.
   - By placing cotton twills in gingival sulcus before starting the operative procedure.
   - Fine cotton twills with ZOE cement are packed in sulcus. It puts GENTLE PRESSURE for some period of time for gingival displacement. It is most effective and conservative of all mechanical methods. But most time consuming (2–7 days).
   - Tissues should be reflected laterally, but not compressed APICALLY.

B. **Surgical removal**
   - Most effective = electrosurgery.
   - Less bleeding.
   - Cutting needle should not contact cementum and bone.

C. **Chemical method**
   - Adrenaline impregnated cord = **0.5 mg/inch adr**.
   - Should not be used in heart patients.
   - Causes vasoconstriction and tissue shrinkage.

CHEMICAL TISSUE RETRACTION

- For impression of finish lines.
- But can damage the attachment of junctional epithelium.

- Cords = knitted/braided/loosely woven made of COTTON.
- May be plain/chemical.
- 2 types of drugs used = vasoconstrictor/astringents.
- **Vasoconstrictors** = Epinephrine; ***0.5 mg/inch of racemic epinephrine***; its causes shrinkage of tissues by constriction of blood vessels and thus decreasing local tissue contour.
- But C/I in HT/heart disease/DM/hyperthyroidism.
- **Astringent** = especially aluminium chloride, or ferric sulfate solutions. Its effect is shrinkage of tissues by decreasing flow of fluid and by coagulation and precipitation of thin surface films. Should not be used in excess, as can cause chemical burns due to low pH.
- Dry field is required for retraction, so anti-sialogogue drugs may be given.
- Chemical tissue peck should **not be left in sulcus for > 5 min**. It should be of WEDGE shape.

GINGIVAL RETRACTION

Method	Features
Physico-mechanical	• e.g. temporary restorations. • rolled cotton/synthetic cord. • heavy weight rubber dam sheet.
Chemical method	• **vasoconstrictor** = e.g. racemic Adr and N Adr. • **biologic fluid coagulants** = e.g. 100% alum; 15–25% aluminium chloride; 10% aluminum potassium sulfate; 15–25% tannic acid; they are very safe and no systemic effects. • **surface layer tissue coagulants** = 8% zinc chloride; silver nitrate; can produce local ulcerations, etc.

GINGIVAL RETRACTION (*Contd.*)

Method	Features
Electrosurgical means	• **cutting** extremely precise; bloodless; with minimum tissue involvement and after effects. • **coagulations** causes surface coagulation of tissues, their fluids; blood, etc. It occurs due to thermal energy; if overdone it leads to carbonization. • **fulgeration** causes deeper tissue involvement; always accompanied by carbonization; greater energy is used. • **desiccation** involves greater tissue depth and area; it is most unlimited uncontrolled, and unpredictable. • during electrosurgery, use light touches and rapid intermittent strokes. • never involve the crest of the free gingival, but only the internal walls of the sulcus. • probe type electrodes = J—or loop shaped. • **bipolar electrodes** are used for fulgerations and desiccation. • **unipolar electrodes** are used for cutting and coagulation.
Surgical methods	

SEPARATION OF TEETH

- Helps to detect a proximal carious lesion in direct visibility.
- Provides space for finishing, matrix band placement, etc.
- **Methods = active or immediate,** i.e. occurs within 30 sec.; **passive** or **slow,** which requires 24 hrs time.

- **Active** is done by wedge method (**Elliot** separator); or traction (**Ferrier** separator).
- Wedging method is preferred over traction, as wedging is less injurious to PD tissues; and applies less pressure than traction method.

  1. Wedge method = elliot separator; wood or plastic wedges.

  2. Traction method = ferrier double bow separator.
- **Passive separation or slow separation** = by rubber dam separator; separating ligature or brass wires; orthodontic separators; orthodontic appliances, etc. Orthodontic grass line ligature contracts under moisture and leads to separation.

WEDGE

It is defined as the wooden or plastic conical shaped device, which is inserted in the embrasure area in order to attain intimate adaptation of matrix band with the tooth and also to attain some sort of separation of teeth to provide room for the matrix band.

It is of 2 types = wooden or plastic; orange wood stick is the best.

Advantages of wedge

- It prevents the overhang of the filling.
- Helps in effective condensation of the material.
- Helps to attain anatomic contour of the restoration.
- Causes some separation of the teeth.
- Helps in intimate adaptation of the matrix band.
- Is placed below the gingival floor.
- Wooden, triangular in shape; base is placed apically towards the gingival papilla.
- Should be inserted from LINGUAL embrasure because it is wider.
- **Moistened wooden wedge** = better secured position and easier placement.
- **Hard wood wedge** = placed forcefully—separates the teeth due to PDL elasticity and compensates for the thickness of the matrix metal.

- Contact area with adjacent tooth should exhibit the resistance to the passage of dental floss. So the band should be slightly loosened (by 1/4–1/2 turn) after placing the wedge.
- Metal matrix band used is = 0.015″ thick.

Rules for placement

- It is placed from larger to narrower embrasure, i.e. from lingual to buccal.
- It is of triangular shape; the apex faces the occlusal surface and the base towards the gingival surface.
- Should fit snugly in the embrasure without hurting the gingival.
- Wooden wedges are preferred over plastic as they absorb the saliva and further improve the snugness and also easily placed.

MATRIX

It is defined as a thin contoured strip used to substitute the missing wall of a compound or complex cavity in order to attain proper condensation and to restore anatomical contour and contact areas.

Functions = Substitute for lost wall of cavity during restoration.

Ideal requirements of a matrix:

- Should be rigid.
- Arc form is helpful because, when it is tightened, the cervical part becomes constricted and upper part is widened, which conforms the anatomical contour of the tooth.
- Maximum edge strength is required in the cervical region during condensation, so wedge is placed to avoid overhang.
- Restores proper proximal contours. When a band is placed, it separates the teeth as per its thickness; and when band is removed after filling, the teeth come together to make proximal contacts.
- Circumferential band may produce a negative contour and open proximal contact. So the band - CONTOURING should be done to avoid it.
- **Thickness of the band material** = generally ranges from 0.0015 inch to 0.003 inches.

- In **anterior teeth** fillings; the matrix should be transparent to confirm proper adaptation. It also allows passage of light for light curing. Curved **Mylar matrix** strip is used mainly. It helps to make anterior interdental contacts.
- It should extend **1–2 mm below cervical edge** and above the incisal edge.
- Direction of pull of matrix strip is away from access opening of the prepared cavity.
- Matrix should be **pulled towards incisal to tighten the strip at cervical margin** and to minimize overextension of the filling material.
- Wedge helps in close cervical adaptation of material.
- Overfilling should be avoided, as filled CR is difficult to finish.
- Light cure allows more working time and incremental additions to build up proper contours.

Examples of MATRICES

1. Toffelmire matrix = double banded for class I cavity and single banded for class II cavity. It is **in arc form**. The retainer can be placed either from lingual or buccal side; it is also known as **universal matrix band**; it is contra-angled.
2. Ivory no. 1 for **unilateral class II**; band is in curved form.
3. Ivory no. 8 for **bilateral class II cavity.**
4. **Ivory no. 9** is used for compound or complex cavities; MOD cavity; it is a straight metal strip..
5. **Auto-matrix** is in the form of Cu-bands. Used for highly mutilated teeth or for taking impression of inlay cavities.
6. Black's matrix for Class II cavity.
7. Anatomical matrix = for mutilated and Class II cavity.
8. Roll-in-band matrix, i.e. auto-matrix.
9. S-shaped matrix band = for Class II with facial/lingual extensions; for cavity on the distal surfaces of cuspids.
10. Celluloid strips = for silicate cements; for Class III cavity.
11. Cellophane strips = for resins; for Class III cavity.

12. Mylar strips = for resin/silicates, etc.; for class III cavity.
13. Stock crown matrix = for Class IV cavity.
14. Aluminium foil = stock metallic matrix used for restoring incisal corner; it cannot be used for light cure restorations.
15. Window matrix = for Class V cavity.

Circumferential Retainers

- Completely encircle the tooth.
- e.g. Ivory no. 9 and Toffelmires.
- Straight and contra-angle Toffelmires.
- Used in MO/DO/MOD cavities.
- Retainers lie to buccal side, but Toffelmire contra-angle type lies on lingual side of the tooth.
- Are more stable than unilateral types (i.e. Ivory no. 1).
- Thickness of band material used = 0.0015″.

Medicaments

1. **Antisialogogues**
   - Are anticholinergics agents.
   - Decrease saliva secretion.
   - e.g. Propanthelin bromide.
     - C/I in glaucoma/severe cardiac diseases.
2. **Antianxiety** drugs
   - Control apprehensions (anxiety).
   - e.g. Benzodiazepines, e.g. Diazepam 10–15 mg, 1 hr before.
   - Barbiturate sedatives act at CNS, e.g. Pentobarbitol sodium; 50–100 mg 1 hr before the appointment.
3. **Antibiotics**
   - To avoid transient BACTEREMIA.
   - Penicillin–V 2.0 gm orally 1 hr before and 1.2 gm orally 6 hr after.
   - To penicillin–allergics—give Erythromycin.

Dentin hypersensitivity = it is an exaggerated response due to non-noxious sensory stimuli; it is due to dentinal fluid movement stimulating pulpal pain receptors. It has a tendency of spontaneous resolution due to deposition of insoluble inorganic precipitates on exposed dentinal tubules from saliva and due to formation of secondary dentin. Most common agent used for its Rx is potassium oxalate and 5% potassium nitrate.

Other methods of Rx of hypersensitivity

1. Cavity varnish.
2. Anti-inflammatory drugs.
3. Partially obturating the dentinal tubules by = burnishing of dentin; silver nitrate; zinc chloride; potassium ferricyanide; formalin, etc. They form insloluble precipitates or protein precipitates on dentin.
4. Calcium hydroxide.
5. Fluoride compounds.
6. Iontophoresis.
7. Dentin bonding agents.
8. GI cement.
9. Restorative resins.
10. Jacket crown in extreme cases.

Management of hypersensitive dentin

- By sealing the exposed dentinal tubules.
- Sensitivity is due to shifting of dentinal fluid by hydrodynamic forces and stimulation of mechanoreceptors in pulp.
- 33% NaF/kaolin/glycerin paste creates smear layer in dentin.
- **Potassium oxalate** forms insoluble precipitates of Ca-oxalate, which occludes the dentinal tubules.
- K/Sr salts (KNO_3, etc.) = decrease nerve excitability.
- By **iontophoresis** also.
- Fluorides.

- Commercial pastes, e.g. sensodent K; sensodyne; thermoseal–RA, etc.

Anesthetics

- LA, with vasoconstrictor, which prolongs its duration of action and so a lesser volume of LA is required due to vasoconstriction of microcirculation.

Astringents

- Cause constriction of tissues, and so arrest the secretions and hemorrhage.
- Aluminium compounds precipitate the protein in attaining their action.
- Vasoconstrictors constrict the blood vessels and controls tissue perfusion.
- Epinephrine or racemic epinephrine (is 15 times more active) = hemostatic due to vasoconstriction of capillaries.

Organic solvents/for degreasing

- Chloroform, acetone, alcohol but irritate tissue and dehydrate the dentin.
- Petroleum distillate, e.g. soltrol–130 has no above-said effects.

Acid neutralizers

- Sodium bicarbonate in saturated solution is mostly used for neutralizing H_3PO_4 or polyacrylic acid.

DENTAL AMALGAM RESTORATIONS (Also see Dental Materials in Vol. II P 210.)

Classification of dental amalgam

According to the no. of alloyed metals	• Binary = Ag–Sn • Ternary = Ag–Sn–Cu • Quarternary = Ag–Sn–Cu, In • Unmixed • Admixed

Classification of dental amalgam (*Contd.*)

According to shape of particles	• Spherical = smooth surfaced • Irregular = lathe cut • Spheroidal
Powder's particle	• Micro cut • Fine cut • Coarse cut
According to Cu content	• Low Cu alloy = if Cu is < 4% • High Cu alloy = if Cu is > 10%
Generations	• First gen = Ag + Sn = 3:1 peritectically ratio • 2nd gen = Ag + Sn + 4% Cu + 1 % Zn • 3rd gen = Ag 71.9 % + Cu 28.1 %; it is Ag_3Cu eutectic alloy (spherical particles) added to the original alloy powder; mainly Ag_3Sn • 4th gen = up to 29 % Cu is alloyed to Ag and Sn to form a ternary alloy. Here, Sn is firmly bonded to Cu. • 5th gen = alloy of Ag, Cu, Sn, in to form a quaternary alloy; here none of Sn is available to react with Hg. • 6th gen = PD 10%, Ag 62%, Cu 28% eutectic alloy is lathe cut an is blended I 1st/ 2nd/ 3rd generation alloys in 1:2 ratio; has highest nobility.

- Reaction of Hg with silver amalgam is Physicochemical in nature.
- Ag, Sn, Zn, and Au were the constituents of **BLACK's amalgam formula** (rather than Cu) initially. Latest is the high - Cu content in alloys as compared to Black's formula.

- Zn = deoxidiser; scanvenger; decreases brittleness; increases deformability; resistance to oxidation; ultimate strength, but delayed expansion occurs in contact with moisture.
- Cu = increases strength, brittleness and proportional limit and hardness.
- Reaction = Ag Sn + Hg → Ag Hg + Sn Hg + Ag Sn + voids.

4 phases of amalgam mass

Phase	Properties
Gamma	remaining uncreated alloy **strongest, most predominant** phase esp Ag and Sn.
Gamma 1	next most predominant Strongest Ag–Hg phase.
Gamma 2	Sn–Hg phase; **weakest phase.**
Voids/air	Undesirable.

Different phases of amalgam

Phase	Composition	Properties
Gamma	Ag_3Sn	Strongest phase should occupy maximum space.
Gamma 1	Ag_2Hg_3	Noblest phase most resistant to corrosion should have maximum available space in bonding matrix.
Gamma 2	Sn_7Hg_8	Least resistant to corrosion; should occupy least space.
Hg	Hg	Weakest phase of the mass. Decreases strength and hardness. Increases flow and creep.
Voids	Air	Act as nidus for internal corrosion and stress conc.

- Conventional alloy = has Cu < 6% wt.
- Spherical particles are formed by ATOMIZING process.
- High-Cu content alloy = Cu-tin compound eliminates/decreases the WEAKEST and most corrodible phase of amalgam (gamma 2). Cu is up to 30 wt %.
- High Cu = less susceptible to corrosion.
- Compressive strength of amalgam = 5 × greater than tensile strength. So the thicker parts are stronger.

Strength

- Amalgam has a very weak tensile and a very high compressive strength.
- Amalgam looses 15% strength, when its temperature is increased from room to mouth temperature.
- 50% strength is lost if temperature is increased to 60°C.
- 50% compressive strength is lost, when Hg content is increased from 53 to 55 %.
- **Increase in strength** depends on:
  (a) reduction in particle size.
  (b) regularity and smoothness of particle shape and surface.
  (c) more trituration energy.
  (d) more condensation.
  (e) homogenization heat Rx of powder alloy.
  (f) minimum amount of Hg in the mix.
  (g) constituents on original alloy, which have good affinity to Hg, e.g. gamma phase.
  (h) spherical alloy attains strength quickly.
- Thermal conductivity is high, so base should be placed below silver.
- Galvanism and metallic taste can occur with different metal, but PASSIVITY soon takes place on the restorations surface.

Dimensional changes in amalgam: It occurs in 3 stages.

- **Stage 1** = is initial contraction occurs from the absorption of Hg in the inter-particular space of alloy powder.
- **Stage 2** = expansion, it is due to formation and growth of matrix crystals.
- **Stage 3** = limited delayed contraction due to the absorption of unreacted Hg.
- according to ADA–1 = –20 to + 20 micron/cm of D-change is acceptable.
- **Moisture contamination** = in Zn containing alloys, H_2 gas is produced. It occurs after 24–72 hrs and up to **2000 psi pressure** is created. Most obvious detrimental change is a **delayed expansion up to 400 micron/c.c**.

MAIN FEATURES OF CAVITY DESIGN FOR AMALGAM RESTORATION

- If grooves/fissures penetrate less than half the thickness of enamel —then it may be removed by ENAMELOPLASTY.
- **Enameloplasty** is the conversion of shallow fissure into a smooth based groove by removal of enamel; it becomes a part of the tooth surface.
- Unsupported enamel and opaque enamel should be removed.
- Buccal/lingual/cervical clearance of the adjacent. tooth should be 0.5 mm or less.
- Conservative cutting should be done. Latest in this methods is the ART, i.e. atraumatic restorative technique.
- While replacing any old restoration—keep in mind that cavity size is increased on an average by 0.6 mm each time a restoration is removed.

Reverse curve

- Used to conserve the tooth structure.
- Normally, it is a straight/convex curve where isthmus joins the bucco-proximal flare.
- It preserves the triangular RIDGE of the affected cusp.

Internal outline form

- Pulpal floor is placed 0.5 mm in dentin; it gives 1.5–2.0 mm of bulk of amalgam for adequate strength.
- Axial walls are placed into dentin for placing RETENTIVE grooves without undermining the enamel.
- **Isthmus width** = 1/3rd of intercuspal distance.
  - 1/5th of BL dim of the tooth.
- Depth is = 0.6–0.7 mm from DEJ.
- Depth of axial wall is less at axio-gingival line angle than at pulpo-axial line angle, because thickness of enamel is LESS cervically.
- Proximal walls should meet the outer tooth surface at right angle to remove all unsupported enamel.
- **Less chances of tooth fracture** are there in cavities—with narrow isthmus and shallow pulpal floor than with wide isthmus and deep pulpal floor; on longer teeth than the smaller teeth; with rounded internal line angles as it help in better force distribution.

Effect of crossing the marginal ridge during cavity preparation:

By 1/4th of intercuspal distance	Decreases the strength of the tooth by 15 %.
By 1/3rd distance	Decreased by 30 %.
By 1/2 distance	Decreased by 40 %.

Effect of crossing the oblique ridge during cavity preparation:

If crossed by 1/4th	Strength decreased by 20 %.
If crossed by 1/3rd	Strength decreased by 35 %.
If crossed by 1/2	Strength decreased by 45 %.

Cement base

- To insulate the pulp against the thermal stimuli.
- Objective = to restore the lost dentin thickness with the cement.

RESISTANCE FORM

- To withstand the stresses of mastication.
- Pulpal and gingival walls should be perpendicular to long axis of the tooth.

RETENTION FORM

- Prevents the filling from being displaced.
- Proximal box = has truncated form or inversely tapered walls to resist occlusally directed tensile forces.
- Grooves are placed in dentin in the proximal box; should be parallel to the PULPAL TISSUES.
- **Dovetail** = resist proximal displacement.

Removal of remaining carious dentin = should be done after staining with **0.5% basic fuchsin,** i.e. caries detection dye; use slow speed bur/sharp excavator.

Finishing

- Cavosurface for amalgam should be = BUTT joint, i.e. at 90 degrees; it provides maximum bulk for strength.
- Leave no unsupported enamel.
- Cavosurface should be parallel to enamel rods direction.
- Pulpal floor should be 0.5 mm beyond DEJ. It is done to pass the zone of maximum innervation of odontoblasts cells extensions. It helps to prevent the sensitivity.

ISTHMUS WIDTH

- Narrower the isthmus width of a cavity (1/4th the intercuspal distance) = enamel rods are more convergent towards the occlusal.
- Isthmus width = 1/3 ICD = E rods on the occlusal wall will be more nearly parallel.
- If isthmus width = 1/2 ICD = rods become divergent towards occlusal surface.
- Enamel rods = apically directed near CEJ, so gingival wall more near to CEJ should be reclined slightly apically.

Class V cavities

- Axial wall depth at occlusal wall is greater than at cervical, because enamel is thicker towards occlusal surface.
- A CURVED AXIAL wall is formed parallel to the pulpal contour to avoid over-cutting and encroachment of the pulp.
- Diverging walls are formed due to the direction of enamel rods and so retention grooves are placed in occlusal and cervical walls in the dentin.
- Retention grooves should not be placed in the mesial and distal walls of the cavity to avoid undermining the enamel at line angles.
- Occlusal stops should be on natural tooth surfaces and not on porcelain or porcelain–metal junction.

Class II cavity

- Dental caries starts just cervical to the contact area.
- Proximal margin of cavity should be cleared by 0.5 mm from the adjacent tooth and should be placed in self-cleansing area.
- Walls should be parallel with direction of enamel rods.
- Width of isthmus should be 1/4 to 1/5 of the intercuspal distance.
- Cavosurface angle/ideal flare = 90 degrees/butt joint.
- Retention should be placed in SOUND tooth tissue.
- Gingival floor should incline apically if it is more near to the CEJ, to avoid unsupported enamel rods.
- Proximal box is triangular in shape, with its base at the gingival area, which is self retentive and exposes less area of the marginal ridge to the masticatory forces.
- Pulpo–AXIAL LINE angle should be ROUNDED/BEVELLED to avoid conc. of stresses in the amalgam.
- Retention should always be located in DENTIN, away from pulp; without undermining the enamel.

Tunnel approach = to interproximal caries via occlusal or buccal side; keeping marginal ridge intact; suitable for small lesions only.

Class 6 lesions, i.e. 2 class II lesions on the same tooth, which are to be restored with a single restoration, e.g. MOD cavity.

Class 3 lesions = on distal surfaces of canines = should be filled with AMALGAM for better load bear; not of esthetic concern.

- It is a smooth-surface lesion–like class II lesion.
- Starts just apical to contact area in anterior teeth.
- Lesion is entered from LINGUAL side for restoration.
- Proximal box with triangular shape and retention groove is formed.
- Lingual dovetail for retention is formed.

MERCURY TOXICITY

Mercury alloy ratio

- **Eames' technique** = 1:1 ratio so , 50% Hg in the final restoration.
- **High Hg technique** also known as **increasing dryness technique**; Hg is 52–53%.

METHODS TO PREVENT HGG TOXICITY

- Hg is volatile at room temperature; and is 14 times denser than the water.
- Greatest risk to Hg is by **inhalation**. During removal of old restorations OR during polishing of the restoration, a heat generation of 60°C leads to evaporation of Hg. So use adequate **water-cooling**.
- **Threshold limit volume** of Hg for producing Hg toxicity is = 50 micro-gm/cubic metre of the environment. Well ventilated operatory should be made.
- Waste amalgam **should be stored under old x-ray fixing solution or potassium permanganate** solution.
- Avoid spilling **Lead** from RG packets can be **used for absorbing small spillages** along with a paste of equal parts of $Ca(OH)_2$ and flowers of sulfur and water.
- Mercury suppressant powders are also available.
- Waste Hg/amalgam should be sealed in screw top bottles.
- Use **high volume aspiration** during removal of silver fillings.
- Use impervious containers, gloves, masks, etc.

- Hg may cause hypersensitivity/allergy/contact dermatitis (< 1%). Wash the skin with soap and water after contact.
- No significant effect on pregnant females, but avoid.
- Amalgam scrap should be stored in tight bottle and covered with **Sulfide-solutions**.
- ADA 1 = deals Ag–alloy.
- ADA 6 = deals with Hg–purity.

Mercury-alloy ratio (Also refer to section on DM in Vol. II, III roles of Hg.)

1. Hg is necessary reactant with alloy particles for developing suitable physical properties of restoration.
2. Hg helps trituration/wetting of alloy particles.
3. Hg influences the plasticity of amalgam and its adaptability to the cavity.
   - M/A are determined by wt-to-wt basis, (wt% of Hg).
   - In pre-weighted capsule, there is < 50% of the Hg.
   - Pre-weight capsule of M and A are best for dispensing.
   - Smaller particle size has more surface area and so trituration is more rapid and rapid setting occurs.
   - Lathe cut alloy particles are ROUGH/irregular; require more Hg.
   - Spherical alloy particles are smooth/regular; require less Hg.
   - Spheres provide MINIMUM SURFACE AREA per unit wt. so less Hg is required.
   - Plasticity of amalgam depends on M/A = higher the Hg more is plasticity. Higher residual Hg content in mix leads to poor properties.
   - Spherical particles exhibit GREATEST PLASTICITY > admixed > lathe cut type.

TRITURATION

- Wets all surfaces of alloy with Hg.
- Rubbing of alloy particles ABRADES AWAY the OXIDE FILM on them, which can be easily attacked by Hg.

- Trituration can be done by amalgamator; mortar and pestle; capsule and pestle.
- Mixing should produce a smooth, non-granular plastic mass of amalgam.

Mulling—helps to enhance the uniformity/plasticity of the mass.

Condensation

- Any delay in condensation decreases plasticity and increases residual Hg in final restoration.
- Helps to minimize Hg content as low as possible.
- Force of condensation should be perpendicular to walls of the cavity.
- Avoid voids in the filling; they weaken the mass.
- Mix should be condensed within = 3–3.5 min.
- At least 6 pounds force should be used.
- A minimum thickness of 1.5 mm of amalgam is required for proper strength.
- **Axio-pulpal line angle** has to be beveled **to avoid stress concentration** in class II cavity.
- Width of isthmus should be 1/4th–1/5th of intercuspal distance.
- Ideal length to width ratio of a cuspal wall surrounding a Class II cavity should be 1:1 or less in dimensions.
- Cavity varnish should be applied on all walls and floor to avoid microleakage and to seal the dentinal tubules.

During condensation—the excess Hg tends to migrate to the surfaces. Hg rich surface should be removed before placing additional increment. This surface Hg helps to bond the subsequent layer of amalgam to the previous one.

(a) Over-filing is done s.t. Hg-rich layer can be removed from final restoration contour and gains UNIFORMITY.

(b) Weakest phase of amalgam = gamma–2 = Sn–Hg

(c) **High Cu alloys** = Cu is 6–25%; are of 2 types = 1. Single composition, i.e. Ag, Sn, Cu these are most resistant to corrosion. 2. Dispersion mix of Ag, Sn, and Cu; Ag.

(d) **Microleakage** with amalgam decreases with time by corrosion products; can be decreased **by varnishes; by a bonding agent,** e.g. amalgam bond or **panavia**—21, which has a resin adhesive, which also bonds to set amalgam; and also **by fissure sealants** over the filled restorations.

Condensers—can be smooth/serrated.

- Force of condensation varies inversely with the area of the condenser face.
- If bigger restoration is to be done = then 2–3 fresh mixes should be used, to avoid loss of plasticity and for better condensation.
- Condensers of amalgam differ from those of gold-condensers.

Burnishing

- Helps further condensation and adaptation of amalgam at margins and surface of restoration.
- Helps in making surface strong.
- Adjustment of Marginal Ridges should be done prior to removal of the band.
- A premature contact on the filling should be removed to avoid fracture and Peri-Apical inflammation.

Polishing and Finishing

- Silex slurry with unwebbed rubber cup or soft cup.
- Tin oxide slurry and a soft cup brush used.
- Use low rotation speed with water spray and light intermittent forces to avoid heat production and so as to prevent leaching out of Hg.
- Silicone rubber points and cups.

Refilling (Replacement)

1. Mostly due to secondary caries, which are:
   - Mostly on proximal occlusal lesions, which are
   - Mostly on proximal surfaces of the tooth.

DIRECT ESTHETIC RESTORATIONS DIRECT TOOTH COLORED RESTORATIONS

- Silicate cement
- Unfilled resins
- Filled resins
- Composite resins
- GIC; aluminosilicate polyacrylate cements ASPA

For interdental lesions on 2 adjacent incisors = the larger lesion should be prepared first; but the smaller lesion should be filled first.

First translucent cement used = silicate cement by Fletcher.

Silicate cement = causes severe pulpal irritation, which is due to highly acidic H_3PO_4.

- Gel like matrix is formed to bond the unreacted powder particles.
- Gel matrix is **sensitive to early moisture contamination** and dehydration, which may cause severe CRAZING; increased solubility and opacity. So cavity varnish/coca butter/silicane grease is applied on the surface.
- **Fluoride released** = so decreases caries activity.
- High solubility and disintegration in oral fluids and so short clinical life.
- **Contraindicated in mouth breather** patients, otherwise crazing occurs.

Types of GI cements

Type	Features
I	Luting cements for crown/bridge orthodontic bands
II	Restorative cements = are of 2 types • esthetic • reinforced used also as fissure sealants.
III	Fast setting lining material
IV	Light cure and dual cure GI cements

Cermet = i.e. GI in which ion–leachable glass is fused with fine silver powder, held together by metal–salt matrix.

Resin-modified GI = in it, 5% resin (HEMA bis–GMA) is present; initial set of material is by formation of polymerization matrix; which is strengthened by acid–base reaction.

Compomer = i.e. GI with composite resins; composed of single hydrophobic resin filled with acid leachable glass particles.

Resin material

- Chemically activated.
- Lack colour stability.
- High degree of shrinkage during polymerization.
- High coefficient of thermal expansion and so poor marginal adaptation.
- Resilient and lack of abrasion resistance.
- INCREMENTAL METHOD of filling of resin = decreases initial shrinkage, by overcoming the shrinkage by successive increments.

TYPES OF COMPOSITE RESINS

Generation	Features
First	• Consists of macro-ceramics phases in the resin matrix. • Have **highest surface roughness.**
Second	• Have colloidal and micro-ceramic phases in a continuous resin phases. • Have **best surface texture.**
Third	• Is **hybrid composite,** i.e. have micro and macro ceramics as reinforcers in a suitable resin matrix in a **ratio of 3:1**.
Fourth	• Are **hybrid types.** • Contain **heat cured**, highly reinforced composite macro-particle with a reinforcing phase of micro-ceramics.

TYPES OF COMPOSITE RESINS (*Contd.*)

Generation	Features
Fifth	• **Hybrid system.** • Continuous resin phase is reinforced with micro-ceramic and macro, spherical highly reinforced heat cured composite particles. • Improved workability. • Improved wettability; and chemical bonding of the particles.
Sixth	• Continuous phase is reinforced with a combination of micro-ceramics and agglomerates of sintered micro-ceramics. • Have **highest percentage of reinforcing particles.** • Exhibit **least shrinkage.**

Composite/filled resin system—By Bowen 1962.

- It has a polymeric, reactive phase (which is continuous) and an INERT phase of grand ceramic particle, is DISCONTINUOUS in nature.
- Ceramic decreases polymerization shrinkage and coefficient of thermal expansion.
- More stiff, durable.

Acid etched tip, i.e. for class IV lesions; the composite resin is the material of choice.

Posterior composites

- Hybrid material with more than 75% fillers should be used.
- Centric stops should be on sound tooth structures.
- Pre-wedging of teeth helps in creation of contact points. It helps in creation of the gap with wedge, which gets closed by bouncing back of the tooth after wedge removal.
- Incremental additions help to compensate for polymerization shrinkage.

Composite/filled resin: It has a 2-phase system

- Dispersed phase = ceramic particles as fillers.
- Continuous = polymer matrix.
- Silane coating on ceramic filler particles enhances bonding between 2-phases.
- Filler = 70–80% by wt.
  - Ductile resin matrix helps the STRESS TRANSFER between the particles.
  - e.g. BIS GMA or urethane diacrylates.
  - Setting reaction = free radical polymerization, which is initiated by BENZOYL PEROXIDE and is accelerated by TERTIARY AMINE.
  - Photo initiator = DIKETONE.
  - Visible LC = Blue light, 480–500 nm, for 20–30 sec.
  - Not soluble in oral fluids.
  - Silane bonding of particles decreases water sorption, and increases colour stability.
  - Filled resin are better able to withstand masticatory stresses.
  - Dimensional stability is more.
  - Shrinkage on polymerization is decreased to 1/4th as compared to unfilled resin.
  - Thermal coefficient of expansion is decreased by = 60%.
  - Low THERMAL conductivity and so insulates from thermal changes.
  - Loss marginal leakage.
  - Drawback = low resistance to ABRASION.
  - Functional Abrasion on contact area may occur, which is due to break down/hydrolysis of silane bond between filler particles and polymer.
  - Macrofilled resins (i.e. larger filler particles) rough surfaces texture and so more stainings.
  - Setting reaction of CR decreases in air or **with eugenol**.

- Pulpal irritation may occur in deep cavities due to penetration of low viscous resin or monomer in dentinal tubules.
- Cement base of liner should be placed as chemical barrier.
- **Dual cure composites** = first, light curing is done for 10 sec; and the final setting occurs chemically.

Microfilled resin

- ♦ Has microfine silica particles—55% by wt.
- ♦ Has smoother surface.
- ♦ Have better gingival response due to smoothness.
- ♦ Size of particles = 0.04 mm.
- ♦ Properties are not as desirable as for CR systems.
- ♦ Base resin is = BIS-GMA.
- ♦ Resin is impregnated with COLLOIDAL SILICA of submicron particle size.
- ♦ Its values for water sorption are higher than CR due to colloidal silica filler and so poor colour stability and marginal adaptation as compared to CR.

Hybrid/Blended resin

- ♦ Combination of micro filled particles.
- ♦ 1–5 μ size filler particles; radiopaque.
- ♦ Smoother surface finishing.

SHADE

- ♦ Vita shade guide is mostly used.
- ♦ Shade should be selected before rubber dam placement and before the eyes become fatigued.
- ♦ Operating **light should not be focused** while selecting the shade. Translucency and depth of chroma vary among the shades.
- ♦ Should be selected against **2 light sources**, one should be natural light.

Acid etching

- Preferential dissolution of interproximate (inorganic part) enamel followed by top surfaces of prisms.
- Surface area is increased by approx **200 times**.
- Micro-irregularities develop with an average **depth of 25 microns**.
- It exposes proteinaceous organic matrix of enamel, which adds to retention of restoration (Primer).
- It **increases the surface energy** of enamel.
- Phosphoric acid adds a highly polar phosphate group to enamel surface, which increases the adhesive ability of enamel surface.
- A **micro-mechanical bonding** is achieved.
- ***Microleakage is zero***.
- 37% ortho phosphoric acid (30–50%).
- Low viscosity unfilled resin is used as the BONDING AGENT to gain retention (PRIMER).
- Etching causes
  - Removal of debris/pellicle from surfaces.
  - Increases surface energy of enamel, making it more reactive.
  - Ends of enamel rods are dissolved, which forms surface irregularities and increases the surface area for bonding.

Mechanical bonding occurs

- Primer (unfilled resin) goes into surface irregularities by CAPILLARY ACTION to form polymer tags.
- Re-mineralization of etched enamel occurs from saliva and after 24 hrs, it is not distinguishable form untreated enamel.
- Etched enamel is porous and has high surface energy. It has 3 zones from surface inwards:
  - Etched zone — 10 microns
  - Qualitative porous zone — 20 microns
  - Quantitative porous zone — 20 microns
  - So the resin tags are of approx — 50 microns long

Depth of micro-pores = approx 20–50 microns

- Acid etching is less effective on PRIMARY teeth = due to LESS (INORGANIC) PRISMATIC STRUCTURE.
- Acid etching is difficult on acid resistant fluorosed teeth also, so repeated etching may be required.
- Polymers = cross–linked BIS-GMA resin.
- Exposed dentin should be protected from acid.
- Acid applied for 60 sec. (latest = 15–30 sec).
- Washing = 30 sec.
- Drying = 15 sec.
- Apply BONDING agent immediately to avoid contamination of etches area.
- **Total etch concept** = enamel and dentin are etched.

Crystal growth bonding technique

It is the latest concept in which tooth surface is treated with a solution of polyacrylic acid containing SO_4^- i.e. sulphate ions. The liberated Ca ions will react with these sulfate ions forming $CaSO_4.2H_2O$. These crystals start growing outwards with irregular rough surface and are similar to etched enamel without loss of tooth structure. On it, primer and resin may be applied for restorations.

Class III cavity

- Dentin contains greater amount of ORGANIC material and has higher moisture. They interfere with wetting by resin bonding agent and formation of polymer tags.
- Acid etching of dentin opens the tubules, releases capillary fluid, contaminating the exposed surface during bonding.
- Cervical and gingival walls should converge towards the opening of the cavity for retention; lingual access is preferred; the walls should be parallel to the enamel rods.
- Retention grooves are placed in DENTIN, but should not encroach the pulp. Most prominent retention is formed in = CERVICAL WALL due to greater bulk of dentin.

- Mechanical bonding with acid etching is not a major retentive factor here because = E rods are etched in a LONGITUDINAL DIRECTION.

Class V cavity: Placed on gingival 3rd of the tooth.

- Due to enamel rod direction; the occlusal and gingival walls are parallel and the mesial and distal walls diverge outwards.
- Found more in old age due to gingival recession.
- Composite resin for esthetic purpose = use dentin bonding agents if cavity margin is not entirely on enamel.
- GIC is the material of choice.
- Wall direction should be parallel to enamel rods and the cavosurface margins should form right angles.
- Incisal enamel cavosurface margin should have a LONG BEVEL to improve retention by acid etching. It also helps in a BETTER COLOUR TRANSITION. The bevel of 1.0–1.5 mm is adequate.

Root caries = caused by **actinomyces viscosus**; GI cement is material of choice; occur after gingival recession; in older age group and due to decreased salivary flow, e.g. in irradiated patients;

Class IV cavity: i.e. caries of anterior teeth.

- Involves incisal edges also.
- Retention is mainly gained by placing CERVICAL RETENTION groove in dentin.
- Cavosurface margins should be BEVELLED to increase surface area.
- Incisal margin is not bevelled = because it will give a thin resin layer, which gets # ed under masticatory loads.
- 1–2 mm long bevel is given.
- A chamfer of 2 mm length in enamel, increases the surface area for bonding and improves plane of orientation of etched enamel rods.

PULPAL PROTECTION BELOW CR

- Placed on axial wall only.
- Liners/bases are used as thermal insulators below CR. But liners act as:
  - Barrier to irritating chemicals.
  - Help in attaining a healthy pulpal response.
  - GI liner in Class A, B, C depth cavities.
  - $Ca(OH)_2$ +GI liners in class C and D depth cavities.
  - Class D cavity = i.e. < 0.5 mm thick dentin remains. $Ca(OH)_2$ helps formation of secondary dentin.
  - GI cement bonds well to the dentin and prepares a seal vs etchant/monomer.
  - $Ca(OH)_2$ has **an air inhibited surface layer,** which can bond with resin, but not with dentin and so will not seal this interface (but GI can do).
  - But light-activated $Ca(OH)_2$ base is inert and will not interfere with resin polymerization.
  - Poly carboxylate cements = can bond with dentin as GI, but not with resin.
  - CR results in discontinuous film of the liner, making it ineffective.

Eugenol results in incomplete setting of resin materials

- Chemicals containing BENZENE RING, e.g. phenol, eugenol inhibit polymerization of resins.

LIGHT CURED RESINS

- No mixing required, so very less chances of air voids.
- Working time is under control = is greatest advantage.
- Better surface texture, strength, etc.
- Incremental filling is possible, which also decreases air, increased strength and compensates polymerization shrinkage.

- Chair light should be kept away from the material, as it may loose their flow properties.
- Composition–(Refer to section of dental materials).

HOW DOES THE BOND OCCUR

- Air inhibited, unpolymerized layer of a cured increment ACTS as a BONDING AGENT, which later cures when it is covered with the fresh resin and unites the 2 increments together.
- Conc. of light beam is greatest at the surface and so the polymerization is faster and more complete here.
- Smaller **increments of < 2.0 mm** should be used, for better curing.
- **Darker shades should be placed in THINNER increments =** because, they have more CHROMA and opaque and so have great difficulty in curing light rejection.
- Microfilled resins have smaller filler particles and less filler content = it does not cure to as great a depth as with longer filler particles.
- An unfilled resin boding agent is applied to etched enamel GI cement. Light cure it for 10–15 sec for optimum bond strength for resin tag formation.
- 450–500 nm, **blue light**, for 20–30 sec.
- Light source should not touch the resin, but should be away by 1 mm only.
- By finishing agents = the softer matrix is abraded at a relatively faster rate and the ceramic particles get projected on the surface, causing rough surface.
- Finishing discs of CR have Al_2O_3 particles on it.
- Abrasive strips = for I/d and gingival smoothening, has Al_2O_3 particles.
- Microfilled CR has better surface smooth finish.
- Etching for 60 sec washing for 30 sec.
- Etched surface appears FROSTY.

- Air inhibited surface of bonding agent becomes the bonding surface for first layer of the veneering resin.
- Darker/more chromatic layer should be placed first; should be 0.5 mm thick; should be thinned out as it approaches the incisal part of the tooth.
- A final increment of lighter shade is placed INCISALLY to make it translucent.
- Final curing is done for 60 sec to cure at all depths.
- Heavily filled hybrid material should be used in areas of FUNCTIONAL STRESSES.
- Hybrid resin veneer cementing surface should be ACID etched for 60 sec to clean it with debris and bonding agent should be applied.
- Porcelain veneer-internal surface should be etched with HF acid and a silane coupling agent is placed before final cementation to strengthen the polymer bond to porcelain.

GI CEMENT

Powder = Ion-leachable calcium aluminosilicate glass and fluoride.

Liquid = Solution of polyacrylic and itaconic acids.

Initial setting reaction = Ca^{++} ions migrate in hydrated siliceous gel and form bridge between polycarboxylate ions (GEL MATRIX).

- **Final setting** = Aluminum salt bridges develop, cross linking occurs; F-complexes formed.
- **Anhydrous GI cement** = dehydrated polyacrylic acid is included in powder; its liquid is composed of distilled water and other additives.
- If dentin in < 0.5 mm thick, a protective layer of $Ca(OH)_2$ should be placed for formation of secondary dentin.
- High M. wt. of poly acrylic acid molecules - can't penetrate dentin tubules and so least pulpal irritant.
- GI gel is SENSITIVE to moisture, so should be protected during setting by varnish or LC unfilled bonding agent/vaseline.

- Low resistance to abrasive wear = so should not be used in areas of functional stresses, e.g. contact areas, centric stops, etc.
- So GI should be limited to class 3, 5 cavities.
- Esthetic qualities and surface polish are inferior to CR. So GI is less preferred than CR in esthetic zones.
- It is the material of choice for class 3 caries extending on root surface.

Class V, e.g. cervical abrasion.

- Usually found in patients with HIGH CARIES RISK.
- If on cementum also = GI is better for adhesion as it decreases microleakage.
- If lesion is surrounded by enamel = CR is better for surface finish.

DENTIN BONDING AGENTS (DBA)

- Dentin has high water and organic content.
- **Smear layer** = has amorphous layer of organic and inorganic debris; decreases dentin sensitivity and prevents loss of dentinal fluid; has more inorganic content as cp to dentin.
- They aim to modify and partially remove the smear layer by acidic primer, which exposes collagen and opens dentinal tubules; then a resin with bifunctional ends is placed, i.e. one end is hydrophilic which bonds with wet collagen and dentin and the hydrophobic end bonds with composite resin.
- Gets bond to dentin through CHEMICAL reaction.
- Bond is a WEAK POLAR BOND, which bonds the phosphate in Bis-GMA to Ca^{++} in tooth.
- Bond is also known as **SCOTCH BOND**.
- Bond strength to etched enamel = 3000 psi.
- Bond strength to dentin = 800–1000 psi.
- Better bond strength to dentin with either OXALATE pretreatment or a GLUTERALDEHYDE base resin.

Generations of dentin bonding agents

I	Phosphate ester of BIS-GMA.
II	Chlor–phosphate ester of BIS-GMA.
III	GLUMA and 4-META.
IV	Moist dentin bonding; moist bonding technique; no air drying required.
V	Primer and adhesive agents combined; one-component system.
VI	Etching eliminated: No etch, no rinse, no cure technology.

GI with CR to restore cervical lesion

- GI is combined with micro-filled CR as 2-step procedure, using DBA.
- Dentin is conditioned with polyacrylic acid.
- GI lining is placed, i.e. GI is placed first as liner and then the CR is filled for bulk.
- Etching of GI and enamel is done for CR.
- It is also known as **SANDWICH TECHNIQUE**
- **Advantages**
  - GI provides chemical barriers to monomer of CR.
  - Provides seal at dentin.
  - Fluoride from GI is anti-caries.
  - CR gives improved esthetics smooth surface and greater durability

CR for posterior teeth

- Are hybrid CR, with greater strength and less dimensional changes.
- But have inadequate wear resistance.
- So it should be limited to those teeth where occlusal support is on sound enamel.

- Dentin should be protected from etchant to avoid pulpal irritation.
- Internal line angles **are more rounded** than for amalgam.
- Occlusal walls should have divergence toward occlusal.
- No BEVEL is placed on cavosurface margin, as it provides a thin filling margin susceptible to fracture.
- Proximal box has convergence towards occlusal, with no cavo surface bevel.
- As cp to $Ca(OH)_2$, GIC bonds to dentin; prevents microleakage. It can also be acid etched for 20 sec to provide porous surface for mechanical bonding to CR.
- Filling is done in INCREMENTS, for proper curing of materials and to decrease total polymerization shrinkage and the internal stresses.
- Time of exposure of light beam should be increased to 40 sec when the distance from tip of light is more than 1.0 mm or the resin increment is > 2.0 mm thick.

Differences between light cure and chemical curing bonding

Light cured	Self/chemical cured
Less wastage of material	More
Filling/curing is done in increments	In one phase
Finishing is good	Poor
Strength is higher	Lesser
Controlled setting time	Starts setting with mixing of primer and adhesive
Working time is long	Less
No mixing is required mixed	2 components are to be
Colour stability is better	Poor
Wear resistance is better	Lesser
In orthodontic bonding, it gives adequate long time for adjusting the bracket position	This freedom is not allowed.

Fused porcelain: By Byram 1908.

- Better esthetics, durability, D-stability.
- But problem with proper marginal adaptation and so tinting agent is visible at cavosurface margin. (BRITTLE).
- It can be prevented by acid itching and bonding with CR.

Porcelain veneer: The fitting surface is roughened with sand blasting, cleaned with alcohol and coated with silane–coupling agents, and then a dentin bonding agent is placed. The veneers are 0.5–0.7 mm thick.

All ceramic crowns: e.g. Empress, etc. are built on high strength alumina cores.

DIRECT GOLD RESTORATIONS

Are the only type of restoration which use pure gold, with the exception of electralloy.

2 types = precipitated gold; gold foils.

PRECIPITATED GOLD

- Gold is precipitated by atomization.
- Spherical particles are produced; of 5–75 microns size.
- 3 forms.

Form	Features
Powdered gold	• e.g. **goldent**; the precipitated gold particles are wrapped in cohesive gold foil to make balls of 1–4 mm diameter. Ratio of precipitated powder and cohesive gold foil is **19:1**.
Mat gold	• Gold is precipitated through electrodeposition. • **Mat foil** = mat gold strips wrapped in cohesive gold foil. • **Electralloy** = is an alloy of **gold with calcium**. The calcium content is in 1% range.

Gold foils

- It is the oldest and most durable direct gold.
- Prepared by cold working/strain hardening of the ingot.
- Thickness range = 0.001–0.007 mm.
- 4 forms.

Form	Features
Plain gold foil	
Corrugated foils	Are more cohesive than plain foil.
Platinum gold foil	Used in areas of stress conc for improved mechanical properties.
Laminated gold foils	It has directional properties. It is much stronger and more resistant to stresses.

Pure cohesive gold foils restorations will be strongest; densest; hardest of all types of direct gold restorations, due to greater **cohesion** between foils.

Cohesive gold

- Surface is protected by chlorine or ammonia gases, which can be removed by degassing just before use.
- It can be done by **3 ways**.
- Heating by an open alcohol flame.
- Heating on a mica sheet over a flame.
- **Electric degassing**

Gold (Direct Filling)–(DFG)

Cohesion: i.e. force which bonds 2 similar molecules.

Forms of cohesive gold.

1. Fibrous gold foil = OLDEST
   - It is a wrought material.
   - Gold sheet formed are of **4″ size.**
   - Sizes vary from to 1/128.

2. **Mat gold**
   - Is a **crystalline deposit** deposited by **electrolytic process.** Extremely pure.
   - **Mat foil** = mat gold wrapped in a thin sheet of fibrous gold foil, which decreases its friability is known as mat foil.
3. **Encapsulated powdered gold**
   - Contain **organic annealing** indicator.
   - Better handling and little waste.
4. **Alloyed filling gold**
   - **Crystalline** structure.
   - **Ca^{++}** is the alloying agent.
   - Produces **Hardest surface** of all direct filling gold.

Type: Cohesive/Semi-cohesive/Non-cohesive

- Cohesive gold material has no surface contamination.
- The **ammonia compound** acts as adsorbent as **a protective covering** to prevent adsorption of nonvolatile substances. It can be removed by heat for making it cohesive.
- **Annealing** = is the cleansing of gold by heating. Contaminants can be sulfides, oxides, etc.
- **Methods** = 1. **Bulk method**—foils placed on MICA Sheet on the open gas/flame, till the gold becomes DULL RED colour.
- DFG should never be annealed directly in open gas flame to prevent its contamination.

2. **Piece method** = most practical method; done on simple alcohol lamp; acetone–free alcohol should be used; it is known as DEGASSING; helps in selecting gold foil of desired size and avoids contamination of foil between annealing and use.

Storage of foils—with ***ammonia vapors***, which get adsorbed on surface and prevents contamination.

- Anneal all direct filling golds before use, to make it cohesive.

Condensation of pure gold

- Hand instrument condensation.
- Pneumatic condensation = i.e. by air pressure.
- Electronic condensation = at 2 ounces–15 lbs force; with 360–3600 cycles/min.
- Hand condensation and mallet.
  - Avoid voids/pits in the filling.
  - **Wedging principle** = condensation should begin at a central area and work towards the walls.
  - Gold foil should overlap each other.
  - Stepping of condenser point necessary over entire surface.
  - Gold is always worked from centre of restoration towards the margin (during finishing).
  - Silex + Tin oxide is used for polishing.
  - A tight proximal contact should be developed with adjacent teeth.
  - Hand pressure condensation-minimum pressure required is **15 psi**; sustained force is employed; condenser face is serrated and of **smaller diameter** than required for Ag-Hg; serration are CONICAL in shape to apply heavy localized, concentrated forces.
  - **Hand malleting** = helps in adapting denser cohesive golds into retention areas; 5 oz mallet is used.
  - **Mechanical method** = pneumatic; electro-mallet; lighter blows with high frequency are preferable.

Types of condensers

1. **Round** = used in retention grooves.
2. **Parallelogram** = used for BULK.
3. **Foot type** = used at cavosurface.

Only fibrous gold foil is of fibrous/wrought nature, rest 3 are of crystalline nature.

Fibrous gold foil: Best suited for small pits and fissures and conservative cavities; on restricted surfaces.

- Gives excellent surface.
- Used to veneer other forms of cohesive gold.
- Used in cavities not having proper convenience form.

Mat foil: For BULK filling of **single surface** restorations, e.g. class I, V.

- Density greater than gold foil—so LESS TIME is required to fill the cavity.
- Not used on SURFACE, as pitting may occur due to its peculiar inadequate subsurface condensation.
- So restoration should be VENEERED with fibrous gold foil to maintain a good surface.
- Heavy hand force is required.

Encapsulated powdered gold

- Used both as a BULK filler and for surface restoration.
- Greater density than mat gold.
- Used **to fill all classes of cavities,** where cohesive gold may be indicated.
- Sustained hand pressure is required.

Alloyed filling gold

- Used **in all classes of cavities** especially, 1, 2, 3, 5.
- Heavy hand pressure is required for good surface.

Indications of DFG

1. Conservative cavities only.
2. No heavy biting stress areas.
3. Should be enclosed with in the cavity walls.

C/I: Should not be used if isolation is not proper; with larger cavities, etc.

CAVITY PREPARATIONS

1. Angular undercut placed in dentin walls of conservative class I cavities = permits easy placement for fibrous gold foil.
2. If more dense gold is to be used = the less angular or a rounded groove should be placed.
3. Fibrous gold foils are WEDGED in the angular retention grooves = wedging helped by ELASTICITY OF DENTIN.
   - Bevel = short cavosurface bevel is required for condensing fibrous/wrought gold foil, as it provides adequate margin strength in thinner cross section.
   - Bevel is protective, as it removes unsupported enamel.
   - It should be at 45 degrees ard 0.5 mm in length.
   - Bevel should not be placed for crystalline gold as it will get fragmented in thinner layers under masticatory pressure.

Filling

1. Thin layer of varnish applied, should not block the retention grooves; should be on DENTIN only.
   - Condensation is started in retention points for fibrous gold.
   - Condenser is stepped in an overlapping manner.
   - Periphery is built slightly ahead of central area of the cavity.

Veneered gold foil restoration = i.e. combined use of alloyed filing gold/mat gold and gold foil on the surface. It is used if SIZE of cavity is LARGE. Heavy pressure is used. Walls of cavity are covered ahead of floor/axial walls, till cavity is 95% filled.

Then = a veneer of **fibrous gold** is started at cavosurface bevel, till whole surface is veneered.

- Burnishing should be done from metal towards the enamel; it helps in work-hardening.
- Silex and tin oxide paste in rubber cup is used for polishing.
- Gold is a malleable material and is always burnished TOWARDS the margins of restorations.

Class III cavity

- For mx incisors = lingual approach to make class 3.
- For md incisors = labial approach to make class 3.

Class II cavity

- Alloyed filling gold/encapsulated powdered gold preferred.
- Should be limited to conservative defects
- Proximal box prepared with triangularity slightly more than used for amalgam cavity.
- A 35° short bevel on gingival margin.
- Internal line/point angles should be well defined.

Matrix

- A Cu-band heated to redness and quenched in alcohol to soften it is used.
- Quenching in water allows formation of oxides, which may contaminate the gold.

CAST GOLD RESTORATIONS

- Pure gold is used only occasionally for inlays in LOW-STRESS BEARING AREAS.
- Types = I, II, III, IV gold alloys.
- From Type I to IV alloys.
  - Hardness increases.
  - PL and strength increase.
  - Elongation decrease.

Type I gold

- Soft gold alloys
- For low stress bearing areas, e.g. small Cl I, 3, 5 cavities.
- Direct method of INLAY preparation is used.

Type II

- Medium hard alloys
- Used for majority of castings, e.g. crowns for single tooth.
- Supports occlusal stresses without deformations.
- INDIRECT method casting is used.

Type III alloy

- HARD alloys
- Greater Tensile strength Required, e.g. FPDs, i.e. for abutment crowns.
- Has lesser elongation.

Type IV

- Extra hard alloy.
- For RPD castings.

CAVITY DESIGN

1. Cavity wall should DIVERGE towards the occlusal. (As cp to silver amalgam and DFG, in which cavity walls should converge.)
2. **Line of draw** = is the axis of taper. Taper permits unobstructed removal of wax pattern. Axis of taper for class 1, 2 cavity = Parallel to long axis (LA) of tooth. Axis of taper for class 5 cavity = Perpendicular to LA of tooth.
3. **Cone angle taper** = 10–16 degrees; it is the relation of all prepared walls of the cavity.
4. Longer preparation require taper in higher range; short preparation in lower range.

INLAY CAVITY

- Divergent walls.
- Rounded line angles.
- No undercuts.

- For onlays = a minimum of 1.5 mm reduction of cusps is necessary.
- For porcelain = silane coupling agent is used on the fitting surface.
- Do not use eugenol with composite resin.

TYPES OF BEVELS

- **Partial bevel** = involves part of enamel wall, not more than 2/3rd of its dimensions.
- **Short bevel** = includes entire enamel wall but not dentin.
- **Long bevel** = include entire enamel wall and up to one half of dentinal wall.
- **Full bevel** = includes all of the enamel and dentin walls. But its use should be avoided as it decreases internal resistance and retention.
- **Counter bevel** = it is used when capping the cusps to protect and support them.
- **Hollow ground/concave bevel** = it allows more space.

Bevels

Helps in adaptation of margins; as gold is ductile and malleable.

1. **Butt joint**
   - 90 degrees
   - Most difficult to adapt
2. **Lap joint**
   - 35 degrees metal margin
   - Easy to adapt
3. **Sliding lap joint**
   - 25° margin
   - Margin should be burnished beyond its P.L. for adaptation.
4. Axio-pulpal line angle is rounded to avoid stress and concentration in this area.
5. Flare of proximal walls should form axio-proximal angle of 100–110 degrees.

6. Occlusal dovetail.
7. Pin holes/post holes = to prevent ROTATIONAL displacement.
8. CERVICAL MARGIN bevel—is important feature. For indirect wax pattern–smaller; for direct wax pattern - bevel should be of greater bulk and of greater MD width across the cervical floor. It should be 1/4th–1/3rd the MD width of cervical floor; it helps easy manipulation of wax, and manipulation of gold margins.
   - Also pulpal floor is SLANTED to the lingual side and so cervical floor will not be parallel to the pulpal floor.

Cuspal protection

- 1.5 mm reduction is done for adequate thickness.

Class 3 = Class 3 inlay is best used on the **distal surface of canines.**

Class IV cavity

- is a 2-surface cavity involving incisal and proximal surfaces.
- Retentive pin hole in cervical and incisal areas are placed (approx 1 mm deep).

Class 5

- Trapezoidal smooth flowing shape.
- Walls should be prepared parallel to enamel rods.
- Axial wall must be curved parallel to pulp chamber.
- Walls are made divergent so that they are parallel to enamel rods.

Cervical finish lines may be:

FINISH LINES

Type	Features
Chamfer	• **Most commonly** used. • 0.5 mm is the maximal depth. • Assures bulk and definite margins. • But limited burnishability.

FINISH LINES (*Contd.*)

Type	Features
Knife edge/ feather edge	• **Least tooth structure involvement.** • Should be used only if alloy is very castable–burnishable type, e.g. gold alloy type II. • Its **disadvantage** is = possibility of indefinite termination for the casting; over contoning.
Beveled shoulder	• **Involves most tooth structure** indicated if **maximum bulk** of cast is needed marginally. • It maximally reduces marginal problems of internal spacing. • Ideal design for subgingivally located margins.
Hollow ground	• Is **exaggerated chamfer** tooth involvement is greater than chamfer and less than the beveled shoulder. • Is **superior to chamfer.**
Shoulder	• Finish line **at 90 degrees** to axial wall. • Used for **porcelain** for maximum bulk. • No burnishing is possible or required.

Die (Also refer to section of prostho.)

- Electroformed metal die is better than stone dies as there is minimum danger of abrasion and overfinishing.
- Dies for long and thin preparation especially on anterior teeth are best formed of metal, as it is least prone to fracture.
- Epoxy/resin materials exhibit polymerisation shrinkage.

SILVER ELECTROFORMING of rubber/Impression

- Helps to form metal dies.
- But polysulfide RBM can't be copper plated due to lack of throwing power of $CuSO_4$.
- Silicone impressions can be copper plated easily.

- Ag = plating of dies is also done, esp. of prepared teeth only.
- Alkaline silver cyanide (Ag-CN) solution and pure silver anode are used.
- Current = 10 mA; (low current can lead to formation of gas bubbles and powdery deposits of silver.
- Electroplating is done for > 12 hrs.

ELASTIC IMPRESSION MATERIALS

- First elastic material was = Agar.
- Agar is a reversible gel; due to a physical phenomenon of temperature change.
- Alginates = irreversible gel, a chemical reaction occurs.
- First rubber base impression material was-polysulfide and then silicone and then polyether.

Polysulfide

- Useful for impression of deeper subgingival areas.
- Hydrophilic.
- Dimensionally stable if dies are to be formed even 1 hr after the impression.
- More difficult to mix.
- Least costly.
- But long WT and ST; less cross linked.

Condensation silicones

- Medium WT/ST.
- Mix easily.
- **Hydrophobic**; require dry field.
- More shrinkage due to loss of bye-products.

Addition silicones

- Newest.
- ***Least amount of shrinkage***—no formation of Bye-products.
- MOST ACCURATE.

- If delay in die formation is there—these are the best impression materials.
- Highly cross-linked.
- High hardness-low flexibility.

Polyether

- Short WT/ST.
- Low flexibility, tear strength and flow.
- So LESS VERSATILE than others.

AGAR: Reversible; due to physical change.

- Impression **must be poured soon after** removal from mouth.
- Only stone dies can be made.
- Agar has high water content, so it is dimensionally instable.
- Conditioning and storage:
  - In liquefying bath for 15 min.
  - In storage bath = 150 degrees F.
  - Tempering bath = 115 ± 5 F for 5 min.

Cooling is done under running tap water for at least 4 min. It is a poor thermal conductor and gelation occurs from outside to inside.

SPRUING

- Hollow sprues better than solid sprue, because they carry less heat and so less distortion of wax pattern; also give firm attachment to the pattern.
- Should be attached in the bulky part of pattern in an area least disturbing the contours/margins.
- Slight **funneling** is done at attachment point to decrease heat build up.
- Should be attached at approx **45 degrees** to occlusal plane; while a casting which has to gain its major portion of compensation by hygroscopic setting expansion HSE, should be placed symmetrically in the investment.
- A Y-shaped sprue is made for MOD casting.

- Sprue length above the sprue former should be **6–8 mm** only.
- Most frequently used sprue diameters are 12, 14, 16 gauge.

INVESTING

- Internal stresses in the wax pattern get released and lead to distortion = so should be invested quickly.
- Linear contraction is 0.4% in wax.
- Casting shrinkage occurs on cooling.
- Expansion in investment compensates this by 3 procedures.
  - NSE = due to crystalline growth of gypsum binder
  - TE = when investment is heated to remove wax
  - HSE = when investment sets in contact with H_2O.
- HSE and TE provide larger amount of expansion.
- HSE is also known as **low heat casting technique.**
- TE is known as **thermal technique.**
- HSE = investment is placed in 100 F water bath for 35 min.

CASTING

- Investment is placed in preheated oven at 900 ± 25 F for 1 hr for wax removal.
- Sprue hole should be down for 1/2 hr and then for 30–45 min with hole upright. So O_2 comes in contact with wax for **complete oxidation of residual wax**.
- Metal is heated by, natural gas and compressed air flame.
- Blue flame is used, it is a reducing zone.
- Metal is heated to light red colour with good fluidity.
- After casting, **quench** the casting; it helps in **breakage of investment**.
- **Pickling** = done to remove surface oxides.
- Saturated Sod. Bicarbonate solution is used to remove residual acid.
- Previously cast gold can be reused after adding some new gold to **replenish the ZINC** content.

- Internal surface of casting is etched by **air-abrasive tech** under low pressure.

SOLDERING (Also refer to the section on dental materials Vol. II).

- Done to make proximal contact area.
- Freehand soldering is simple/efficient.
- Anti-flux = carbon pencil; graphite.
- Flux = Borax and Boric acid.
- Type II casting gold, 650 fine, 18 K solder is used to make the contact and other contours.
- If during seating—a heavy consistency of cement mix is placed ON CASTING and tooth, then a saturated solution of $NaHCO_3$ is applied for disintegration of cement and its removal.
- **Proximal contacts are first adjusted before seating.**
- Cervical margin of seated inlay is the **first to be adapted.**

Direct wax pattern—for class II cavity.

- Type I wax is used.
- Matrix adapted = 0.002″ matrix band.
- Wax heated in water at 122 F for 5 min.
- Heavy finger pressure maintained for 3 min.
- 20 gauge hollow sprue placed just inside the Marginal Ridge on occlusal surface for removal of wax pattern.
- Hollow 14 or 16 gauge sprue attached to proximal surface, slightly to LINGUAL SIDE of contact area; should form 45 degree angle with the occlusal plane after investing.
- Type I soft gold is most often used for class 2 casting.
- For class 3 wax pattern = 0.0015″ mylar matrix is selected.
- Soft type I gold alloy is good for class 3, 5 inlays, because of low functional stresses encountered.

PORCELAIN FUSED TO METAL (PFM) RESTORATIONS

- Dicor crown = **cast** ceramic crown.
- Cerestore crown = **injection molded** crown.

- Colour/shade = is produced by the REFRACTION, INTERFERENCE, ABSORPTION.
- **Refraction**-occurs when light passes from one medium to another, in which its velocity is different.
- **Interference** = is by thin transparent films on a surface st light waves travel at different rates.
- **Absorption** = colours of object is the reflection of wavelength (colours) not absorbed.
- UV light produces chemical changes; damages the retina (retional determent) and the infrared is a source of heat.
- **Hue** = describes colour, i.e. red, yellow, blue.
- **Chroma** = describes intensity of colour; it is the strength/ saturation of colour.
- **Value** = describes brightness/dullness of colour. It is determined by amount of gray/white present.
- **Opaque** = blocking the passage of light.
- **Transparent** = permitting the passage of light.
- **Translucent** = permitting the passage of light, but diffusing it.
- For shade selection = both artificial and natural lights should be used.
- PFM crown = it has a cast substructure, of special alloy to which porcelain is fused.
- Feldspathic porcelain = feldspar (81%), quartz = (15%), kaolin (4%) and metallic oxides (< 1%). But it is TRANSLUCENT.
- **Aluminium porcelain jacket crown** = its CORE has 50% high strength alumina + 50% porcelain. It was developed by John McLean. It is OPAQUE.
- Mostly, the failure of porcelain jacket crowns is due to propagation of microcracks, which occur during cooling. This propagation is interrupted by HIGH-STRENGTH ALUMINA CORE.

BONDED ALUMINA CORE

- Stress concentration is high around microcracks on the inner surface of ceramic.

- Metal can relieve stress concentration around the crack, and thus prevents its propagation under loading.
- Aluminous porcelain is bonded to pure Pt foil by first coating the foil with 0.2–2.0 mm of TIN before firing on the porcelain. Then porcelain is CHEMICALLY-BONDED to the metal coping.

CERESTORE CROWN

- It is a ceramic restoration, which uses a ***shrink free alumina ceramic core***, with an ***aluminous porcelain veneer***.
- High strength alumina core, so the crown is **better for posterior teeth**.
- Made by **injection molding technique** and so has an EXCELLENT MARGINAL FIT.
- ***No metal substructure.***
- Has translucency.

DICOR CROWN

It is a truly castable–ceramic restoration.

It is used for posterior teeth.

- ***No metal substructure*** or underlying core.
- Its shade is not durable, because it is applied to the SURFACE of restoration.

Acrylic jacket crown

- Mainly used for PROVISIONAL RESTORATION
- Used for YOUNG patients with large pulpal chambers; and so extensive crown cutting cannot be done for ceramic.
- Colour stability of heat cured is better than the self cured acrylic.

ABUTMENT PREPARATION

- For anterior tooth = the shoulder is extended to lingual line angle of the tooth—for esthetic season.
- For posterior tooth = the shoulder is just beyond the buccal line angle.

- Width of shoulder = 1.5 mm till I/D area and it narrows as it extends toward the lingual for anterior teeth.
- Incisal/occlusal reduction = 2–2.5 mm.
- Lingual surface reduction = 0.5–1.0 mm.
- **Bevel** is placed on labial shoulder = it provides metal collar, which is the most resistant to distortion during the stages of porcelain firing = where esthetics is not of much concern.
- If esthetics is required = than SLOPING SHOULDER provides space for both metal and porcelain.
- A BUTT-JOINT = is best for an ALL-PORCELAIN margin. Strength of porcelain depends on its bulk, and the butt joint provides most bulk in the restoration.
- A 10° convergent taper towards INCISAL.

Die fabrication

- Metal die is preferred for fabrication of PFM crown—as it resists the abrasion.
- Electroformed dies can be formed on rubber base impressions.
- Fabrication of cerestore restoration requires use of **special epoxy die**, for the development of alumina core.
- A ***canine-guided occlusion*** favors the use of porcelain occlusal surface, as there is no facial contact on porcelain in lateral movements.

PIN RETAINED RESTORATIONS

- To enhance retention during filling of extensively decayed tooth.
- Help in transmitting occlusal stresses to the surrounding tissues and so fracture of filling is reduced.
- Pins decrease the TENSILE STRENGTH values of amalgam.

Types of pins

1. Cemented = helpful for non vital teeth.
2. Self-threading pins = also known as TMS pins; best.
3. Friction lock type retained by RESILIENCY OF DENTIN.

Most commonly used pin = self threading type.

Features	Cemented pins	Frictional grip/ friction lock	Threaded
Pin channels	Larger in diameter	Slightly narrower	**Narrower**
Stresses	Little/ no stress	**Maximum**	Intermediate
Retention	**Least**	Intermediate 2–3 times	Most 5–6 times
Crazing	Nil/little	**Maximum**	Intermediate
Retention to restorative materials	More retentive	**Least retentive** to amalgam and resin; **least used pin**	More retentive
Distance from DEJ	0.5–1.0 mm	**> 2.5 mm**	1.5 mm

Basic rules

1. Should be placed in dentin only due to its elasticity. 1–1.5 mm from DEJ.
2. Dentinal engagement : pin protrusion in cavity = ideal is 2:1; for best retention.
3. A minimum of 2 mm distance should be there between 2 pins for better retention.
4. Cemented pin is the only technique to be used for RCT teeth and/ or to be located very close to DEJ. 0.5–1.0 mm.
5. Threaded pin technique is used for vital teeth. Pin is located at least 1.5 mm from DEJ.
6. Staple post = i.e. post in 2 adjacent root canals is continuous.

Guidelines

1. Pins should be placed as close as possible to **the line angle of the tooth**, which is the area of greatest bulk of dentin.

2. Pin holes should be in the dentin, **at least 0.5 mm from DEJ and** no closer than 1.5 mm to external surface of the cavity.
3. If more than one pin is to be placed-the optimum inter-pin distance is 5 mm.
4. Pins should be placed s.t. their axes are not parallel. It helps to increase the retention.
5. Direction of pin holes should be parallel to the external contour of the tooth.
6. Should be placed at least **0.5 mm from the axial wall** of tooth. It allows adequate condensation of restorative material. Smaller size of the condensers are used.
7. Minimum no. of pins should be used to avoid crazing; to maintain inter-pin distance; in general one pin is used for replacing one cusp and marginal ridge.
8. For molars = 1 pin/missing cusp.
9. For premolars = 2 pins/missing cusp.
10. Pin depth of **2 mm into dentin** provides sufficient retention.
11. Optimum length of pin extending **into amalgam is 2 mm**. If more, it can lead to fracture of amalgam
12. Holes are drilled at the speed of 300–500 rpm. It is done in one thrust for uniformity of the hole.

Cemented pins

- Pin holes should be 0.001–0.002 inches wider than the size of the pin.
- Twist drill = 0.021 or 0.0027″ diameter.
- Holes are placed at 3–4 mm depth, at dissimilar angles.
- GI or reinforced ZOE used for cementation, as they have more favorable pulpal response.
- **Least TRAUMATIC to dentin**, as placed in oversized holes.
- Preferred for NON-VITAL TEETH, because no crazing or internal stresses produced.
- RETENTION is LEAS, because cement may be soluble. Microleakage is more.

Friction lock type pins

- Size of the pin hole is 0.001 inches smaller than the size of the pin.
- They are retained by friction.
- Introduce maximum stresses in the dentin.
- Give maximum discomfort to the patient.
- Retention is 2–3 times more than the cemented pins.

Self-threading pins—(also known as TMS = thread made system)

- Best and **most widely used.**
- Mechanical retention due to viscoelastic property of dentin.
- Pin - hole = is 0.0015-0.004″ smaller than the pin size.
- Pinhole size is SMALLER than diameter of PIN.
- No cement used.
- Best retention (5–8 × more than the cemented pin).
- Lesser depth of pinholes is required.
- Least microleakage.
- Disadvantage-rauma to dentin, may lead to CRAZING AND CRACKING AND fracture.
- Less discomfort to the patient.
- **Pin hole perforation**—pulpal perforation is treated by $Ca(OH)_2$ intermediary base into the pin hole.
- Periodontal perforation—is sealed by AMALGAM.

Types of the Pins: Pins are of 3 types:

Pin type	Diameter
Minikin	0.019 inch
Minim	0.024 inch
Minuta	0.015 inch

Amalgapin

- Here pins are not used, but 2–3 mm deep holes are made, in which amalgam is condensed for retention.
- But amalgapin chambers are more wide than pin holes and so more conservative.

Post for restoration of devital teeth

- RCTed teeth are BRITTLE and DRY.
- Get fractured with time, so should be restored.
- Instrumentation of RC leads to weakening of tooth and fracture
- Only 9% loss of free water in a pulpless tooth occurs as cp to vital tooth and there is no change in BOUND water.
- Devital teeth will fracture if they are not restored with CUSPAL COVERAGE.
- Post and core may be placed. The CORE replaces the lost crown structure, the post is used for retention for a core.

Characteristics of a POST

- Minimal length of post should be equal to the clinical crown.
- Apical RC seal should be 5–6 mm (apical 3rd) to prevent microleakage.
- Parallel-sided posts have better retention than TAPERED post, but less than threaded post.
- Internal tooth structure should be preserved to provide maximum resistance to fracture.
- A safe ended GATES-GLIDDEN or peeso reamer is used for preparing the dowel space.
- An external cavosurface bevel is placed to provide a degree of resistance to prevent tooth fracture.
- Anti-rotation lock/keyway placed to prevent rotation.
- On max. first PM-lingual canal is used for POST—as it is STRAIGHTER.
- In max. molars-PALATAL canal is used-as it is largest and widest.
- On mandibular molar-DISTAL canal is used.

- A vent is placed along the length of post for escape of cement during cementation.
- A generally accepted rule for restoring RCTed posterior tooth = MOD protected cusp gold inlay is used as a minimum restoration.
- Types of post and cores: (1) prefabricated/custom made; (2) parallel sided/tapered; (3) threaded/smooth/serrated.
- Parallel sided have better retention; but tapered are less likely to cause apical 3rd perforations of root canal.

Important points

- For achieving proper proximal contact, the best material is = cast gold.
- For thin margins restoration and cusp restoration, the best material is = gold foil because it is malleable and ductile.
- Saliva is cultured upon MSB medium or on 20% sucrose + sulphasomidine at a pH of 5.0.
- Xylitol is the most effective of the sucrose substitutes in reducing decay.
- Maximum fluoride is deposited in = cementum.
- Acid etching cannot be done on cementum, because acid dissolves it uniformly rather than creating the micropores; cementum has only 45–50% of inorganic part.
- **Cusp protection** is required if the occlusal margin of the lesion is more than halfway to the cusp tip.
- **Supporting cusps** require more BULK or thickness of protection than balancing cusp, due to more occlusal load.
- Up to 2 mm should be removed from working cusp, but only 0.5 mm from nonworking cusp for bulk of metal.
- Internal line angles should be rounded for better stress distribution in the tooth and the material.
- Occlusal taper should be approx 5 degrees.
- Retention grooves are placed in the dentin, away from the pulp.
- MTA is the latest material being used as a setrograde filling material after epicoectomy.

2

Pedodontics

- A child's behaviour problem can be handled by familiarization if the basis of problem is = fear.
- The greatest period of growth of cranium occurs b/w = birth and 5 years of age.
- A broad understanding of the development of human behaviour requires a knowledge of basic concepts of = maturation and learning.
- Acute herpetic gingivostomatitis is main cause of generalized acute gingival inflammation in a preschool child.
- Small, irregular bright red spots on child's buccal mucosa with bluish white specks in the centre is of = rubeola.

Mile stones

Age	Milestone
1 month	Holds head up
2 months	Smile with recognition
3 months	Reaches for objects but misses
4 months	Sits up with support
5 months	Sits on lap grasp with support
6 months	Sits in chair with back rest
7 months	Sits unaided
8 months	Stands with aid
9 months	Stands holding into furniture
10 months	Crawls
11 months	Walk with support

Mile stones (*Contd.*)

12 months	Pulls to standing position using furniture
13 months	Crawls up steps
14 months	Stands unaided
15 months	Walks unaided

Development of different tissues of the body

Age of IUL	Tissues
4 weeks	Thyroid gland
6 week	Parotid and submandibular glands
6–7 weeks	Cleft lip
6–8 weeks	Human face
7 weeks	Muscles of mastication
8 weeks	Sublingual gland
8 weeks	Premaxilla/maxilla
4–8 weeks	Tongue
14 weeks	Bony palate established
32 weeks	Infantile swallowing established
12–15 months of age	Adult swallowing is established.

GROWTH

- RATIO b/w skull and face at birth = 8:1.
- Neurocranium = desmocranium + chondrocranium.
- Desmocranium = cranial vault; formed by intra-membranous ossification.
- Chondrocranium = base of skull; formed by endochondral ossification.
- Viscerocranium = i.e. bones of facial skeleton; formed by intramembranous ossification.

FONTANELLES: 6 in no.

1 Frontal/ anterior	b/w 2 parietal and frontal bones	Close at 8–12 months
1 Occipital/ posterior	b/w 2 parietal and occipital bones	Close by 2 months
2 Sphenoid/ antero-lateral	paired; b/w frontal, parietal; temporal and sphenoid bones	Close by 3 months
2 Mastoid/ postero-lateral	paired; b/w parietal; occipital and temporal bones	Close by 12 months

- Cephalocaudal gradient of growth.

Head circumference at birth = 35 cm approx.

Head size

At birth	22 % of the total body length.
10 yrs	95 % of total head growth completed.
15 yrs	98 % of total head growth completed.
3 yrs	Width of head completed.
17–18 yrs	Length of head is completed.

Mandibular foramen

- Lies below OP = in very young child.
- At OP level = during primary dentition phase.
- Above OP approx 7 mm = in adults.

Height and weight predictions

	Boys	**Girls**
Adult height Adult weight	2 × height at 8 yrs 5 × weight at 2 yrs	2 × height at 7.6 yrs 5 × the weight at 1.6 yrs

Height and weight charts

Age	Increment	Height
Birth	–	20 inches
0–6 months	1 inch/month	26 inches
6–12 months	0.5 inch/month	32 inches
1–7 yrs	3 inch/year	50 inches
8–15 yrs	1 inch/year	62 inches

Weight chart

Age	Increment	Weight
Birth	–	7–8 lbs
0–4 months	2 lbs/month	15–16 lbs
4–12 months	2 lbs/month	23–24 lbs
1–2 yrs	1/2 lbs/yr	29–30 lbs
2–10 yrs	5 lbs/yr	69–70 lbs

Changes from birth to adulthood

Head	2 × that of birth size
Trunk	3 × that of birth size
Arms	4 × that of birth size
Legs	5 × that of birth size

Tonsils/adenoids

At birth	Very small; may regress after few days
First few months.	Growth occurs
6 mos–2 yrs	Maximum growth occurs known as primary physiological enlargement
6 yrs	Hypertrophy occurs known as secondary physiological enlargement
Puberty	Regression and atrophy occurs

According to **Scammon's growth curve**

Growth of lymphatic tissues > neural > somatic > genital tissues.

Later on, lymphatic tissues start regressing.

PHYSIOLOGY OF GROWTH (Also refer to orthodontics in Vol 1.)

Effect of hormones

- GH, thyroxine, corticosteroids and insulin = bring changes in growth rate.
- PTH, vitamin D, calcitonin = affect skeletal maturation and pubertal growth.
- GH and insulin = stimulate stomatomedin release and cause cartilage growth.
- Pubertal growth spurt is enhanced by steroids and GH and helps in accelerated bone maturation.
- PTH = osteoclastic activity.
- Calcitonin = bone deposition enhancer.

Methods of growth assessment

- **Biometrics** = i.e. a science of statistical biology in which collection and statistical analysis of data regarding a living being is considered, e.g. cross-sectional study; longitudinal study; semi-longitudinal study.
- **Craniometry** = is the measurement of cranial dimensions in dry skulls.
- **Somatometry** = is the measurement of facial dimensions on a living person. Only soft tissues measurement can be done.
- **Cephalometry** = measurements of craniofacial complex made on a standardized x-ray plate. It is a 2 D picture of a 3 D figure.
- **Implant metals indicators** = by Bjork; metal acts as a reference point and so growth of bone is studied on x-ray.
- **Superimposition** = of a series of x-rays on some reference points and comparing.
- **Stereo-pair images** = 3 D computer analysis is done by digital imaging method.
- **EMG.**
- **Animal experiments.**

- **Vital staining = alizarine dye** is found in **madder plants**; which gets deposited in the areas of active growth. But animal has to killed for studying.
- **Radioisotopes** = get collected in the areas of growth. Growth is measured with Geiger-Muller counter by studying the emission of radiations. Mainly **99 m Tc** is used.
- **Natural markers** = certain developmental features of bone act as reference markers.
- **Anthropometry** = certain landmarks on soft tissues corresponding to bony landmarks are studied and measured, e.g. data by Farkas.

AGES AS THE GROWTH DETERMINANTS

1. **Chronologic age** = is calculated from child's Date of birth. It is not a good predictor of growth.
2. **Somatotypic age** = 3 somatotypes exist according to Sheldon. Ectomorphics are late maturers, i.e. growth in them continues for longer time. Endomorphs are early maturers. It is also not a good predictor of growth.
3. **Height and weight ages** = height and weight are affected by genetic and environmental factors and cannot be used as a sole predictor of developmental age of child.
4. **Dental age** = is calculated by observing the state of dental development and teeth eruptions. It is simplest but least accurate method. Calcification of a tooth is also an indicator of somatic maturation, e.g. mandibular canine calcification stages.
5. **Sexual age** = pubertal changes are observed in males and females due to hormonal changes. Peak height velocity PHV occurs early in females than in males. Maturation occurs early 2–3 yrs in females than the males. Onset of menstruation indicates completion of pubertal growth spurt.
6. **Facial age**
7. **Skeletal age** = most reliable method; many methods can be used, e.g. hand wrist x-ray; CVMI; (cervical vertebra maturation indicator); SMI (skeletal maturation indicators), etc.

Influence of deciduous tooth morphology on cavity design and restoration placement

Anatomy of deciduous teeth	Implication for cavity design and tooth restoration
Enamel thinner than in permanent teeth	Dentin involved more rapidly
Crowns more bulbous than permanent teeth	Influences placement of floor of i/d box in class II cavities
Primary molars are narrower occlusally, esp Ds	Adaptation of matrices is more difficult Cusp strength is influenced by width of occlusal restoration
Broad contact points in molars	In proximal caries diagnosis; so bitewing r/gs are required for detection
Pulp chambers are larger; pulphorns are more pointed; pulpal outline follows DEJ	Cavity size must be restricted. Limited space for sufficient bulk bulk of restorative material to resist fracture.

Atraumatic caries treatment ART = here, caries is removed using the hand instruments and restored with GI cements.

Non-mechanical caries removal/chemical caries removal = carious dentin is removed by using ***N–mono-chloro-amino-butyric acid NMAB.***

Traumatic injuries

1. Concussion = tooth traumatised but not loosened.
2. Subluxation = tooth is dislocated in the socket but not displaced.
3. Extrusion = tooth displaced in occlusal direction.
4. Intrusion = tooth displaced in apical direction in the socket.
5. Lateral displacement = tooth pushed laterally, buccally, or palatally.
6. Avulsion = tooth totally displaced from socket.

CLASSIFICATION OF TOOTH DISCOLORATION

(I) Intrinsic Discoloration: Occurs following a change in the structural composition of hard dental tissues, e.g.

1. Aging
2. Alkaptonuria
3. Amelogenesis imperfecta
4. Congenital erythropoietic porphyria
5. Congenital hyperbilirubinaemia
6. Dentinogenesis imperfecta
7. Enamel hypoplasia
8. Fluorosis
9. Pulpal haemorrhage products
10. Root resorption
11. Tetracycline staining

(II) Extrinsic Discoloration

1. Metallic
2. Non metallic

(III) Internalised Discoloration: Is due to incorporation of extrinsic stains within the tooth substance following dental development. It occurs in enamel defects and in the porous surface of exposed dentine, e.g. in acquired defects like:

(a) Tooth wear and gingival recession.

(b) Dental caries.

(c) Restorative materials.

- Bitewing r/g is good for the detection of proximal caries lesions.
- Caries lesions always appear smaller on the r/g than it actually is, because the r/g is a 2 D picture of a 3 D object.
- Proximal caries if not restored timely leads to the loss of arch length due to mesial migration of the adjacent tooth.
- Child's first dental visit and oral examination should be at least at 9–12 months of age or as soon as the first tooth erupts in the oral cavity.

- Cleaning of the gum pads of the child should be done regularly by a soft moist cloth.

INFECTION CONTROL PROCEDURES IN A DENTAL CLINIC: As approved by ADA and CDC PHS in US Deptt of health.

1. Obtain a thorough medical history.
2. Clean instruments in an ultrasonic cleaner or soap and water solutions. Wear heavy rubber gloves during cleaning. Adhering blood or tissues do not allow proper penetration of heat and sterilisation.
3. Sterilize all reusable instruments.
4. Monitor the use and functions of sterilizer by using spores test routinely. **Spores of actinobacillus stereothermophillus** bacteria are used.
5. Use gloves during all treatment procedures.
6. Wear surgical masks and protective eyewears to avoid aerosols and splatter.
7. Wear protective gowns and uniforms during Rx.
8. Protect operatory surfaces by protective covers, e.g. plastic wrap, aluminium foils, etc.
9. Use rubber dam and high speed suctions.
10. Require vaccinations vs Hep B, etc.
11. Hand wash between the patients contacts by antimicrobial surgical hand scrubs, e.g. STERILLIUM.
12. Perform waste-disposal properly.
13. Use disposables syringes, etc. where ever possible. Destroy syringes/needles, etc. after use before rejection.
14. Incineration of soiled items should be done at a proper place.
15. Place biopsy specimen in sturdy containers with a tight lid to prevent leakage (10% formalin).
16. Disinfect all contaminated operatory surfaces in b/w the patients, e.g. 1:10 diluted solution of household bleach for nonmetallic surfaces or with Iodophore.
17. Clean and sterilize all handpieces.

18. Clean and disinfect impressions and intra-oral appliances before handling, e.g. glutraldehyde; surgi-scrub; iodophore solutions, etc.

CHILD ABUSE AND NEGLECT

First documented and reported case of child abuse occurred in 1874.

Battered child syndrome term was coined by Henry Kempe in 1962. Its S/S are:

- Fractures of any long bones
- Subdural hematoma
- Failure to thrive
- Soft tissue swelling
- Skin bruising

Types of child abuse

1. Physical abuse/non-accidental trauma
2. Child sexual abuse/exploitation
3. Failure to thrive
4. Health care neglect
5. Dental neglect
6. Safety neglect
7. Emotional neglect
8. Emotional abuse
9. Physical neglect
10. Educational abuse
11. Intentional drugging or poisoning.
12. **Munchausen syndrome by proxy** = i.e. children who are victims of parentally fabricated or induced illness.

Physical abuse = is most important type of abuse; it is the injury inflicted on a person below 18 yrs of age.

Soft tissues injuries esp bruises are most common injury sustained in child abuse.

DATING THE BRUISES

Time elapsed	Characteristics
0–2 days	Swollen, tender
0–5 days	Red, blue, purple
5–7 days	Green
7–10 days	Yellow
10–14 days	Brown
2–4 weeks	Cleared

CHILD PSYCHOLOGY

Pedodontic treatment triangle

- Rx of a child is a one-to-one relationship.
- Triangle consists of the CHILD-DENTIST-FAMILY esp mother.
- Child is at the apex of the triangle and focus of attention of family and dentist.

Developmental milestones = are the physical changes appearing at the specific chronologic ages during the development of the child.

Intelligent quotient IQ by **Binet:**

IQ = mental age × 100/chronologic age.

IQ classification guide.

American association of mental deficiency classification

52–68	Mild	140 and up	Very superior
36–51	Moderate	120–139	Superior
20–35	Severe	110–119	High average
19 and below	Profound	90–109 80–89 70–79 69 and below	Average Low average Borderline defective Mentally retarded

How does the maternal anxiety affects the child's behaviour in the dental clinic? The highly anxious parents tend to affect their child's behaviour NEGATIVELY.

FRANKL BEHAVIOUR RATING SCALE

- Rating 1 = definitely negative
- Rating 2 = negative
- Rating 3 = positive
- Rating 4 = definitely positive

Types of PARENTS

1. **Overprotective parents** = their behaviour often prevents the natural development of the child towards independence.
2. **Manipulative parents** = have excessively demanding attitude.
3. **Hostile parents** = they question the necessity of the Rx. The question is posed in a distrusting manner.
4. **Neglectful parents** = failure of cooperation; miss the appointment, etc.

DEVELOPMENT OF DENTITION (Also refer to the section of orthodontics.)

- Mandibular D = no resemblance to any tooth-primary or permanent.
- Max. D = resembles max 5.
- Max E = resembles max 6.
- Mandibular E = resembles mandibular 6.
- Mandibular D = buccal cervical ridge is MOST prominent; and oblique.
- Mandibular E = MB pulp horn is the HIGHEST.

Eruption sequence = ABDCE.

Calcification sequence of primary teeth = ADBCE.

Evolution of dentition

3 stages of tooth evolution:

- Reptilian stage/haplodont = simplest; single cone type.
- Early mammalian stage = triconodont.
- Triangular stage = tritubercular molars.
- Quadri-tubercular molars.

Characteristics of dentition

Acrodont	Teeth attached to jaws by a connective tissue.
Pleurodont	Teeth are set inside the jaws.
Thecodont	Teeth are inserted in bony socket.
Polyphyodont	Teeth replaced through out the life.
Diphyodont	2 sets of teeth, e.g. human teeth.
Monophyodont	Single set of teeth.
Homodont	Single type of the teeth.
Heterodont	Many types of teeth, e.g. human teeth.
Human teeth are	Heterodont; diphyodont and continuously invested teeth.

Origin of teeth

- Theory of concrescence.
- Theory of trituberculy = widely accepted.
- Theory of multi-tuberculy.

Types of eruption

- Continuously growing teeth.
- Continuously extruding teeth.
- Continuously invested teeth = e.g. human teeth.
- Clinical eruption = i.e. movement of tooth from its position in the socket to the functional position in an occlusal plane.

Stages of tooth eruption

Pre-emergence eruption = occurs when crown formation is completed and root development starts post-emergent eruption.

Theories of eruption

- Root growth theory
- Constriction of pulp
- Pulp growth
- Bone growth
- Tissue fluid pressure
- Shrinkage of collagen

Eruption rhythm = mean daily eruption velocity is approx 71 microns/day.

Accelerated eruption	Retarded eruption
Hyperthyroidism Hyper-pituitarism Turner's syndrome	Hypothyroidism Hypopituitarism Cleidocranial dysostosis Downs syndrome Achondroplasia Hypovitaminosis A, D Amelogenesis imperfecta Osteopetrosis

Special points wrt morphology of primary teeth (Also refer to the section of dental anatomy.)

- **Max CI** = its MD diameter of crown is more than the cervico-incisal length (opposite of permanent max CI).
- **Max LI** = its cervico-incisal dimension is more than the MD width.
- **Max C** = root is more than the twice the length of the crown.
- **Mandibular LI** = is similar to the mandibular CI but is somewhat larger in all dimensions except labio-lingually. Its incisal edge slopes towards the distal aspect of the tooth.
- **Max D** = ML cusp is largest and sharpest. MD dim is greatest and then converges cervically.

- **Max E** = it resembles max 6. Its root bifurcation on buccal side is close to the CEJ. Cusp of Carabelli is on ML cusp. Oblique ridge joins ML cusp to DB cusp.

Mandibular D

- Does not resemble any permanent tooth.
- Distal area of tooth is shorter than mesial area.
- Has prominent buccal ridge.
- Pronounced lingual convergence of the crown on the mesial aspect.
- MMR is so well developed that it appears as another small cusp lingually.
- Cervical line slants upward from the buccal to the lingual surface because crown length is more in MB area than the ML area.

Mandibular E = it resembles mandibular 6.

- 3 buccal cusps are of equal size but in mandibular 6, the distal cusp is smaller than the other 2 buccal cusps.

RADIOGRAPHY

(Also refer to section on radiography in volume I and operative dentistry in Vol. III.)

Primary **biologic effects** of low level radiations are: carcinogenesis; teratogenesis; mutagenesis.

Younger the tissue and more actively it is dividing, the more sensitive it is to the radiations.

Which **stage of mitosis** is affected most by the radiations?

Critical organs = which should be shielded from radiations are:

- Skin
- Red bone marrow
- Gonads
- Eyes
- Thyroid
- Pregnancy
- Breasts

1. Lead apron and thyroid collar should be used to protect from stray radiations.
2. Annual maximum permissible dose/MPD = 5 rem for occupationally exposed person.
3. Cumulative MPD = 5 (N–18) rem, where N = age of the person.
4. Nonoccupational exposure = 10% of that for radiation workers = 0.5 rem.

Size of the x-ray films

For a young child = 2.2 × 3.5 cm IOPA.

For an older child = 3.1 × 4.1 cm IOPA.

Occlusal film = 5.7 × 7.6 cm.

Sizes of the film

No. 1	22 × 35 mm	Pediatric film
No. 2	24 × 40 mm	Adult anterior
No. 3	32 × 41 mm	Standard adult
No. 4	27 × 54 mm	Bite wing
No. 5	57 × 76 mm	Occlusal film
Screen films	4 × 5 inches 5 × 12 inches 8 × 10 inches	

- **ALARA rule** = also known as reasonably achievable.
- **Bite wing** r/g is used to detect the proximal caries lesions when the teeth are in tight contacts.
- **15 IOPA films** are used for full all-around intra-oral examination, i.e. 8 in upper arch and 7 in lower arch. An additional IOPA is required in max incisor region because the teeth are larger in size.
- **SLOB rule** (same lingual, opposite buccal)= as known as **buccal object/CLARK'S rule**, i.e. if the cone of the rays is displaced

while shooting the r/g, the lingual object moves in the same direction and the buccal object moves in the opposite direction.

- Films are available as A to E speed films from lowest to highest speed, the **E-speed films should be used**. These films help in reducing the radiation exposure to the patient.

Suggested R/G protocols for a child patient

Age	R/G survey	Views
3–5 yrs	4 film survey	2 = U and L anterior occlusals 2 = R and L posterior bitewings
6–7 yrs	8 film survey	2 = U and L anterior occlusals/ IOPA. 2 = R and L max posterior occlusals. 2 = R and L mandibular posterior IOPA. 2 = R and L posterior bitewings.
8–9 yrs	12 film survey	4 = U and L, R and L posterior IOPA. 4 = U and L, R and L canine IOPAs. 2 = U and L anterior IOPAs2 = R and L posterior bitewings.
10–12 yrs	16 film survey	12 film survey + 4 = U and L; R and L permanent molars IOPAs.

Positioning the patient

- Sagittal plane must be vertical and perpendicular to the floor.
- **Ala-tragus line** should be parallel to the floor for the maxillary teeth.
- **Angle of mouth-tragal line** should be parallel to the floor for the mandibular teeth.

Tooth	Centering point	Vertical angle
Lower molar region	3 cm anterior to angle of mandible, 1 cm above the lower border.	0–10 degrees
Unerupted 3rd molar	2 cm anterior to angle, 1 cm above the lower border.	0
Lower PMs	Line down from angle of mouth when open, 1 cm above the lower border.	–10–15
Lower	Along the line of tooth.	–20–30
Canine	1 cm above the lower border.	
Lower incisors	1 cm above the lower border in the midline.	–20–30
Max molars	At the intersection of a line perpendicular 1 cm behind the outer canthus of eye crosses the ala-tragus line.	20–30
Max 3rd molar		5–10
Max PMs	At the intersection point, where the perpendicular from the midpoint of infraorbital margin crosses ala-tragus line or above the corner of mouth.	35–40
Max canine	Ala of nose along the inter-dental space b/w canine and first PM	45–50
Upper incisors	Along the I/D area b/w CI and LI. Centering point is along the vertical axis of tooth through the nose to extension of ala-tragus line in incisor region.	50–55

- ♦ Proclined teeth require more degree of angulation than the normal.
- ♦ If high dome of palate/deep palate is there = the small angle between tooth and film is taken.
- ♦ Angle of incidence increases, when alveolar processes get resorbed.
- ♦ Mostly, D and E speed films are used.
- ♦ High kVp helps = decreasing patient's exposure; decreases contrast; decreases exposure time.
- ♦ Anode to film distance is kept = 10–20 cm.
- ♦ Slightly more angle is required for max LI than CI.

GENETIC ASPECTS OF DENTAL ANOMALIES

- ♦ **Differentiation of cells** = is a progressive specialization and hence limitation of cell functions.
- ♦ Protein synthesis is the critical element which determines cell functions and the cell type.
- ♦ DNA is the genetic material which controls the functions and differentiation and protein synthesis.
- ♦ **Gene** = the genetic material DNA controls the production of a single protein/polypeptide chain.
- ♦ **Cytogenetics** = is the study of human chromosomes.
- ♦ **Karyotyping** = is the technique of chromosome analysis.

By karyotyping, the human chromosomal set has been divided in 8 groups as:

Group	Chromosomes	Group	Chromosomes
A	1–3	E	16–18
B	4–5	F	19–20
C	6–12	G	21–22
D	13–15	Sex	XX/XY

- **Deletion** = is the absence of a piece of chromosome.
- **Duplication** = the insertion of an extra fragment into a chromosome from its now deficient homolog.
- **Inversion** = breaking of a chromosome in 2 places and subsequent rejoining with middle piece inverted.
- **Translocation** = attachment of a broken piece from one chromosome to another but non-homologous chromosome.
- **Denver nomenclature** = is the most commonly accepted system for chromosomal identification. It is based on chromosomal morphology.
- **Monogenic trait** = it is produced and regulated by a single gene. It follows simple Mandelian principles.
- **Polygenic trait** = controlled by many genes at different loci, e.g. skin colour, height, etc.
- **Multifactorial inheritance** = i.e. determined by a combination of genetic and environmental factors.
- **Proband/propositus** = is the first affected person in the family who brings that family to attention.
- **Siblings** = i.e. brothers and sisters in a family.
- **Phenotype** = i.e. the clinical appearance of a given trait for an individual.
- **Genotype** = i.e. the specific genetic make up which controls that phenotype.
- **Alleles** = genes at the same locus on a pair of homologous chromosomes.
- **Homozygous** = when both members of a pair of alleles are identical.
- **Heterozygous** = i.e. when the 2 alleles at a given locus are different.
- **Dominant gene** = i.e. a gene which expresses a particular phenotype in single dose.
- **Recessive gene** = i.e. a gene required in double dose to express a phenotype.

CHROMOSOMAL ABNORMALITIES

- **Trisomy** = i.e. when an extra chromosome is present, e.g.
  - Trisomy 21 = as known as Down syndrome.
  - Trisomy 18 = Edwards syndrome.
  - Trisomy 13 = Patau syndrome.
- **Monosomy** = i.e. one chromosome is missing.

SOME INHERITANCE-LINKED DISORDERS

Autosomal dominant inheritance	**Autosomal recessive inheritance**
• e.g. dentinogenesis imperfecta. • **50 % offsprings** affected. • **Both sexes** are equally affected. • Mostly, **heterozygous** individuals.	• i.e. expressed by the individual who has both altered recessive alleles and **Homozygous.** • **25% siblings** are affected. • e.g. **acatalasia,** i.e. absence of enz. Catalase. • So H_2O_2 is not metabolized to H_2O and O_2, leading to gangrenous stomatitis in the absence of O_2 and nutrition. • Incidence = 1:10,000. • Heterozygous parents are **carriers** and unaffected. • Higher frequency of **parental consanguinity.** Other examples are = albinism; juvenil periodontitis; Papillon-Lefevre syndrome; hypophosphatasia; Phenyl ketonuria; sickle cell anemia; fibromatosis gingiva; ectodermal dysplasia.

- **Turner syndrome** = monosomy of X-chromosome, i.e. XO.
  - Missing one X-chromosome.
  - Phenotypic FEMALES.
  - 1:10,000 live births.
- **Deletion** = e.g. short arm of chr. No. 5 = cri-du-chat syndrome
- **Translocation** = **philadelphia chromosome** = T 22, 9. It is related to the aetiology of CHRONIC GRANULOCYTIC LEUKEMIA.

Polygenic traits = are susceptible to environmental modifications, i.e. a multifactorial course, e.g. CLP.

Sex linked recessive inheritance, SLRI	**Sex linked dominant inheritance, SLRI**
Males are hemizygous for all X-linked genes, i.e. they have XY pair.	Gene is dominant, so seen **more in females.**
So in males, even a recessive gene on X-chromosome can express itself.	**All daughters** of an affected father get affected. because of X-chromosome.
So rare SLRI are **practically restricted to males.**	**Affected males do not transfer the trait** to their sons (as seen in SLRI).
Affected father passes genes to all his daughters, who are now carriers and not to the sons. It is known as **criss-cross inheritance**.	It appears about **TWICE in females** than males.
e.g. hypohidrotic ectodermal dysplasia; hemophilia.	Its transmission is indistinguishable from ADI and can be differentiated only by observation of offspring of affected males, not the affected females, e.g. hypoplastic amelogenesis imperfecta.

Environment = is defined as those non-genetic circumstances which render an individual more or less susceptible to a disease state.

Disease **risk to offsprings** of an affected person

Monogenic dominant trait = 50%

Monogenic recessive trait = 25%

Polygenic trait = < 10%

Genetic aspects of dental caries

- **Vipeholm study** = done by Gustafson and associates.
- Because of genetic differences certain environmental factors are more cariogenic for some people than for others.
- Children especially daughters show remarkable similarity in caries to their parents caries' susceptibility esp to mothers.
- **Proline-rich proteins PRP** in saliva have been linked to early plaque/pellicle formation. They bond tightly to hydroxyapatite. They are inherited as ADI trait. Coded by a block of genes known as **salivary protein complex,** which is located on **short arm of Chr 12.**
- Patients with high resistance to dental caries have a specific immunoglobulin in saliva, which lyses the cariogenic bacteria. It is transmitted as ADI trait.
- Caries a **polygenic trait,** i.e. a multifactorial disease.
- Genetic modifications of caries concept, i.e. food, vaccine, etc.
- **BRAX–I gene** is responsible for enamel growth in teeth.

DEVELOPMENTAL/INFECTIONS DISORDERS OF TEETH (Also refer to sec. on oral pathology in volume I.)

Condition	Features
Alveolar abscess	Caused by Strept. Viridans. Localized by fibrous capsule bacteria are not susceptible to TETRA-CYCLINE R/g shows thickened PDL. A gum boil/fistula can be seen in chronic cases.

Condition	Features
Cellulitis	Diffuse and massive swelling of soft tissues, a serious infections may lead to cavernous sinus thrombosis CST. Ka as Ludwig's angina if it involves submandibular, sublingual and sub-mental spaces bilaterally. Caused by streptococci, which produce Enz. hyaluronidase, i.e. spreading factor and fibrinolysins, which help in spread of infections. Some staphylococci may also be present.
Fusion of teeth	It is the union of 2 independent teeth. Have separate pulp chambers and root canals. Mostly involve the **anterior teeth.** May be seen in both deciduous/permanent teeth.
Gemination	It is an incomplete division of a single tooth germ by invagination occurring during proliferation stage. Bifid crown on a single root is present seen in both deciduous/permanent teeth but mostly in deciduous teeth.
Dens in dente	i.e. tooth with in a tooth/pregnant tooth. Mostly seen in permanent max LI. Is a lingual invagination of enamel. Invagination is lined with enamel and the presence of foramen cecum/lingual pit, which may lead to caries and a very early pulp involvement. The enamel is very thin in the depth of pit.

EARLY EXFOLIATION OF TEETH

A variation of 18 months in the exfoliation time of primary teeth is considered normal.

A delay of 6 months in the eruption time of primary teeth is considered normal.

Main **causes** are:

1. Periodontosis
2. Cherubism

3. Acrodynia
4. Hypophosphatasia
5. Pseudohypophosphatasia

Cherubism	As known as familial fibrous dysplasia. Multi-locular areas of bone destruction and thinning of cortical plates esp. mandible. Premature exfoliation of primary teeth due to loss of support and root resorption. Premature loss of permanent teeth due to interference in root development. Conservative approach is taken as they are self-limiting lesions and tend to resolve with maturity.
Acrodynia	As known as pink disease. Due to mercury poisoning.
Hypophosphatasia	Absence of severe gingivitis, but still loss of alveolar bone and teeth; limited to ANTERIOR region only. Low alkaline Pase levels = 7 King-Armstrong units (normal is 13–17 KA units) Hypocementosis of affected teeth.
Pseudo-hypophosphatasia Anomalous dental development	Serum alk. Pase levels are normal. Patients exhibit osteopathy of long bones/skull. Defective root development in dentinal Dysplasia and shell teeth. Absence of cementum from root surface and so loss of PDL support.
Cyclic neutropenia	Decreased no. of PMN neutrophils. Occurs after every 3 weeks cycle. Severe gingivitis and ulceration. Prepubertal periodontitis = due to repeated infections and considerable loss of supporting bones.

6. Anomalous dental development
7. Cyclic neutropenia
8. Acatalasia
9. Hyperpituitarism
10. Juvenile diabetes
11. Progeria
12. Histocytosis X
13. Leukemia, etc.

ENAMEL HYPOPLASIA

- Interference in normal enamel matrix formation and so surface defects appear.
- **Prenatal disturbance** is seen as an accentuated neonatal ring in the primary teeth.
- **Postnatal amelogenesis** is confined to the part of crown located cervically from the enamel are present at birth.
- Lead poisoning as known as **plumbism;** lead can cross placenta. It delays the development and eruption of primary teeth.
- **Turner's tooth** = i.e. due to local infection or trauma.
- Radiations = ameloblasts are resistant to rays, but **dentin is severely affected**; root formation is stunted; development of tooth arrested.
- **Fluoride** = lead to mottled enamel; pigmentation is **limited to outer 3rd of enamel;** nitrogen content of enamel is higher than normal.
- Other causes = rubella/german measles; deficiency of vitamin A, C, D, Ca, P, etc.

DENTINOGENESIS IMPERFECTA

- Its is an ADI trait. It is a MESODERMAL DEFECT.
- Seen with osteogenesis imperfecta.
- Type I = DI + OI.
- Type II = DI only. It is as known as hereditary opalescent dentin.

- Enamel gets chipped off due to **lack of scalloping at DEJ;** exposed dentin gets abraded.
- Pulp chambers are **small or entirely absent.**
- Pulp canals are very small.
- Extraction of affected teeth is difficult due to brittleness of dentin.

AMELOGENESIS IMPERFECTA

- 1:14,000 to 1:16,000 incidence.
- 3 types, i.e. hypocalcified type; hypomaturation type and hypoplastic type.
- Hypoplastic type.
    - Enamel matrix is imperfectly formed.
    - Calcification occurs and enamel is hard.
    - But enamel is defective in amount and has a rough and pitted surface.
- **Hypocalcified type**
    - Matrix formation is of normal thickness.
    - But calcification is defective, enamel is soft and rough.
- **Odontogenesis imperfecta**
    - It is the combination of amelogenesis and dentinogenesis imperfecta.
    - It is as known as enamel and dentin dysplasia.
- **Very large pulp chambers** and root canals
    - Teeth are devoid of enamel.
    - Cementum is normal and acellular.
    - DEJ lacks scalloping.

SHELL TEETH

- **Very large pulp chambers** and root canals.
- Roots are short and early exfoliation of teeth occurs.
- Very small amount of enamel and dentin formed.

Taurodontism = as known as bull teeth:

- Crowns enlarge at the expense of roots.
- **Pulp chambers are elongated** and extend deeply in the areas of roots.
- It is a familial trait.

Conditions having large pulp chambers of teeth

1. Odontogenesis imperfecta
2. Shell teeth
3. Taurodontism

Ankylosed tooth = i.e. lack of PDL in some areas of tooth; mandibular deciduous teeth esp D/E are most common; a solid sound is heard on percussion. Tooth not able to erupt.

Submerged tooth = teeth adjacent to ankylosed tooth are free to erupt and carry the alveolar bone with them, so the occlusal level of ankylosed tooth is at a lower level than the adj. teeth.

Impacted tooth = tooth is not able to erupt due to interference in its path of eruption.

Inostosis of enamel may lead to ankylosis of a permanent tooth. It occurs due to a chronic infection of deciduous tooth, which irritates the follicle of permanent tooth. So the enamel epithelium disintegrates and coronal cementum or bone gets deposited leading to ankylosis.

Anodontia

- Complete failure of teeth to develop is very rare.
- Partial anodontia, i.e. congenital absence of a few teeth is a common condition, e.g. in ectodermal dysplasia.
- Partial anodontia has SLRI pattern and crisscross inheritance occurs.
- Partial anodontia is as known as oligodontia or hypodontia.
- There is lack of alveolar growth as the teeth act as the functional matrix for its growth.
- But skeletal structures/jaw bases are normal.
- Lack of sweat glands and so no sweating.
- Pt is uncomfortable in hot weathers.

- **Induced anodontia** = is due to extraction of teeth.
- Every distal tooth of a group is missing, e.g. 2nd premolars; 3rd molars and max LI, except in lower incisor region, where central incisors are congenitally are missing.

DOWN SYNDROME: Also known as mongolism/trisomy 21.

- Delayed tooth eruption.
- Prolonged retention of primary teeth.
- Defect gets initiated b/w 6–8 weeks IU.
- It is linked to **increased age of mother.**
- Depressed nasal bridge; maxillary growth deficiency; skeletal class III relation.
- Increased periodontal diseases; high prevalence of bacteroides melaninogenicus.
- Low susceptibility to dental caries = due to increased salivation.
- Large fissured tongue; protruded.

Hypothyroidism

- Delayed eruption of teeth.
- Cretinism = congenital hypothyroidism; it is present at birth; short arms and legs; dwarf; head is disproportionately large.
- Delayed primary/permanent dentition.
- **Macroglossia** = so anterior open bite.

Hypopituitarism

- Decreased/retarded growth.
- Delayed dentition and eruption; prolonged retention of deciduous teeth.
- Is due to decreased growth hormones.
- Usually does not appear before 4 yrs of age.

Achondroplasia: Autosomal dominant

- Growth of limbs is limited due to lack of calcification in cartilages of long bones.
- Head size is large.

- Nasal bridge and maxilla is deficient.
- Skeletal Class III relation; due to early closure of synchondroses in the base of skull and so limited growth of maxilla.

Delayed dentition is also seen in following:

1. Fibromatosis gingiva.
2. Rickets.
3. Gardener syndrome.
4. Chondro-ectodermal dysplasia/Ellis Van Creveld synd.

INTRINSIC PIGMENTATION OF TEETH

Erythroblatosis fetalis

- Dentin is affected; it is due to excessive destruction of RBCs.
- Colour of teeth is blue-green due to deposition of bilirubin and biliverdin in dentin which are the products of Hb.
- Mother's blood is Rh –ve with a Rh +ve baby.

Porphyria

- It is due to increased production of porphyrin pigments in the body.
- Patient is **hypersensitive** to light.
- Red colour urine.
- Porphyrins get deposited in the teeth giving them purplish brown colour.

Cystic fibrosis

- Teeth are yellowish gray to dark brown.
- Patients are given TETRACYCLINE during childhood for its Rx, which causes discoloration of teeth.
- Mouth breathing and open bite due to nasal obstruction.
- Delayed dental development and erup.
- Seat the patient in an upright posture during treatment as in asthma.
- Low dental caries.

- Abnormal water and electrolyte transport across the epithelial cells.
- Involvement of multiple systems, e.g. pancreas, sweat glands, liver, GIT, respiratory system, etc.

Tetracycline Rx

- Teeth are yellow to brown in colour.
- Dentin is affected more as compared to enamel (9:1).
- Tetracycline forms chelate-complexes in the calcifying tissues which get deposited.
- Exposure of teeth to light causes oxidation and so colour changes from yellow to brown.
- Fluorescence occurs under UV light.
- Tetracycline can cross placenta and can affect the developing teeth.
- **Most critical period** = 4 to 9 months of age for the primary anterior; and 3–5 months to 7 yrs of age for permanent anteriors.
- Rx = is by vital bleaching; done by 35% H_2O_2 + ethyl ether solution (5:1) at 120°F for 30–40 sec. It decreases the oxidation process and so discoloration of teeth under light.

CONDITIONS OF TONGUE

Circumvallate papillae	Are 10–15 in no. Largest size, have taste buds, are vascularized.
Fungiform/mushroom shaped papillae	Present on the dorsum of the tongue esp. tip and lateral margins vascularized.
Filiform	Most numerous thin and hair like evenly present on dorsal surface of tongue no vascularization.

CONDITIONS OF TONGUE (*Contd.*)

Foliate	Arranged in folds along the lateral margins of tongue taste sensation is associated with them.
Macroglossia	Is over-development of lingual ms, e.g. in cretinism/hyperthyroidism in infants in Downs syndrome. Abnormal growth of jaws with class III m.o. and flared lower incisors and generalized spacing tongue is fissured and crenated due to continuous pressure of teeth on the lateral border of tongue.
Ankyloglossia	i.e. tongue tie due to forward attachment of the lingual frenum on the ventral surface of tongue. Speech problems due to restricted tongue movement. Stripping of lingual tissues may occur in anterior region. Nursing problems in infants. Partial ankyloglossia is more common. Rx = lingual frenectomy.
Fissured tongue	e.g. seen in cretinism, Downs syndrome. Vitamin B deficiency.
White straw berry tongue	Enlargement of FUNGIFORM PAPILLAE, e.g. in scarlet fever.
Black hairy tongue	Enlargement of FILIFORM PAPILLAE in middle 3rd of tongue due to prolonged antibiotics Rx.
Geographic tongue	Also known as benign migratory glossitis due to lack of FILIFORM PAPILLAE.

CONDITIONS OF TONGUE (*Contd.*)

	H/E = desquamation of keratin layers of papillae and inflammation of corium.
Medial rhomboid glossitis	Seen immediately anterior to circumvallate papillae. No FILIFORM PAPILLAE, due to *Candida albicans* infections.

ABNORMAL LABIAL FRENUM

- Labial frenum has 2 layers of **epithelium** enclosing **loose vascular connective tissue. Muscles fibres are absent**, but if present, the fibres are from orbicularis oris m.
- Arises at the midline on the inner surface of lip and inserted in the midline in the outer layer of periosteum and in the connective tissue of internal maxillary suture and alveolar process.
- It is attached to palatine papilla at birth and **recedes with the growth** of alveolar process.
- Diagnosis = by BLANCH TEST.
- It causes midline diastema if remains attached to palatine papilla, as it does not allow the approximation of max CIs after eruption of permanent canines.
- Orthodontic closure of midline diastema = **wait till eruption of permanent canines**. Then close the spaces. Frenectomy/ **Wanton's clipping** is to be done only after orthodontic closure.
- If frenectomy is done before ortho Rx = the **elastic scar tissue** formed will not allow the closure of space and will lead to relapse.

ERUPTION OF TEETH (See ortho section and oral path section also in Vol. I)

1. Max teeth are ahead of mandibular teeth in the development.
2. Teeth of females erupt earlier than males.
3. Mandibular teeth erupt earlier than max teeth.

4. First clinical sign of tooth eruption in a child is increased salivation and a habit of poking finger in the mouth.
5. A variation of 6 months of the usual eruption time is considered normal for primary teeth.
6. Teeth start moving in the bone when 1/2–2/3rd root has been formed and erupt in the oral cavity when 3/4th root has been formed.
7. Teeth move 1 mm in 3–4 months period in bone during eruption under normal eruptive forces.
8. Enamel calcification requires 2 more yrs to be completed after eruption in p.o. saliva.
9. Development of tooth starts at 11 weeks, i.e.
10. No tooth erupts in oral cavity during 9 yrs of age, i.e. a period of quiescence.
11. Hammock–ligament theory is the most important theory for eruption. Changes occur in the intermediate layer of PDL.
12. Interval between crown completion and until the tooth is in full occlusion is approx 5 yrs for the permanent teeth.
13. Mandibular 6 is often the first permanent tooth to erupt in oral cavity.
14. Sequence of eruption in mandibular arch is 6 1 2 3 4 5 7 8; in max arch is 6 1 2 4 5 3 7 8 or 6 1 2 4 3 5 7 8.
15. It is desirable that mandibular 3 erupts before 4, 5. It helps in maintaining adequate arch length and prevents lingual tipping of incisors.
16. If 7 erupts before 5 in any arch, it may lead to loss of arch length as it may push 6 mesially and loss of E-space occurs.
17. If lower incisors erupt lingually and slightly crowded (< 2 mm), before 7½ yrs age—then no intervention should be done, as it may resolve itself by tongue forces, alveolar and basal growth of jaws.
18. **Natal teeth** = i.e. which are present at birth.
19. **Neonatal teeth** = erupt during first 30 days of life.
20. 85% of natal/neonatal teeth are lower deciduous incisors. They should not be removed if not supernumerary.

21. **Epstein's pearls** = along the midpalatine raphe. It is the remnants of epithelial tissue trapped along the raphe.
22. **Bohn's nodules** = present along the buccal and lingual aspects of dental ridges. These are remnants of mucous glands tissues.
23. **Dental lamina cysts** = present on the crest of U/L ridges. Arise from remnants of dental lamina.
24. **Eruption cysts** = bluish purple fluid filled area; esp. in E and 6 regions.

DEVELOPMENT OF DENTITION

A. Gum pads: Dental arches till no teeth erupted are known as gum pads.

- Touch in future primary first molar region only.
- Anterior open bite is present which helps in tongue positioning during suckling.
- Anterior overjet due to smaller lower jaw.

Gum pads

Transverse groove	Divides the pads in 10 segments.	Correspond to the deciduous teeth.
Lateral sulcus	Lies b/w C and D.	
Gingival groove	Separates the gum pad from palate.	
Dental groove	Starts in incisive papilla region; extends backwards to touch gingival groove in canine region and then laterally to end in molar region.	
U and L gum pads contact	In D region only.	Overjet all around.
Shape	U = horse-shoe shaped. L = U-shaped.	

- Posterior overjet due to wider upper arch than lower.
- Intercuspation of occlusal height in primary dentition establishes for the first time = at eruption of primary first molars only.
- Tongue lies in b/w the gum pads and helps in suckling.
- Upper gum pad is horseshoe shaped and lower is U-shaped.

B. Baume's classification of PRIMARY MOLARS occlusion.

- Flush terminal plane 76% (to be observed most critically).
- Mesial step 14%.
- Distal step 10%.

- **Distal step** = (a) changes to Class II, if minimum growth differential is there. (b) changes in end-on, by loss of leeway space and forward mandibular growth.
- **FTP** = (a) end-on if minimum growth differential is there.
  (b) in Class I, due to loss of leeway space of mandibular E.
  (c) in Class II, if maxillary E is lost before mandibular E.
- **Mesial step** = (a) to Class I, if minimum growth differential is there.
  (b) to Class III, due to loss of leeway space and forward mandibular growth.

Spacing in deciduous dentition = if present, it is known as **open dentition.** If absent, it is known as **closed dentition.**

Class	If deciduous teeth	Crowding chances in permanent teeth
I	Crowded	10 in 10
II	No spaces	7 in 10
III	< = 3 mm spacing	5 in 10
IV	3–6 mm spacing	2 in 10
V	> 6 mm spacing	None

Primary spacing/physiological/developmental spacing = occurs due to growth, helps in proper alignment of bigger size permanent teeth, 70% in maxilla and 63% in mandible.

Primate/simian/anthropoid spaces are found mesial to primary maxillary canines and distal to primary mandibular canines, named as it is found in primates, i.e. between BC/CD.

C. Mixed dentition period

- Begins with the eruption of first permanent molars at 6 years of age, generally in end-on relationship, marks the Stage I of natural bite opening.
- **First transitional period/early MDP** = eruption of 6, 1, 2, mostly lower erupt first, 6–8 years age.
- Correction of FTP/end on relation to Class I occurs by utilisation of physiologic space, leeway space and differential forward growth of the mandible.
- **Early mesial shift** occurs in **open dentition at 6–7 years**, due to closure of primate spaces by pressure of erupting molars.
- **Late mesial shift** occurs **in closed dentition at 10–11 years**, due to closure of leeway spaces after shedding of primary second molars.
- **Incisal liability** = difference between sizes of primary and permanent incisors, 7 mm in upper and 5 mm in lower arch: overcome by—utilisation of interdental spacing, incisor inclination labially, increased intercanine width.

(Warren Mayne's principles)

Method	**Maxilla**	**Mandible**
I/D spacing	0–10 mm, av = 4 mm	0–6 mm, av = 3 mm
Increase in intercanine width	4.5 mm	3 mm
Incisor position	2.2 mm	1.3 mm

- **Incisor liability** = difference in sizes of permanent and primary teeth, space comes from 3 sources.
  1. Increase intercanine width = 2 mm, M > F, U > L.

     Girls have greater liability to incisor crowding.
  2. Labial positioning of permanent incisors = 1–2 mm.
  3. Repositioning of mandibular, canines distally in primate spaces when mandibular LIs erupt = 1 mm space. (But not in (U) Arch, as primate space is between B and C.
- If a child has FTP in MDP, then approx 3.5 mm of movement of mandibular first molar forward with respect to maxillary first molar is required for smooth, transition to Class I relation in permanent DP (i.e. a one half cusp transition in molar relation).
- **Inter-transitional period** = is a quite period, 8–10 years of age, no change in dentition occurs.
- **Late mixed dentition/second transitional period** = eruption of 3, 4, 5, leeway space of Nance is the difference between MD sizes of CDE and 345; 1.8 mm in maxilla and 3.4 mm in mandible; mostly due to primary mandibular second molar known as **E-space** (2–3 mm), helps in late mesial shift to achieve Class I molars.
- **Significance of pronounced attrition** in MDP is observed to help in—decrease in deep bite, prevent interlocking and thus, paving way to unhindered forward growth of mandible.
- **Deep bite decreases** by—eruption of permanent molars, attrition of incisors, and forward movement of mandible due to growth.
- **Intercanine width** increases more in spaced dentition, more in maxilla, up to a later age in maxilla.
- **Secondary spacing** occurs in closed dentition, with eruption of lower incisors, which pushes primary mandibular canine laterally. It creates space for proper eruption of maxillary lateral incisors. It helps to increase the intercanine width in both arches and increase in arch circumference in maxilla.

- **Ugly duckling stage of broadbent** = in maxillary, 8–9 years age, canines pressing roots of laterals, root crowding, crowns move distally, spaces develop should not be disturbed till eruption of canines, is a self correcting anomaly.
- Arch length decreases by 2–3 mm when MDP changes to PDP, both from anterior and posterior sides. Also posterior teeth move mesially throughout life due to attrition and anterior component of force.
- **Largest arch length = is before eruption of first permanent molar.**
- **Signs of incipient malocclusion** are = lack of interdental spacing in primary dentition, crowding in permanent incisors in MDP and premature loss of primary canines esp mandibular.
- Transition in chewing pattern develops in conjunction with eruption of permanent canines at age 12 years.

Self-correcting anomalies

Gum pads Stage	Primary D P	Mixed DP
Open bite	Deep bite	End–on molars
Increased overjet	FTP	Ugly–duckling stage
Tongue in between gum pads	Primary spacing Primate spacing Small mandible More upright incisors	< 2 mm of lower incisors crowding

- According to Owen, the Space loss (due to caries) is most likely in mandibular deciduous second molar area.
- Arch length decreases during change from the mixed dentition to permanent dentition. It is mainly due to loss of E-space.
- Arch circumference and width increase with growth of [illegible] bases.

- **Chewing pattern of child vs adult** = adult opens straight and then lateral/child moves laterally.

Natural bite opening: Occurs at 6, 12, 18 years of age, with eruption of permanent molars.

- 3 periods of bite opening (Schwarz).
- 6 years = when Ist molar erupts, 12 years = 2nd molar erupts, 18 years = 3rd molar erupts. It is due to that soft tissues covering the erupting molars touch each other and so patient feels pain and he keeps then in non-occlusion. So a gap is created anterior to them, in which the premolars are free to supra-erupt.
- U/L permanent incisors erupt lingual to primary teeth and move forward under tongue pressure as they erupt.
- 7-8 years age = critical period.
- Sudden change during the eruption of the CI and LI is shown by = **1.5 mm crowding** in both M and F. Average females recovers slightly better than males.
- No great relief of crowding in incisor region is expected after full eruption of LI.
    - Maxillary CI seem to erupt from LABIAL.
    - Mandibular CI, LI seem to erupt from LINGUAL.
    - Maxillary LI = no labial gingival bulge.
    - Maxillary second molar erupts D and F.
    - Maxillary third molar erupts D and B and outward.

DENTAL CARIES

(Also refer to the sections in oral pathology and in operative dentistry.)

3 theories of caries:

1. Proteolysis theory (Gottlieb and Frisbie).
2. Proteolytic chelation theory.
3. Acidogenic/chemo-parasitic theory (Miller).

Proteolytic chelation theory

First, organic component of enamel is attacked and then the breakdown products make chelates with the tooth minerals.

Acidogenic theory: Is most popular.

Acid produced from carbohydrates first causes the DECALCIFICATION OF inorganic part and then the DISINTEGRATION OF organic part of the tooth.

- **Main bacteria** = *S. mutans; S. sanguis; S. salivarius.*
- *S mutans* is not present in oral cavity of infants at birth and is detected only after primary teeth begin to erupt.
- **Sucrose** is the main culprit sugars for caries.
- **pH** of acid produced = 5.5–5.2.
- 0.2% **chlorhexidine gluconate** is an antiplaque, antibacterial and antiseptic agent.
- Acid diffuses in enamel surface through organic inter-prismatic material and starts demineralising outer edges of HA crystals.
- Outer surface of enamel is more resistant to demineralization so the greatest amount of demineralization is seen **10–15 microns** below the enamel surface. It forms **incipient subsurface** caries and is seen as **white spot.**
- Remineralization of subsurface incipient lesion is possible only if the surface layer is intact. Saliva and fluorides help in it.

Incipient caries

- Early lesion seen as white spot. Due to subsurface demineralization.
- Intact surface layer; can be remineralised under saliva.

Occult/hidden caries

- These cannot be diagnosed clinically but detected by R/G, etc. only, e.g. bite wing or OPG.
- Associated with low caries rate due to F exposure; hidden lesions also known as fluoride bombs/or fluoride syndrome.

- Other methods of detection are FOTI (fibre optic transillumination); ERM (electrical resistance method).

Arrested caries

- i.e. progress of lesion is stopped; open to oral environment.
- Also known as **eburnation of dentin.**
- Yellowish brown colour.

3 peaks of new caries lesions are seen at = 4–8 yrs; 11–19 yrs; 55–65 yrs ages.

In **rampant caries** = lower incisors (teeth/parts of teeth considered to be resistant to caries) are attacked.

In **nursing bottle caries** = upper incisors esp **labial surfaces** are attacked; the milk gets collected in this area.

Linear enamel caries = also known as **odontoclasis;** it occurs in neonatal line of max anterior primary teeth.

Grading of root caries (acc. to Billings 1986)

Property	Grade 1	Grade 2	Grade 3	Grade 4
Surface texture	Soft	Soft, irregular	Soft	Deeply penetrated
Dental explorer	Penetrable	Penetrable	Penetrable	Deeply penetrated
Surface defect	No	< 0.5 mm deep	> 0.5 mm deep	Deeply penetrated
Pigmentation	Light tan to dark brown	Tan to dark brown	Light brown to dark brown	Brown to dark brown
Synonyms	Initial	Shallow	Cavitation	Pulpal

- First national oral health survey done by IDA was in = 1984.
- Since the enamel calcification at the time of eruption of teeth is incomplete and requires 2 years for its completion by saliva; so

the teeth are more susceptible to caries during 1st 2 years after eruption.

- Environmental factors have greater influence on caries than the genetic factors.

CARIES PROCESS

Demineralization = occurs at critical pH of 5.5 or below (5.2– 5.5).

Remineralization = can occur if pH is neutral by buffering action and ions, e.g. Ca and PO_4 in saliva can inhibit the process of demineralization by COMMON ION EFFECT.

Buffering action of saliva is due to = Ca and PO_4 ions.

3 primary factors (given by KEYES 1960) for initiation of caries are = susceptible tooth; microflora and the local substrate.

4th factor added to above list by Newbrun, 1982 = time.

Ions like Se, Cd, Pb, Mn, Ba = increase caries.

Caries susceptibility of primary teeth = EDCBA.

Caries **susceptibility** of permanent teeth = first molars are most and the lower 1, 2, 3 are least susceptible.

Sequence of caries attack in primary teeth is = mandibular molars; max molars; max anteriors.

D are the less susceptible to caries than E.

Mandibular 6 are more susceptible to caries than max 6.

CARIES ACTIVITY TESTS

1. **Lactobacillus count** = by dentocult test.

   If count is > 10,000 cfu/ml = high caries.

   If < 1,000 cfu/ml = low risk. (cfu = colony forming unit).

2. ***Strept. mutans* count** = it is not a reliable test. Based on the fact that bacitracin inhibits growth of all other strept except *S mutans*.

3. **Cariogram** = 5 sectors of pie diagram have been noted as:

Colour	**Significance**
Green	Chance to avoid caries
Dark blue	Diet
Red	Bacteria
Light blue	Susceptibility
Yellow	Circumstances

4. Snyder test = bromocresol green is used.
5. Salivary reductase test = diazoresorcinol dye is used.
6. Enamel solubility test.
7. Alban test.
8. *S mutans* adherence test.
9. *S mutans* screening test.
10. Buffer capacity test.
11. Dewar's test.
12. Fosdick calcium dissolution test.
13. Viscosity measurement.

Sugar substitutes

1. Caloric sweeteners = sugars and sugar alcohols.
2. Non-caloric sweeteners = aspartame; acesulfamate potassium; saccharin; sucrolose; neotame.
   - Glucose/dextrose; fructose/levulose and invert sugars are caloric sweeteners.
   - Sorbitol is less cariogenic than sucrose.
   - Xylitol has antimicrobial, antiplaque properties; and is sugar substitute for diabetics.
   - Sucrose, maltose; fructose are cariogenic sugars.
   - Cane sugar contains which carbohydrate = ?

Diagnosis of caries: Besides clinical examination; exploration; radiographs, the latest methods are:

1. **FOTI, fibre optic transillumination** = decayed part of the tooth has a lower index of light transmission than the sound tooth part, it appears as darker shadow. It is good especially for the anterior teeth.
2. **Fluorescence** = in the carious teeth, the emission spectra shifts towards RED range, i.e. more than 540 nm under UV light. With argon laser light, carious tissue appears dark, fiery, orange, red. Diagnodent is based on fluorescence.
3. **ERM, electronic resistance measurement** = increased conductance or decreased resistance show the p.o. hypo or demineralisation. It occurs due to increased pore volume in enamel.
4. **Ultrasonic** = i.e. using sound waves for caries detection. At the cavity site, a higher amplitude echo is produced.
5. **Dyes**
   - For enamel caries = calcein; zyglo ZL-22.
   - For dentin caries = fuschin, acid red system, 9-aminoacridine.

Nursing caries = maxillary anterior teeth are carious due to accumulation of milk.

Mandibular anterior teeth are spared due to tongue coverage and salivary action.

C/f = neck of the tooth is involved in a ring like pattern along the gum line.

Rampant caries = is an acute, wide spread caries with early pulpal involvement of the teeth, which are usually **immune to caries**. Massler defined it as suddenly appearing, rapidly burrowing, wide spread and uncontrollable caries causing early involvement of pulp and involves those teeth/surfaces, which are immune to caries.

Caries rate = 10 or more lesions per year.

Proximal surfaces of lower anteriors involved.

Especially mandibular incisors are affected.

Rapid appearance of new lesions occurs.

PIT AND FISSURE SEALANTS (Details in sec on dental material also Vol. II and operative dentistry in Vol. III)

Proposed by Hyatt 1923.

Fissures are filled with silver or cement as soon as the teeth erupted.

Fissure eradication: Deep retentive fissures are converted in cleansable areas.

Mainly, **BIS-GMA** is the material used as sealants.

Types of fissures: V, U, I, K types (given by Nango 1960).

U, V types are wide and self-cleansable; non-invasive technique is used to remove them.

I, K types are narrow and caries prone, so invasive techniques are used.

Sealants can be of = self curing type and light curing types.

1st generation	Cured by UV light
2nd generation	Self cure
3rd generation	Visible light
4th generation	Fluoride releasing

Age at which P and F sealants are used:

3–4 yrs	For primary molars
6–7 yrs	For first permanent molars
11–13 yrs	For 2nd permanent molars

Viscosity of sealants should be less, so that it may penetrate the deep and narrow fissures and in etched surface micro-porosities by CAPILLARY ACTION.

FLUORIDES (Refer to Vol. II sec on Fluorides.)

History

Year	**Investigator**	**Inference**
1901	McKay enamel	**Colorado stains**; mottled
1933	Dean	**Shoe leather** survey
1939	Dean and McKay	Dental fluorosis
1944–1959	Knutson, Arnold	Grand Rapids = muskegon study of water fluoridation. Grand Rapids = experimental town; NaF added at 1 ppm level muskegon = control town

History (*Contd.*)

Year	Investigator	Inference
1946–1960	Blayney, Hill, Zimmerman	Evanston = Oak Park study 40% reduction in caries noted
1961	Backer Dirks, et. al.	Dutch study 88% decrease in smooth surface caries, 43% decrease in P and F caries
1965	Ludwig	New Zealand study 69% decrease in smooth surface caries, 43% decrease in P and F caries
1969	**WHO**	**Recommended 1 ppm F in drinking water**

- Maximum F concentration is in the first formed enamel, near the incisal edges and in the enamel layer located at or near the tooth surface.
- Maximum fluoride is accumulated in cementum.
- F conc is very less near CEJ. So in young children, the enamel is more susceptible to demineralization around the neck of tooth.
- So topical F Rx in young children is better for prevention and also for remineralization of incipient caries.
- F inhibits enz **enolase activity** in bacteria and so inhibits bacterial metabolism and acid formation.
- Tea = has 97 ppm F.
- Fishes = 84.5 ppm F.
- F is completely and passively absorbed from stomach.
- F absorption is inhibited by the p.o. calcium or Al compounds.
- Principal route of F excretion is urine.

- F is deposited in hard tissues of the body.
- In bone, it is deposited in the area of most active growth.
- In enamel, it forms fluorapatite and fluor-hydroxy apatite crystals, which are more resistant to acid attack.
- Highest F in dentin is adjacent to odontoblastic layers.
- In blood, 75% of F is in plasma and 25% in RBCs.
- In saliva, the F is = 0.02–0.03 ppm average.

Percentage of caries reduction with various forms of fluorides

Procedure	% reduction in caries
Community water fluoridation	50–60
Salt fluoridation	40
Dietary supplements	50–85
Fluoride dentifrices	20–30
Topical fluoride/professionally	30–40
Topical fluoride/self-application	20–50

METHODS OF FLUORIDE ADMINISTRATION

- F from saliva decreases acid production in plaque by **inhibiting the activity of enz glucosyl transferase** and so the metabolism of sucrose/glucose, etc.
- F at higher conc is bact E and so multiple F therapy should be done for each patient.
- **Fluoridation** = i.e. systemic application of F, e.g. through water fluoridation. NaF was the first compound used for water fluoridation.
- **Fluoridisation** = i.e. topical application of F.
- **Topical Fluoride application**

2% NaF	0.91 ppm F available
8% SnF_2	1.95 ppm F
1.23 % APF gel	?

Compound	**Properties**
SnF_2	Bad taste, stains arrested lesions stains silicate cements, but not harmful to procelain, low pH = 2.1–2.3; should be freshly prepared; applied for 4 min once/twice per year.
APF; as known as **Brudevold**	Does not stain or cause pigmentation, but damages the porcelain restorations applied for 4 min, 2 times/year. APF is a mix of NaF, HF acid, H_3PO_4 acid. PH = 3–3.5 more effective than NaF.
2% NaF	Neutral apH acceptable taste, does not damage/discolour the restorations, but multiple Rx are required. NaF was the **first compound used** for water fluoridation.
Knutson technique	NaF is used. Apply at 3, 7, 11, 13 yrs of age, as at these ages, the new teeth also erupt. Apply for 4 min. Applied 4 times at one week interval, so total 4 × 4, i.e. 16 applications.
Natural defense mechanism of saliva	Lysozymes and other antibacterial factors. Salivary pH to neutralize the acid, Ca and P contents of saliva.

- **Para-sympathetic stimulation** causes flow of watery and profuse saliva.
- **Sympathetic stimulation** causes flow of scanty and thick saliva.
- **Choking-off phenomenon** = after application of NaF, a layer of CaF_2 is formed which interferes with further diffusion of F ions in enamel surface.

- **Systemic fluorides** = get incorporated in developing enamel, also have topical effects as it gets secreted in saliva and gingival fluid.
- **Recommended dose** of F for children above 3 yrs of age is = 1 mg/day.
- F makes the P and F more shallow and self-cleansing.
- **Halo–effect or diffusion** = beverages bottled in fluoridated areas get supplied to other fluoride-deficient areas and pass on the beneficial effects.
- **Recommended level** of F ions in water according to WHO 1971 = 0.7–1.2 ppm; WHO 1994 = 0.5–1.0 ppm.
- **Calculation of F levels** = ppm F = 0.34 E; where E = 0.38 + 0.0062 × temp in F°. E is the estimated water intake by the residents of that area.
- **Salt fluoridation** = mostly KF (250 mg/kg salt) and NaF (225 mg/kg salt) are used.
- Only 6 countries have set specific policies for salt fluoridation = Belgium; France; Germany; Spain; Swiss; Hungary.
- **School-water fluoridation** = higher conc of F is required in school water, because children are there in school for small no. of hours and consume less water during that period. 4–6 times more conc of F than community water is used.

DIETARY Fluoride SUPPLEMENTS: (revised 1999)

Age yrs	Conc of F in drinking water ppm		
Yrs	< 0.3 ppm	0.3–0.6 ppm	> 0.6 ppm
0–6 months	–	–	–
6 months–3 yrs	0.25 mg/day	–	–
3–6 yrs	0.5 mg/day	–	–
6–16 yrs	1.0 mg/day	–	–

FLUORIDE VARNISHES

- e.g. bifluoride; duraphet (21000 ppm F); fluorprotector (7000 ppm F); fluoritop.
- Applied twice/year.
- Forms a water tight film on tooth surface, stays for many days and action of F occurs on the enamel surface.
- **Iontophoresis:** a small electric current helps to drive F ions into the enamel.
- **Fluoride dentifrices:** have 1000–1500 ppm F.

Age yrs	Use of F tooth paste
< 4 yrs	No
4–6 yrs	Once/day
6–12 yrs	Twice/day
> 12 yrs	Thrice/day

Safety features of F

Lethal dose	35–70 mg of F/kg body wt, i.e. • 5–10 gms of NaF for adult of 70 kg. • 1–2 gm of NaF for a child of 15 kg. • Rx = induce vomitting; gastric lavage; milk; hydroxides of Al/Mg/Ca; milk of magnesia. • Calcium gluconate i/v to prevent shock.
Certainly lethal dose CLD	5–10 gm of NaF or 32–64 mg F/kg body wt.
Safely tolerated dose STD	1/4th of CLD, i.e. 1.25 gm NaF or 8–16 mg F/kg body wt.

DEFLUORIDATION

- **Ion exchange method** = by using bauxite; zeolite; charcoal; clay; magnesite, etc.

- **Precipitation method** = by alum; alum and lime; calcium chloride, etc.
- **Membrane separation method** = i.e. by reverse osmosis.
- **Nalgonda technique** = uses lime and alum.
- Calcined magnesite and Nalgonda tech combined.
- **Prasanti technology.**

RECENT METHODS OF CARIES PREVENTION

1. **Antiplaque agents** = interfere with enz. Glucosyl transferase.
2. **Altering surface morphology**/increasing tooth resistance = i.e. by using surface-active polymers, acidified calcium phosphate solution applied and then a fluoride solution is applied.
3. **Lasers** = CO_2 laser is used.
4. **Bacterial replacement Rx** = i.e. by genetic engineering of the bacteria, e.g. **Strept. gordoni** are being produced which produce enz. Mutanase and decrease the acidogenic potential of *S mutans* and decrease plaque adhesion.
5. **Self-assembling polypeptides/SAP** = are protective; help in enamel remineralization.
6. **Chewing gums** = are sugar free; contain xylitol, lacititol; and urea.
7. **Tooth friendly sweets** = are non-cariogenic sweeteners, e.g. lacititol.
8. **Microdentistry.**
9. **Teledentistry.**
10. Indigenous products, e.g. neem; mango leaves; tea, etc.
11. **Caries vaccine** = can be given by either oral or systemic routes; oral route stimulates secretory IgA antibodies via MALT/GALT; systemic route is concerned with the production of IgG antibodies; these antibodies act vs *S mutans* and prevent its colonisation; they give secondary immune response.
12. **Genetically modified apple** = they contain a fragment of peptide which prevents the *S mutans* from sticking the teeth.

ROLE OF CHLORHEXIDINE AND ITS MOA IN DENTISTRY

0.2% of chlorhexidine gluconate is used.

It is bacteriostatic at low conc and bactericidal at high conc.

It is antiplaque; antiseptic and antibacterial.

ROLE and MOA of ZOE (Also refer to the section of operative dentistry Vol. III.)

It arrests the progress of a disease.

Transforms soft; painful carious dentin into hard; leathery; arrested lesion under ZOE.

Decreases the bacterial count.

Has soothing effect on pulp and decreases inflammation.

Bacteriostatic and cariostatic.

ROLE and MOA of $Ca(OH)_2$ (Refer to the section of operative dentistry Vol. III.)

Moller's index for the dental caries (1966)

Grade	Smooth surface caries	Pit and fissure caries
0	Sound surface	Sound
1	White opaque areas with loss of luster catching of probe	Discoloration of P and F with slight or no
2	Slight discontinuity in enamel	Definite sticking of probe in P and F
3	A definite cavity with dentinal involvement	– do –
4	Probable pulp involvement	– do –

Moller's index for the dental caries (1966) (*Contd.*)

Grade	Smooth surface caries	Pit and fissure caries
Modification of moller's index		
5	Filled tooth	– do –
6	Tooth indicated for extraction	– do –
7	Tooth extracted due to caries	– do –
8	Unerupted tooth	– do –
9	Tooth missing due to other reasons	– do –

Dean's index for fluorosis

Index	Features
0	Normal enamel
0.5	**Questionable mottling** **Few white flecks/**spots
1	**Very mild mottling** Small opaque paper white areas scattered over the teeth involving < 25% tooth surfaces. Summit of cusps of premolars and 2nd molars are affected commonly.
2	**Mild mottling** More extensive **white, opaque areas** involving < 50% tooth surfaces
3	**Moderate mottling** All enamel surfaces affected **Attrition** with marked wear Brown staining

Dean's index for fluorosis (*Contd.*)

Index	Features
4	**Severe mottling** All enamel surfaces affected Marked enamel hypoplasia Discrete or confluent pitting **Corroded appearance** of tooth

Disclosing agents: e.g. erythrosin (FDC red); bismarc brown; mercurochrome; alpha-plac.

Disclosing solutions: (1) basic fuchsin + 95% ethanol; (2) KI + I_2 crystals + water + glycerine (3) wafers.

DENTIFRICES

Composition (Also refer to perio section in Vol. III.)

Abrasives	Dicalcium phosphate, ca—pyrophosphate, ca, mg carbonates, etc.
Foaming agents	Sodium laruryl sulfate.
Flavoring agents	Peppermint, spearmint, cinnamon, etc.
Humectants	Sorbitol, glycerol, propylene glycol, they prevent the hardening of pastes.
Binders	Natural gums, seaweed colloids, cellulose, etc. act as thickening agents.
Sweetening agents	Saccharine, sorbitol, etc.
Therapeutic agents	Fluorides.
Colouring agents	
Preservatives	
Anti-plaque agents	Triclosan, etc.
Medicines	Potassium nitrate as desensitising agents.

ORAL HYGIENE AIDS

Tooth brushes; floss; tooth picks; mouthwashes; dentifrices; datun; irrigation machines.

Types of tooth brushes: manual/powered; super soft/soft/medium/ hard; straight/angled; small/medium/large; orthodontic brushes; interdental; proxa brush.

Style of bristles: pointed, straight, oblique, curved.

FLOSS: unitufted/multi-tufted, waxed/unwaxed.

METHODS OF TOOTH BRUSHING

According to 4 basic motions, there are:

1. Horizontal reciprocating = e.g. scrub method.
2. Vertical sweeping = e.g. roll and physiologic methods.
3. Circular motion = e.g. fones method.
4. Vibratory = Charters; Stillman; Bass methods.

A few **important points** regarding tooth brushing:

- Time taken for tooth brushing.
- Frequency of brushing.
- Force used during brushing.
- Most common and best method of brushing for a child.
- Surfaces to brush.
- No. of strokes.
- Age at which the child should see a dentist first.

Classification of children according to age.

- Infant
- Toddler
- Preschool child
- Early school age child
- Pre-adolescent
- Adolescent

NUTRITIONAL ASPECTS

Weight gained during pregnancy.

1. 1 pound/month for first 3 months.
2. 1 pound/week for next 6 months.
3. Total weight gained = 25 lbs.
4. Average weight of infant at birth = 7.5 lbs.

- Alcohol intake during pregnancy causes fetal alcohol syndrome/ FAS.
- Ca and Mg interfere with Fe absorption.
- Most rapid period of growth in humans life = during first 6 months of life.
- Original birth weight of infant doubles at 6 months and triples at 1 yr of age.
- Breast feeding is best food till 4–6 months of age.
- Meat is best source of iron, as hemi iron.
- Milk is very poor in iron.
- Dietary calcium may protect against colon cancer.
- Carotene rich foods protect vs lung cancer.
- Hypertension is known as silent killer; it is associated with less calcium intake.
- Vitamin C = essential for collagen formation; decreases permeability of sulcular epithelium.
- Vitamin A = helps to maintain the integrity of epithelial tissues.
- Folic acid = required for the formation and maturation of RBCs and WBCs. It decreases permeability of sulcular epithelium and so decreases the inflammation.
- Vitamin E = acts as antioxidant; prevents free-radical formation; increases cell membrane resistance and inhibits prostaglandins formations.
- Calcium and phosphorus = adequate dietary ratio of Ca and P is 2:1.

- In hyperparathyroidism = minerals get lost from bones, leading to osteoporosis and reduction in density and trabeculation of bones especially of alveolar bones.
- Periodontal disease may result from a low Ca or high P intake.
- Artificial sweeteners = e.g. saccharin; aspartame, etc.

LOCAL ANAESTHESIA (Refer to Vol. I also.)

- Local anaesthesia is defined as a loss of sensation in a circumscribed area of body caused by a depression of excitation in nerve endings or an inhibition of the conduction process in peripheral nerves.
- **Esters of benzoic acids** = e.g. butacaine, cocaine, ethyl amino benzoate, benzocaine, hexylcaine, piperocaine, tetracaine.
- **Esters of PABA** = chloroprocaine, procaine, propoxycaine, etc.
- **Amides** = articaine, bupivacaine, dibucaine, etidocaine, lidocaine, mepivacaine, prilocaine.
- **Quinolone** = centbucridine.
- LA prevents the normal passage of ions through the nerve membrane thus preventing the conduction of nerve impulses.
- Nerve membrane is a lipoprotein membrane; with resting potential at 70 mV.
- Intracellular fluid has mainly K^+ and extracellular fluid has Na^+ ions.
- Inside of resting nerve membrane is **negatively charged.**
- On stimulus, the transmembrane potential increases to firing threshold, i.e. 40–55 mV, due to entry of Na^+ ions inside, and so **partial depolarization** occurs.
- LA stabilises the nerve membrane and blocks the normal passage of ions through the membrane.
- **Surface charge theory** = suggests that LA may increase binding of Ca^{++} to nerve membrane. Ca^{++} is normally displaced from membrane during impulse transmission allowing increased access of Na^+ ions.
- **Membrane expansion theory** = LA binds to receptors on membrane thus increasing membrane stability and prevents opening of channels for passage of electrolytes.

Configuration of LA molecule

- Hydrophilic amide part helps its diffusion through interstitial fluid to reach at the nerve.
- Lipophilic aromatic part helps LA diffusion in lipid rich nerve membrane.
- Intermediate chain determines it as an ester or amide.
- Amide LA are metabolised in liver.
- Ester LA are metabolized by enz. plasma cholinesterase.

Composition of LA

LA agent **Vasoconstrictor**	Adrenaline.
Reducing agents	Sodium metabisulphite; it protects vasoconstrictor from oxidation.
Preservatives	Methyl paraben, capryl hydrocuprienotoxin, it stabilises the LA.
Fungicide	Thymol.
Vehicle	Ringer's solution.

- Methyl paraben may cause hypersensitivity/allergy.
- All LA except cocaine have vasodilating effect.
- Vasoconstrictors are contraindicated in thyrotoxicosis.
- Prilocaine undergoes more rapid biotransformation than other amides.
- Warning against lip biting should be given immediately and repeated to the parents and patient before sending them off the clinic.

Theories of mechanism of action

1. Acetylcholine theory	Discarded	Dett Barn 1967
2. Calcium displacement theory	Discarded	Goldman 1966
3. Surface repulsion theory	Not credible	Wei 1969
4. Membrane expansion theory	Especially for benzocaine	Lee 1976
5. Specific receptor theory	Most accepted	Strichartz 1987

Specific receptor theory: according to it, the LA binds on receptors present on Na^+ channels and prevents entry of Na^+ into the cell.

TECHNIQUES OF LA

Local infiltration

- Given supra-periosteal.
- Small nerve endings in area of surgery.
- 0.6–1.0 ml solution only is used.
- Can be used for deciduous molars also, because cortical plate is less dense in children than in adults.

Field block

- LA is given near the large terminal nerve branches.
- e.g. injections above the apex of the tooth in maxilla.

Nerve block

- LA is given near the main nerve trunk, e.g. inferior alveolar block.
- 1.8–2.0 ml solution is used.

Intraligamentary

- Used for a single tooth.
- LA is injected under high pressure.
- e.g. by peri-press or ligamaject syringes.

- 30 gauge needle is used.
- 0.2 ml solution is used.

Interseptal

- Used to reinforce infiltration analgesia.
- Esp used for primary mandibular molars.
- 0.1 ml solution is used.

Intrapapillary

Intrapulpal

Intra-osseous

Topical anaesthesia = e.g. benzocaine; action is in within 30 sec.

Pressure injection/jet injection = e.g. syrijet; at 2000 psi pressure and 0.05–0.2 ml amount of LA injected; produces surface anaesthesia.

Peri-press syringe = used for PDL injections; 0.14 ml solution is deposited; no vasoconstrictor is required in LA solution; useful in **bleeding disorders, e.g. hemophilia.**

Inferior alveolar injection

1. in < 5 yrs age child = 0.5 cm below the level of OP.
2. in 6 yrs child = at the level of OP.
3. in > 6 yrs age child = above the level of OP.
4. Terminal ends of inferior alveolar nerves cross the midline to opposite sides to provide the double innervation to the incisors; so local infiltration in that area is also required. Labial cortical plate in lower incisor area is very thin.

Mandibular conduction anaesthesia = also known as **Gow Gates** technique.

- Here, extra-oral landmarks are used.
- LA is deposited at the base of neck of condyle.
- Wider area is anaesthetised.

Nerve fibres of greater/anterior palatine nerves usually extend to the canine area.

In the area of max primary molars—there is a plexus formation of middle and posterior superior alveolar nerves.

Infiltration for primary teeth should be made closer to gingival margin as compared to permanent teeth, because roots of primary teeth are shorter.

RECENT METHODS

1. Iontophoresis = i.e. for surface anaesthesia.
2. Intra-oral lignocaine patch.
3. Jet injection = surface anaesthesia.
4. Computer controlled injection system = e.g. wand LA system.
5. Electronic dental anaesthesia = e.g. TENS.
6. **Topical anaesthesia.**

Sprays	10% lignocaine	e.g. nummit spray
Ointments	5% lignocaine	
Emulsions/ jellies	2% lignocaine	
Ethyl chloride	Volatile	Produces anaesthesia **by refrigeration**
Benzocaine	As topical LA; safest	Ethyl ester of PABA
EMLA	Eutectic mixture of LA; by Clark 1986	Has lignocaine and prilocaine mixture

ORAL SURGERY/EXTRACTIONS IN CHILDREN

- **Cowhorn forceps and elevators are C/I** in children to avoid damage to the permanent tooth buds.
- Young and elastic bone of child and incomplete root development makes extraction easy.
- Anterior primary teeth should be luxated to labial—because permanent tooth bud is present on its lingual side.
- Posterior teeth should be delivered to lingual.
- Fissural cysts are rare in children.

- Dentigerous cysts are most common.
- Traumatic cyst = no lining or soft tissue contents are found in the cyst cavity.
- Eruption cyst = occurs on the alveolar ridge.

PHARMACOLOGIC MANAGEMENT OF PATIENT BEHAVIOUR

Conscious sedation

- Only patients who are ASA Class I or II are routinely acceptable for conscious sedation.

Inhalation sedation: Also known as **relative analgesia.**

- Most frequently used method.
- Nitrous oxide gas is used.
- Gas has a partition coefficient of 0.47 in blood.
- It must be coupled with > 20% oxygen during sedation.
- Absorbed from lung alveoli; no biotransformation; gets rapidly excreted by lungs, when conc gradient is reversed.
- May lead to **diffusion hypoxia** when the sedation is reversed, so patient should be maintained at 100% oxygen for 5–10 min at 5 liters/min and also keep N_2O conc as low as possible.
- It is a CNS depressant; causes altered state of awareness.
- Prolonged exposure may lead to spontaneous abortions, hepatic diseases, etc.
- It is stored in BLUE cylinders.

Plane I	Moderate sedation and analgesia	5–25% N_2O
Plane II	Dissociation sedation and analgesia	25–45% N_2O
Plane III	Total anaesthesia/analgesia	45–65% N_2O
Plane IV	Light anaesthesia/contact with the patient is lost	65–85% N_2O

DOSE CALCULATION FORMULAE

Young's formula	CD = age × AD/(age + 12)
Dilling's	CD = age × AD/20
Augsberger's	% of AD = 0.7 × wt in lbs of child
Clark's rule	CD = wt of child in lbs × AD/150
Individual dose	CD = wt in Kg × AD/70
Individual dose	CD = surface area × AD/1.7
Bastedo's	CD = AD × (child's age + 3)/30

(CD = Child's dose; AD = Adult dose)

Oral sedation drugs

- Midazolam; phenergan.
- Most universally accepted method and easiest.
- Effects are dependent on absorption of drugs in GIT.
- At least 30–45 min are required before the procedure.

Intramuscular

- Best area is upper outer quadrant on gluteal region.
- Anterior lateral aspect of thigh in vastus lateralis m.
- Middle of the posterolateral aspect of deltoid m.

Rectal route

- Enterohepatic system is bye-passed.
- Drugs enter the circulation directly through intestinal mucosa.
- Drugs through this route are excreted slowly and so a longer duration of effect is there.

Intravenous

Most rapid, most efficient and reliable and safest route.

Agents used.

GENERAL ANAESTHESIA (See pharmacology section.)

- **Halothane** is the most common agent used of the inhaled halogenated anaesthetics agents; others are N_2O, enflurane; isoflurane, etc.
- PAC, i.e. **pre-anaesthetic check up** of the patient is a must to rule out any contraindication.
- **Pre-anaesthetic medications/PAM** to allay anxiety and fear of the patient; to relax him; to decrease the secretions; and to decrease unwanted autonomic reflexes.
- Anti-cholinergics = most commonly used is atropine and recently the glycolpyrrolate.
- Sedatives = e.g. benzodiazepines; barbiturates; chloral hydrate and meperidine; midazolam, etc.
- Anti-emetic agents = hydroxyzine, metaclopramide.
- Fentanyl and droperidol are used.

Intravenous induction

- Most common agent used is 2.5% thiopental sodium.
- Pre-oxygenation with 100% O_2 for 2–5 min is done.

Important points

- Maintenance of GA is by inhalational agents, e.g. diethyl ether; halogenated hydrocarbons; they are generally combined with N_2O gas.
- Semiclosed system is most commonly used technique for inhalational GA; other techniques are insufflation; semi-open; open and closed systems.
- An anaesthetic's potency is defined as the concentration of the agent required to inhibit response to a standard surgical stimulus. It is expressed in terms of MAC, i.e. minimal alveolar concentration; MAC values are additive, when different agents are used in combination.

DENTAL MATERIALS

(Also refer to Vol. II for dental materials and operative in Vol. III.)

Etching patterns: Are of the 3 types, i.e.

1. Type 1 = generalised roughening of enamel surface occurs; hollowing of prism centres; intact peripheral regions of enamel rods, i.e. **honey-comb appearance** occurs.
2. Type 2 = prism peripheries removed or heavily damaged.
3. Type 3 = mixed type 1 and 2.

Etching in deciduous teeth

- A **longer etching time;** approx. 120 sec, is required for primary teeth, because of the lower mineral content and higher internal pore volume and so a larger amount of exogenous organic material than in the permanent teeth.
- Retention of sealants is better in permanent teeth than the deciduous teeth, because deciduous teeth have some **prism-less enamel** mainly in cervical region and so no resin tags are formed.
- Layer of P and F sealants is felt by an instrument known as THYMOZIN or by a blunt probe after polymerisation.

Advantages of acid etching

- Increases the surface area by 200 times; depth of grooves formed is around 20–50 microns.
- Micro-mechanical bonding; stronger bond.
- Proper surface cleaning occurs.
- Decreased/zero microleakage.

Restorative dentistry

(Refer to the sections of dental material in Vol. II and to operative dentistry in Vol. III).

Chemical removal of caries

- By CARIDEX.
- N-monochloro-DL-2-aminobutyrate/NMAB.

Morphologic considerations of deciduous teeth

- Crowns of deciduous molars are bell-shaped, with a definite constriction in CEJ.
- Due to sharp constriction of neck of primary teeth = special precautions in forming the GINGIVAL FLOOR in class II cavity preparation.
- Pulp horns of deciduous teeth are sharper and longer, so deeper cavity should be made with precautions.
- Greater buccal and lingual extensions at cervical area is required in proximal box due to broad-flat contact areas of the deciduous molars and distinct buccal bulge in gingival 3rd.
- Width of isthmus should be = 1/3rd of inter-cuspal distance or less.
- Axio-pulpal line angle should be bevelled to avoid stresses in the material.
- Contact areas between primary molars are broader and flatter and situated gingivally; but on permanent molars these are present occlusally.
- Furcation of primary molars is towards cervical areas.
- Reparative dentin formation in primary teeth is more than the permanent teeth.
- Innervation in primary teeth is less, so primary teeth are less sensitive to operative procedures than the permanent teeth.
- Inorganic content of primary teeth is less in enamel and dentin.
- Primary cementum is abundant; secondary cementum is absent.

Cavity varnish = it is placed before placement of amalgam to help in.

- Prevents/Decreases marginal leakage.
- Decreases discoloration of dentin.
- Decreases sensitivity.

Functions of cavity liners

- Protects the pulp from thermal shock.
- Insulates vs galvanic actions.

- Inhibits mercury penetration in dentin.
- Anodyne effect on pulp.
- Antibacterial.
- Neutralizes acid of cements, e.g. of silicates; zinc phosphate.
- Decreases marginal leakage, etc.

Classification of rubber dam sheets

- Thin = 0.15 mm.
- Medium = 0.20 mm.
- Heavy = 0.25 mm.
- Extra-heavy = 0.30 mm.
- Rubber dam sheet size = 5 × 5 inches.
- Main clamp for a first permanent molar = ivory no. 7.
- For distal surfaces of canines-silver amalgam is the best choice, because it is a stress bearing contact area.
- If porcelain laminates are used—the inside surface of laminate is etched with HF acid and then coated with silane.

Bonding agents: i.e. primer.

- Contains thinned BIS-GMA resins without fillers; hence having lower viscosity.
- So penetrates the etched surface by **capillary action.**
- Produces good wetting.

Dentin bonding agents (Refer to section of operative dentistry in Vol. III.)

- To bond with dentin, e.g. phosphorus esters of BIS-GMA; polyurethanes.
- GLUMA; 4-META, etc.

Black's concept of cavity designing

1. Outline form = the cavity should extend to 0.5 mm depth in dentin and 0.2–0.3 mm clearance from the adjacent tooth.
2. Resistance form.
3. Retention form.

4. Convenience form.
5. Removal of remaining carious dentin.
6. Finishing and detailing of cavity.

Recent concept of cavity making

- Minimal invasive technique.
- Remineralisation of early caries lesions.
- Reduction in cariogenic bacteria.
- Repair rather than replacement of existing restorations.
- Disease control.

How to avoid iatrogenic damage to the pulp?

Dehydration	Avoid it to prevent the displacement of the nuclei/cells of dentinal tubules.
Depth of cavity	Minimum of 2 mm thick dentin is required for pulp protection.
Heat production	Avoid it.
Nature of cutting	Use carbide burs with coolants esp water.
Polishing	Use wet field to avoid heat production. At temp > 46° C = stasis and thrombosis of blood occurs. At temp > 55° C = necrosis occurs.
Pressure	At low speed = < 4 oz. At high speed = < 12 oz.
Speed of rotation	> 1.5–2.5 lac rpm with coolant is safest.

Class II cavity design in primary molars: Typical points are:

- Gingival floor of proximal box is wide due to broader contact areas.
- Box converges occlusally.
- Isthmus should not be > 1/3rd the inter-cuspal distance.

- Axio-pulpal line angle should be bevelled and rounded to avoid the stress concentration.
- Gingival seat should not be bevelled because enamel rods in cervical areas are oriented occlusally.
- Axial wall should follow contour of the external surface to avoid the pulp exposure.
- Avoid the MB pulp horn in D tooth.
- Young permanent teeth esp first molars are not mineralized properly; the P and F are deeper and not united completely, so they are more susceptible to caries.
- Kinetic Cavity Preparation: It uses **fine abrasive particles** at high speed and pressure. Dimensions/type/material of particles and pressure and speed.
- Only materials with polyacrylic acid can adhere to the tooth, e.g. GIC, polycarboxylate cement.
- **GIC powder** is calcium fluoro- alumino silicate glasses and GIC liquid is polyalkenoic acid.
- Classification and generations of GIC, i.e. cermet; miracle mix; reinforced; water setting and light cure types.
- **Anhydrous GIC** = in it, liquid used is either clean water or dilute tartaric acid. Polyacrylic acid is incorporated in powder.
- **Resin–modified** = 15–25% of HEMA is incorporated in liquid and < 1% of photo-initiators are added.
- **GIC** is bonded chemically to enamel through ION-EXCHANGE METHOD.

COMPOMER = i.e. GIC + composite resin.

- Has dehydrated polyalkenoic acid also.
- Complete absence of water, so **no ion exchange** possible.
- In it, no fluoride uptake possible so compomer **is not a fluoride reservoir.**
- It adheres by **acid etch-resin bond system** to the tooth.
- Setting reaction of GIC is ACID-BASE TYPE, with the formation of calcium poly-acrylate chains through ion-exchange method.

- Before filling GIC in the cavity — the cavity should be conditioned with 10% polyacrylic acid for 10 sec to remove the smear layer and to increase the surface energy.
- **SMEAR LAYER** (Refer to operative in Vol. III).
- Always prevent the setting GIC from water contamination and so use varnish to cover it. Otherwise the ions formed will get washed away with saliva, etc. and no adhesion with tooth will occur.
- GIC has a low pH.
- ABC of GIC = adhesion; biocompatible; anti-caries.
- GIC is biocompatible because polyacrylic acid/polyalkenoic acid has larger molecules with high m wt. and complex chains, which cannot penetrate the dentin and pulp.
- Also, free F prevents *S. mutans* to make the enamel surface resistant and harder.
- Also Ca and PO_4 ions exchange occurs and help in remineralization.

RECENT METHODS OF RESTORATIONS

1. Preventive resin restoration
2. **ART technique,** i.e. atraumatic restorative treatment.
   - Uses GIC.
   - Originated in Zimbabwe and Thailand.
   - Ion-exchange adhesion with walls of cavity.
   - Only hand instrumentation is used for removal of caries.
3. **Lamination technique—Sandwich technique**
   - GIC as base/dentin substitute = ion–exchange and adhesion to dentin.
   - CR as enamel substitute = for strength and aesthetics; enamel and GI are acid etched with 37% phosphoric acid for 15 sec; fill and light cure for 40 sec; use increments if required to build up the restorations.
   - Light should be held close to the material without touching it.

4. Other latest and conservative methods for Class II cavity making are = tunnel cavity; slot cavity/minibox; proximal approach.
5. **BRAX-1 gene** = is responsible for the control of **enamel growth;** can be used as bio-mimetic dental material.

Important points

- Surface energy of enamel is low and fluoride decreases it even more; so the surface does not easily attract plaque and other molecules.
- Surface energy of all restorative materials especially the metallic ones is higher and so more debris accumulates; it may lead to marginal deterioration and secondary caries.
- Cavity varnish and etching can help decrease the microleakage.
- During restorations, the shade of resin should be selected before rubber dam placement, because dehydration of tooth causes it to appear lighter than normal.
- A calcium hydroxide liner should be placed on dentin before acid **etching.**

Cavity varnish

- It is a natural rosin/synthetic resin dissolved in a volatile solvent, e.g. chloroform, ether or acetone.
- Leaves a thin film on the surface of approx. 4 micron thick.
- 2–3 applications are done for making continuous film.
- Reduces microleakage.
- It is not a thermal insulator.
- Prevents discoloration of teeth by preventing diffusion of metallic ions from amalgam into enamel and dentin.
- It prevents the acid from $ZnPO_4$ cement from penetrating the dentin.
- It should not be used with composite resins, as the resin gets softened and with ZOE cement as the eugenol prevents the polymerisation.

- Microleakage in amalgam decreases with age, due to accumulation of corrosion products in the interface between cavity and restoration.

Cement bases

- Main function is to replace the lost thickness of dentin.
- It promotes the recovery of injured pulp and its protection.
- Is a thermal insulator and barrier to acid penetration.
- **At least 0.5 mm thick** it should be, to properly bear the loads.
- It should support the condensation and masticatory load.
- **Material of choice** = GIC with its obvious advantages of biocompatibility; anti-caries and strength. Other materials used are $ZnPO_4$, Calcium hydroxide, etc.
- If zinc phosphate is used as a base, the varnish should be applied.
- If ZOE or Calcium hydroxide is used as base, then the varnish is used above the base.

Mercury toxicity

- M: A ratio = 6:5, i.e. Hg should be = 54.5%.
- Eame's technique or minimal Hg technique = Hg is approx. 40% or in 1:1 ratio.
- Primary risk to a dental person is through INHALATION OF Hg VAPOURS.
- Maximum safe level = 50 micro gm/cubic meter of air.

Preventive measures

1. Well ventilated operatory.
2. Waste Hg/amalgam should be stored in sealed container under sulphide solution.
3. If spilled, then clean as soon as possible.
4. Do not use vacuum cleaners.
5. Mercury suppressant powders.
6. Wash the skin with soap and water.

7. Use water spray and suction while grinding amalgam.
8. Do not use ultrasonic condensers.
9. Periodic monitoring of exposure levels.
10. Remove gold jewellery while using Hg.
11. Do not mull amalgam on palm as Hg may penetrate through skin.
12. Avoid heat generation during polishing; use coolants.

Delayed expansion

- It is seen after 4–5 days of placement; amount.
- In Zn containing alloys (Zn > 0.01%) amalgams.
- Moisture contamination, e.g. by saliva contamination or mulling on palm; leads to formation of H_2 gas and cause expansion.
- May lead to extrusion of fillings, margin breakage, voids and pain on mastication.
- Use Zn-free alloys to avoid it.
- Do not mull amalgam on palm.

Silicate cements

- It releases **fluoride;** which is an **enzyme-inhibitor** in carbohydrate metabolism and so anti-cariogenic; it increases enamel hardness.
- It gets stained and **disintegrated in oral environment.**
- Average life = 4 yrs.
- It is C/I in **mouth breathers.**
- Acidic pH even after a longer period of placement = leads to pulp irritation.
- Its strength is less.

Zinc phosphate cements

- Acidic pH so pulp irritation.
- Cool mixing slab and wider area of mixing is used.
- Incremental addition/6 increments of powder during mixing is done.

- Mixing time = 90 sec.
- Good strength, used as bases below amalgam restorations.
- Use varnish below it to prevent acid penetration towards pulp.
- Acid base reaction is **exothermic.**

TREATMENT OF DEEP CARIES

INDIRECT PULP THERAPY/indirect pulp capping:

- As known as gross caries removal.
- Teeth with deep caries, which are free of symptoms of pulpitis should be selected.
- A bactericidal dressing of Calcium hydroxide is placed at the base and cavity is closed with ZOE mix.
- Leads to sclerosis of dentin and formation of reparative dentin and arrested caries.

Uses of calcium hydroxide	**Uses of ZOE**
Indirect pulp capping	Provides healing atmosphere to pulp
Direct pulp capping	Decreases pulp inflammation/ anodyne effect
As base/liner in deep cavity	Decreases the bacterial count
Apexification	Germicidal
Intra-canal medicament	Neutralize irritants
Weeping canal Rx	Arrests caries
Apexogenesis	Reparative dentin formation
Perforated RC	Sclerosis of dentin
Pulpotomy	Decreases acid penetration towards pulp
Internal resorption	Has a very good marginal sealing ability of cavities and so prevents marginal leakage
Crown/root fracture Rx	
During the acid etching	
Can promote osteogenesis within 2 days	

- Kept for 6–8 weeks, the dentin formation starts after approx 21 days.
- Also helps in neutralizing the irritants and reducing the pulpal irritations.
- It decreases the risk of direct pulp exposure and preserves pulp vitality.

ROLE/MOA of Calcium hydroxide (Refer to sec on operative in Vol. III.)

Calcium hydroxide in contact with pulp immediately causes severe pulpal inflammatory response. It causes **4 stages:**

1. Localised necrosis of pulp.
2. Inflammatory cells come there.
3. Undifferentiated mesenchymal cells proliferated and form odontoblasts.
4. Dentin formation occurs.

DIRECT PULP CAPPING

- Should be done for pinpoint, small accidental exposure of pulp during cavity preparation under isolated sterile conditions; it should not be of long duration.
- Exposure should be surrounded by sound dentin.
- Pain should be absent.
- No bleeding should be there.
- Calcium hydroxide is the material of choice for capping, e.g. dycal.

PULPOTOMY

- Removal of coronal pulp, which is inflammed.
- Vital normal pulp left in root canals for healing and growth of the roots.
- **Calcium hydroxide pulpotomy** = is used in the Rx of permanent teeth esp with immature root development for apical closure/ apexogenesis; there should not be any symptoms of painful pulpitis.

- **Formoa-cresol pulpotomy** = use in deciduous teeth; Calcium hydroxide should not be used in deciduous teeth as it cause internal resorption and so early exfoliation of teeth occurs. 1:5 conc of formoa-cresol is placed for 5 min only. It causes fixation of pulpal tissues. Seal the cavity with ZOE, etc.
- **If pulp** tissue of RC appears hyperemic then RCT is indicated, as it shows that the pulp inflammation has spread to RC also.
- Pulpotomy is done for **posterior teeth only,** because anterior teeth have **no sub-pulpal wall.**

Formoa-cresol has = 19% formaldehyde + 35% cresol in a solution of 15 % glycerine and water.

MOA of formoa-cresol

- It has germicidal action and fixation properties.
- It prevents tissue autolysis by bonding to proteins.
- Pulp becomes fixed and fibrous and acidophilic within few minutes of application.
- After a few days of application 3 zones are seen:
  1. Zone of fixation.
  2. Zone of atrophy/cells and fibres decrease.
  3. Zone of inflammatory cells diffusing to the apex.
- No reparative dentin formation occurs.

GLUTRALDEHYDE

- 2% glutraldehyde is better than formoa-cresol.
- Bactericidal; superior fixative properties
- **Better than formoa-cresol,** because
  - Its action is irreversible.
  - It has larger molecules which do not penetrate beyond apical foramen (self–limiting penetration).
  - It fixes the pulp instantly with lower doses.
  - Lesser amount is absorbed systemically.

- Initial zone of fixation of pulp does not migrate apically and so pulp remains normal and vital, below fixed zone.

Capping materials containing antibiotics

When mixed with calcium hydroxide:

- The antibacterial activity of penicillin is entirely destroyed.
- Chlortetracycline retards proliferation of fibroblasts and interferes with pulp healing.
- Vancomycin is compatible and helps in stimulating the formation of reparative dentin.

TRAUMATIC INJURIES

ELLIS' CLASSIFICATION

Class	Features
I	Fracture crown involving little or no dentin.
II	Fracture crown involving dentin but no pulp.
III	Fracture of crown involving pulp.
IV	Non vital tooth with/with out loss of crown structure.
V	Tooth loss due to trauma.
VI	Fracture of root with/without loss of crown structure.
VII	Displacement of tooth without fracture of crown/ root.
	VIII Fracture of crown en-masse.
IX	Injury to the deciduous tooth.

- **Contusion** = injury due to **blunt** trauma.
- **Abrasion** = injury due to **friction.**
- **Laceration** = injury which causes discontinuity in skin or mucous membrane.

- **Avulsion** = loss of tissue due to trauma.
- **Avulsion flap** = undermined laceration.

WHO CLASSIFICATION?

Classification by Andersen (1981)

A. Injuries to the hard dental tissues and pulp

1. Crown infraction (N 873.60): An incomplete fracture (Crack) of the enamel without loss of the tooth substance.
2. Uncomplicated crown fracture: A fracture contained to the enamel (N 873.60) or involving enamel and dentin, but not exposing the pulp (N 873.61).
3. Complicated crown fracture (N 873.62): A fracture involving enamel and dentin and exposing the pulp.
4. Uncomplicated crown root fracture (N 873.64): A fracture involving enamel, dentin and cementum but not involving the pulp.
5. Complicated crown-root fracture (N 873.64): A fracture involving enamel, dentin and cementum and exposing pulp.
6. Root fracture (N 873.63): A fracture involving dentin, cementum and the pulp.

B. Injuries to the periodontal tissues

1. Concussion (N 873.66): An injury to the tooth supporting structures without abnormal loosening or displacement of the tooth, but with warded reaction to percussion.
2. Sub luxation (N 873.66): An injury to the tooth supporting structures with abnormal loosening, but without displacement of the tooth.
3. Intrusive luxation (central dislocation) (N 873.67): Displacement of the tooth into the alveolar bone. This injury is accompanied by communication or fracture of the alveolar socket.
4. Extrusive luxation (peripheral dislocation) partial avulsion (N 873.66): Partial displacement of the tooth out of its socket.

5. Lateral luxation (N 873.66): Displacement of the tooth in a direction other than axially. This is accompanied by communication or fracture of the alveolar socket.

6. Exarticulation (complete avulsion) (N 873.68): Completed displacement of the tooth out of its socket.

C. Injuries of the supporting bone

1. Communication of alveolar socket (mandible N 802.20, maxilla 802.40): Crushing and compression of the alveolar socket. This condition is found together with intrusive and lateral luxation.

2. Fracture of the alveolar socket wall (mandible N 802.20, maxilla N 802.40): A fracture contained to the facial or lingual socket wall.

3. Fracture of the alveolar process (mandible N 802.20, maxilla N 802.40): A fracture of the alveolar process which may or may not involve the alveolar socket.

4. Fracture of the mandible and maxilla (mandibular N 802.21, maxilla N 802.42): A fracture involving base of the mandible or maxilla and often the alveolar process/jaw fracture). The fracture may or may not involve the alveolar socket.

D. Injuries to gingiva or oral mucosa

1. Laceration of gingiva or oral mucosa (N 873.69): A shallow or deep wound in the mucosa resulting from a tear and usually produced by a sharp object.

2. Contusion of gingiva or oral mucosa (N 902.XO): A bruise usually produced by an impact from a blunt object and not accompanied by a break of the continuity in the mucosa, causing submucosal haemorrhage.

3. Abrasion of gingiva or oral mucosa (N 910.00): A superficial wound produced by rubbing or scraping of the mucosa leaving a raw bleeding surface.

Injuries to hard dental tissue and pulp		**Injuries to PDL tissues**	
N 873.60	Crown infarction	N 873.66	Concussion
N 873.60	Uncomplicated crown fracture/ enamel	N 873.66	Subluxation
N 873.61	Uncomplicated crown fracture/ dentin	N 873.67	Intrusive luxation
N 873.62	Complicated crown fracture/pulp	N 873.66	Extrusive luxation
N 873.64	Uncomplicated crown-root fracture	N 873.66	Lateral luxation
N 873.64	Complicated crown-root fracture	N 873.68	Exarticulation
N 873.63	Root fracture		

Injuries of the supporting bone		**Injuries to gingiva oral mm**	
Comminution of alveolar socket	Md = N 802.20 Mx = N 802.40	Laceration	N 873.69
Fracture of alveolar socket wall	Md = N 802.20 Mx = N 802.40	Contusion	N 902.x0
Fracture of alveolar process	Md = N 802.20 Mx = N 802.40	Abrasion	N 910.00
Fracture of max and mandibular	Md = N 802.21 Mx = N 802.42		

Vitality tests

1. Heat test with gutta percha stick.
2. Ethyl chloride spray, conc., pressure, time.
3. Ice.
4. EPT.
5. CO_2 snow.

Electric pulp test EPT (Also refer the section of endodontics in Vol. I and operative in Vol. III.)

- A negative response is not reliable indicator soon after the injury, because the tooth is in a state of shock and may recover vitality after some time.
- If injured tooth requires more current than normal tooth—it shows that pulp is undergoing degeneration.
- If less current is required—it shows pulpal inflammation.
- EPT is frequently unreliable on normal teeth also with open apices.

Thermal tests: More details/temp/time/response, etc. (Also refer the section of endodontics in Vol. I and operative in Vol. III.)

- It is more reliable in testing primary incisors in young children.
- Failure of tooth to respond to heat shows pulpal necrosis.
- If less heat is required—it shows pulpal inflammation.
- More painful response to ice shows pulpal pathosis.
- A traumatized tooth may be in a state of shock and may not respond immediately. So tooth must be re-tested in 7–10 days for vitality.

Pulp capping/direct pulp therapy

- Done within 1–2 hrs of injury and the vital pulp and the exposure is small.
- Calcium hydroxide is the material of choice.
- Adequate seal against leakage is must.

- Exposure should be < 1 mm, i.e. minimal exposure, with minimum haemorrhage; and of < 24 hrs duration.
- Agents used = calcium hydroxide is the best; isobutyl cyanoacrylate; resin bonding agent; hybridization; e.g. by 4-META; laser (CO_2), etc.

Pulpotomy

- **Apexogenesis,** i.e. physiologic root end closure/development and formation.
- If pulp exposure is larger and the tooth is permanent with open apices; and/or root fracture.
- Done for a injury after several hrs-days, i.e. 72 hrs.
- Calcium hydroxide is the material of choice.
- Formoa-cresol can also be used.
- It helps in normal root end closure of an immature tooth, because pulp in the root canals is vital.
- Access to RCs is easier with formoa-cresol pulpotomy as compared to calcium pulpotomy.
- Best for Class III and IV fractures of young permanent teeth with vital pulps and open apices.
- Laser pulpotomy = by Nd–YAG laser.
- Electro-surgical pulpotomy = it carbonizes and the heat denatures the pulp and bacterial contamination.

Pulpectomy = i.e. complete removal of pulp from the tooth; as known as root canal treatment.

Blunderbuss canals = i.e. RC is funnel-shaped; the lumen of RC is largest at the apex and smallest at the cervical part. These are very difficult to obturate esp in children, as there is no apical base against which the obturation can be done.

Apexification: Suggested by Frank.

- Is the process of stimulating the root growth/apical closure after pulpal necrosis in young permanent teeth.

- Based on normal physiologic root development pattern to help apical development.
- Often a calcific bridge develops just coronal to the apex, against which obturation can be done.
- Calcium hydroxide is the material of choice, mixed with CMCP.
- At least 6 months time is required.
- Rxed teeth are brittle due to non-vitality and thin dentinal walls of the roots.

RC obturating materials for deciduous teeth

- ZOE paste = it is resorbable with the root resorption of deciduous teeth.
- Calcium hydroxide.
- KRI paste.
- Iodoform paste.
- Vitapex.
- Gutta-percha is C/I in deciduous teeth as it does not resorb with the deciduous tooth roots.

External root resorption

Starts from without and pulp may not be involved. It is of **3 types:**

1. Inflammatory.
2. Traumatic.
3. Replacement = leads to ankylosis.

Internal resorption = also known as **pink tooth of Mummery.**

- Starts within the pulp.
- It requires **3 factors** for perusal, i.e. constant source of irritation/ vital pulp/denudation of dentin, i.e. removal of predentin layer.
- If any of the above 3 factors is removed, then it can be stopped.
- Rx = RCT.
- Calcium hydroxide is the material of choice.

TIME OF STABILISATION

Injury type	Period of stabilisation
Avulsion	1 week
Subluxation	2 weeks
Extrusion	2–3 weeks
Intrusion	6–8 weeks
Lateral luxation	6–8 weeks
Root fracture	2–3 months
Periodic follow up	Every 6 months

INTRUSION OF DECIDUOUS TEETH: It may cause:

- Damage to labial surface of permanent tooth known as Turner's hypoplasia, because the permanent tooth bud lies lingual to the deciduous tooth.
- It may deflect the path of eruption of permanent tooth.
- May cause dilaceration of root of permanent tooth.
- Intruded deciduous teeth are watched as they tend to re-erupt in 3–4 weeks. No attempt is made to reposition them.
- Root resorption and pulp necrosis are most common sequalae of intrusion.
- Deciduous teeth which are displaced but not intruded should be repositioned.

INTRUSION OF PERMANENT TEETH

- The prognosis of pulp is more favourable if root formation is incomplete.
- Teeth with complete root formation undergo root resorption more rapidly than with incomplete root formation.
- Root resorption if occurs is more extensive and progressed rapidly in incomplete root developed teeth.
- Have poor prognosis than deciduous teeth. The Rx is gradual orthodontic repositioning in 3–4 weeks and then stabilising them for 3–4 weeks.

- RCT within 2–3 weeks should be done to prevent inflammatory root resorption.
- Immature teeth RCT should be done with calcium hydroxide.

AVULSION

- Rx is replantation as soon as possible.
- Root resorption of the tooth occurs.
- Ankylosis may occur; also known as replacement resorption.
- Success of replanted tooth depends on length of the time the tooth was out of the socket.
- For success, the PDL should be viable and undamaged.
- Most common tooth = maxillary CI especially in Class II div 1 m.o., and Class I type 2 m.o., it is more common in boys.
- If time gap is < 30 min the prognosis is more favourable.
- If open apex, the prognosis for revitality is more favourable; the RCT should be done if closed apex.
- **Storage media** = for transportation, the best medium is ISOTONIC SALINE; or milk; the acceptable medium is saliva, buccal sulcus of the patient. It helps to keep the PDL vital and prevents the dehydration of the PDL. **Heck's medium** is one of the best synthetic medium for storage and carrying the avulsed tooth.
- Cleaning = wash with isotonic saline or milk.
- Socket wall should not be scraped.
- Root of the tooth/PDL should not be abraded.
- Proper stabilisation 7–14 days during healing is required; it should allow some mobility of implanted tooth.
- Rigid stabilisation leads to ankylosis.
- RCT should be done during 1st week of injury and RC should be filled with calcium hydroxide only. It helps to avoid root resorption.

ROOT FRACTURE

- Is uncommon in deciduous teeth due to more pliable alveolar bone.
- Pulp in permanent tooth with root fracture as better chance to recover than non-fracture. It is because the force of trauma gets distributed during root fracture.
- Fracture in apical half gets repaired with good prognosis. Fracture in cervical part has poorest prognosis.
- **4 types of healing** is expected after root fracture.
  - Healing with calcified tissue = most favourable.
  - Healing with interposition of connective tissue.
  - Healing with interposition of connective tissue and bone.
  - Interposition of granulation tissue = it is least favourable.
  - It requires 2–3 months of rigid stabilisation for healing.
  - RCT with placement of intra-canal implants is a good procedure for treatment.

Important points

1. Periodic follow up of traumatized tooth = every 6 months.
2. RCT is must for displaced teeth.
3. Calcium hydroxide is the material of choice for RC fillings for at least 1 yr after, which obturation with gutta-percha is done.
4. Calcium hydroxide prevents the root resorption in traumatized teeth.
5. Calcium hydroxide helps apexification in immature teeth.

Speech sounds

Sibilants	S, Z
Linguo palatal	T, D
Labiodental	F, V
Linguo-dental fricatives	TH, CH, SH
Linguo-alveolar continuants	L

MEDICAL CONDITIONS RELATED TO DENTAL CONDITIONS

DISABLED CHILD

Horizontal scrub method of brushing is recommended.

Fluoride rinsing.

Topical vancomycin = is plaque reducing agent.

Mental retardation

- Idiot IQ < 25.
- Imbecile IQ 25–50.
- Moron IQ 50–70.

Downs syndrome

- Head is brachycephalic.
- Tongue = macroglossia; scrotal tongue.
- Teeth = microdontia; over-retained deciduous teeth; oligodontia.
- Short stature.
- **Class III m.o**; maxillary hypoplasia.
- **Brushfield spots** are present in eyes as the specking of iris.
- Incidence of **leukaemia** is 10–20 times more than the normal patient.
- Septal cardiac defects.
- Incidence = 1.5:1000; more in older females.

With a Deaf patient

1. Speak at natural pace and directly to the patient.
2. Do not use exaggerated facial expressions.
3. Use tell-show-do approach or/and sight-taste-touch approach.

Cerebral palsy = patient has motor disability as a loss of impairment of voluntary ms control.

Intra-oral findings = caries; PD diseases; malocclusion; bruxism.

1. Monoplegia = involvement of one limb only.
2. Hemiplegia = involvement of one side of body.

3. Paraplegia = involvement of both legs only.
4. Diplegia = involvement of both legs with minimal involvement of both arms.
5. Quadriplegia = involvement of all 4 limbs.

1. **Spastic cerebral palsy** = 70% cases.
   - Involvement of **cerebral cortex.**
   - Increased motor tone, **stiffness** and difficulty in moving limbs.
   - Lack of control of neck ms/**head roll.**
   - Difficulty to maintain upright posture.
2. **Athetosis/dyskinetic** = 15%.
   - Involvement of **basal ganglia.**
   - Uncontrolled voluntary ms contraction.
   - Hypertonic neck ms; open mouth; **protruded tongue;** hypotonic perioral ms.
   - **BRUXISM.**
3. **Ataxia** = 5%.
   - **Cerebellar** involvement.
   - Involved ms **unable to contract** completely.
   - Lack of balance and staggering gait.

RHEUMATIC FEVER

- It is due to group A streptococcal pharyngeal infections.
- Most common in 6–15 yrs age group.

Jone's criteria

Major criteria	Minor criteria
• Carditis	• Fever
• Poly-arthritis	• Arthralgia
• Chorea	• Prolonged PR interval in ECG
• Subcutaneous nodules	• Increased ESR; + ve CRP test
• Erythema marginatum	• Previous history of Rheumatic fever

INFECTIVE BACTERIAL ENDOCARDITIS

- Is a microbial infection of heart valves/endocardium.
- Acute form = by Staph; group A strept; *Pneumonococcus*.
- Subacute form = by **strept viridans.**
- Embolization is a characteristic feature due to bacterial vegetation.
- Transient bacteremia is important cause of SABE.
- Prophylactic antibiotics Rx is must before any invasive procedure to control bacteremia esp in prosthetic heart valves.
- RCT in esp deciduous teeth and/or permanent teeth should not be done.

HEMOPHILIA

- **Hemophilia A** = factor 8 deficiency/classical hemophilia.
  - X-linked recessive.
  - In males only.
  - Females are carriers.
- **Hemophilia B** = factor 9 deficiency/Christmas' disease.
  - In hemophilia, there is **normal fibrinolytic mechanism,** but thrombin production is inadequate.
  - Also inhibitor antibodies are formed vs the host clotting factors and so patient has decreased ability to respond to replacement therapy.
  - DDAVP/**desmopressin** is an extremely useful adjunct for haemostasis in mild hemophilia–A.
  - Oral intubation is preferred oven nasal if GA is required.
  - **Von-Willebrand** disease = is autosomal dominant.
  - Pt have decreased factor 8 activity and abnormal platelet functions.
  - **Hallmark of hemophilia** = haemorrhage in joints and ms.

Hemophilia classification

Degree	% of factor 8 or 9
Severe	< 1 %
Moderate	1–5 %
Mild	5–35 %

Treatment

- Factor replacement therapy = purified concentrates of missing factors are given.
- Epsilon-amino caproic acid.
- I/v DDAVP = desmopressin acetate in mild hemophilia is given. It is an antidiuretic hormone and it increases the factor 8 activity and releases endogenous factors normally bound to vascular basement membrane.
- Cryoprecipitate transfusion.

During extractions

- Intraligamentary LA injections can be given.
- Local infiltration can be given when haemostatic level is > 25–30%.
- **Block anaesthesia should never be given**, as if bleeding occurs in deeper tissues, it is difficult to control by pressure.
- **Replacement therapy** should be given before subgingival scaling.
- Conventional **RCT is preferred** over extraction.
- **Intrapulpal injections** are safer.
- **Electro-surgical procedure is not recommended** in the absence of replacement Rx. It may cause spontaneous bleeding after several days due to clot lysis.
- **No suturing** should be done.
- **Minimal traumatic** procedure should be used.

Local haemostatic agents

- Pressure pack.
- Bovine thrombin/avitene.

- Chromostat; adrenaline pack.
- Stomadhesive = local intra-oral bandage.
- Oxidised cellulose.

Haemorrhage associated with lacerations of mucosa

- Single dose of factor concentrates to increase the levels to 50%.
- E-ACA infusions continued till epithelialisation is complete.
- No need of more infusion of factor concentrates.

Lacerations requiring suturing

- Repeated doses of factor concentrate.
- Level = 25% of normal is maintained.
- EACA continued to healing of wound.

For extraction of deciduous/permanent teeth

- Factor 8 levels required = approx 100%.
- Loading dose of EACA.
- Maintenance dose of EACA for 7–10 days postoperative.
- Extraction should be atraumatic.
- Avoid suturing.

LEUKAEMIA (Also refer oral pathology in Vol I.)

- Proliferation of abnormal leukocytes, which appear in blood as immature and undifferentiated blasts cells.
- ALL = most common in children.
- Common in Downs Syndrome and Bloom synd.
- Commonest in 2–5 yrs age.
- AML = bone marrow transplantation is the Rx of choice.
- **Erythroleukaemia** = is as known as **DiGuglielmo.**
- S/s = pt has anemia, thrombocytopenia and granulocytopenia, tachycardia, hepatosplenomegaly, petechia, gingival bleeding, infections, vague bone pains.

Chemotherapy = multiple drugs given.

- First phase known as induction = given for 4 weeks.
- Cranial vault and testes are irradiated at 28th day to prevent relapse.
- Anti-leukemic drugs do not cross blood-brain barrier, so intrathecal methotrexate is given; it is known as CNS-intensification stage.
- 3rd stage = maintenance; for 2–2.5 yrs.
- Follow up every 3rd month by bone marrow aspiration.
- Prognosis of non-lymphocytic leukemia is poor.

Oral S/S

- Gingival bleeding and **hypertrophy;** common in non-lymphocytic leukemia.
- Cranial N palsies; jaw pains.
- Regional lymphadenopathy (LAP).
- Petechiae and ecchymosis = common in ALL.
- Stasis in small vessels lead to anoxia and ulcerations and necrosis.
- Thrombocytopenia = vascular integrity decreases and so petechia/ ecchymosis occur.
- **Gingival hyperplasia** = due to infiltration of leukemic cells.
- **Strangulation of pulp and necrosis and pus** formation.
- **Necrosis of PDL** = loosening of teeth.
- Generalized osteoporosis due to enlargement of Haversian canals and Volkmann's canals.
- Osteolytic lesions due to focal areas of necrosis and haemorrhages.
- **Generalised loss of trabeculations,** loss of lamina dura; widening of PDL; destruction of crypts of developing teeth.

Dental Rx

1. Preventive Rx = is the best.
2. All elective procedures should be deferred in an uncontrolled or relapse case.

3. Pulp Rx of deciduous teeth is C/I.
4. RCT of permanent teeth of a chronic granulocytic suppressed patient is C/I.
5. A platelet count of 1,00,000/cubic mm is adequate.
6. If platelets are < 20,000/cubic mm, no elective dental Rx given, as there is a high risk of bleeding.
7. If absolute granulocytic count is < 1000/cubic mm, then all elective dental Rx should be deferred.
8. Infections is the **primary cause of death** in leukemia.
9. **Most common cause of death** after bone marrow transplantation = infections.
10. Immature WBCs cannot fight infections and signs of inflammation are also suppressed.
11. **Candidiasis** is very common due to immunosuppression. Its Rx is nystatin (dose = 1 lac units/ml).
12. **Avoid aspirin** (anti-platelet functions).
13. Use soft nylon brushings.

ANEMIAS

Iron deficiency anemia	Microcytic, hypochromic anemia
Vitamin B_{12} deficiency anemia	Macrocytic anemia; seen in strict vegetarians
Folate deficiency anemia	Macrocytic anemia: Found in malabsorption syndrome Lack of folic acid intrinsic factor
Pernicious anemia	Due to lack of Vitamin B_{12} intrinsic factor Atrophy of filiform papillae Hunter's glossitis Beefy red tongue Painful glossy tongue

ANEMIAS (*Contd.*)

Hemolytic anemia	Premature destruction of RBCs Rx = by **splenectomy**; folic acid
Aplastic anemia	Due to bone marrow dysfunction Fanconi's anemia is of congenital type Neutropenia causes infections Rx = by antibiotics; bone marrow transplantation;immuno-suppressive drugs, etc.
Sickle cell anemia	**Autosomal recessive** Abnormal Hb is +nt known as Hb–S Occurs in reduced O_2—tension. Sickel shaped RBCs can lead to infarctions and tissue damage due to vaso-occlusion. Skeletal deformities Jaw pains, labial anesthesia Hypercementosis; dense lamina dura. Osteoporosis due to bone marrow hyperplasia Hypomeneralised dentin; calcifications in pulp. Multiple systems get involved. **Dental Rx** = antibiotics to prevent infections. If GA is used, then at least 30% O_2 is required inhalation sedation is safe. **Desferrioxamine mesylate** S/C and **hydroxyurea** given to increase the levels of HbF and to avoid vaso-occlusive crisis. Conservative and stress-free methods.

ANEMIAS (*Contd.*)

Thalassemia	An autosomal recessive trait **Decreased synthesis of alpha/beta globin** chains. **Decreased Hb** production. **Hypochromic, microcytic** anemia **Thalassemia–major is most common form**.S/S = appear **within first yr** of life. Hepatosplenomegaly, folate deficiency; and growth retardation. Hemosiderosis due to iron overload. **Oral S/S = chipmunk facies =** enlargement of maxilla and spacing of teeth and increased overjet. **Chicken wire appearance** of alveolar bone. **Hair-on-end appearance** of skull Large medullary cavities, thin cortices and generalized osteoporosis.

CLEFT LIP AND PALATE

(Also refer to the section of oral surgery in Vol. III; and orthodontic and oral pathology in Vol. I).

Causes are = multifactorial; polygenic; hereditary; rubella infections; Downs syndrome, Treacher-Collins syndrome, Pierre, Robin syndrome; fetal alcohol syndrome, etc.

Primary palate = includes philtrum and alveolus bearing 4 incisors and palate anterior to incisive foramen. It develops from fusion of MNP and maxillary process b/w 4–7 weeks of IUL.

Secondary palate = fusion of palatal shelves from maxillary process; occurs b/w 7–12 weeks of IUL.

Cleft lip = failure of fusion of MNP and maxillary process.

Cleft palate = non fusion of palatal shelves.

Incidence = CLP more in males.

Isolated CP more in females.

Unilateral is more common than bilateral.

Left side is more than right side.

Classifications: Veau's system:

- Group I = cleft of soft palate only.
- Group II = cleft of hard and soft palates till incisive foramen.
- Group III = unilateral complete cleft lip and palate.
- Group IV = bilateral complete cleft lip and palate.

Facial growth in unrepaired cleft cases

- Occurs normal.
- Only local bony defect is present.
- Abnormal development of dento-alveolar segment near cleft lip due to absence of normal lip pressure.

Facial growth after CL repair

Maxillary growth in anterior direction is inhibited by tight upper lip scar and so maxillary hypoplasia and skeletal Class III relation.

Mandible is free to grow due to anterior crossbite and so unimpeded mandibular growth may cause mandibular prognathism.

Effect of CP repair

Scar causes contracted maxilla and so posterior cross bite.

Scar has red elastic tissue, which leads to relapse of orthodontic Rx/expansion.

Problems associated with CLP

1. Speech problems and nasal twang = especially BDKPTG consonants are affected.
2. Middle ear infections.
3. Nasal regurgitation and feeding problems.

4. Esthetics.
5. Psychological.
6. Respiratory.
7. Asymmetry and deviations.
8. Malocclusions and periodontal problems.
9. Velopharyngeal incompetence.

Management

By interdisciplinary approach.

Feeding advice and feeding plates.

Pre-surgical orthopedics in only selected cases.

CL repair = rule of 10, i.e.

- 10 gm % Hb.
- 10 week age.
- 10 lbs wt.
- 10,000 WBCs.

CP repair

For adequate speech development.

Controls nasal regurgitation and feeding.

Early repair = maxillary growth is retarded.

Late repair = 4–5 yrs age; speech problems develop; but can be controlled by giving obturators to the patients to cover the defect.

Alveolar graft = at 9–10 yrs age; provide bony medium for the proper eruption of maxillary canines.

Management

Stage I = maxillary orthopedic stage; 0–18 months.

1. **Obturator** = to improve feeding problems; cross-cut nipple is used; orthopedic molding of cleft segment is done.
2. **Premaxillary orthopedics** = 0–4–5 months; esp bilateral CLP with premaxillary protruded; and posterior segments collapsed. It helps in preventing lip dehiscence after surgery.

3. **Chieloplasty** = surgical lip repair; helps in suckling; improves esthetics; has molding action on maxilla.
4. **Maxillary orthopedics** = 3–9 months; obturator; prevents constriction effect of lip closure; patient is ready for primary cleft bone graft at 6–9 months.
5. **Bone grafting**

Primary bone graft	In patients < 2 yrs of age
Early secondary bone graft	B/w 2–4 yrs
Secondary bone graft	B/w 6–15 yrs
Late secondary bone graft	In adults

But, primary bone graft leads to anteroposterior deficiency of maxilla and crossbite; limitation of maxillary growth.

6. **Palatoplasty** = surgical palatal closure; at 1–2 yrs age; helps in development of normal speech; but scar formed interferes with the transverse growth of maxilla and so narrow maxillary arch; posterior crossbite; red elastic scar tissue leads to relapse of expansion.

Stage II = primary dentition stage; no particular Rx required except crossbites; growth assessment; oral hygiene; speech development; obturator can be given if palatal defect.

Stage III = mixed dentition period; very crucial stage; skeletal and dental conditions Rx is required; crossbite treated by expansion. Delaire's face mask and chin cap for control of skeletal conditions.

Secondary alveolar graft = gives medium for the erupting maxillary canine; gives bony support to lip and ala of nose; placed at 9–11 yrs age when canines root is 1/4–1/2 formed. Expand the arches before grafting so that adequate bone graft may be placed and to avoid future defects problems during expansion if done later.

Stage IV = permanent dentition; 12–18 yrs; surgical option for skeletal discrepancy; cosmetic surgeries.

Over-denture = is a complete or partial removable denture supported by retained roots to provide support, stability and tactile and proprioception and to reduce ridge resorption.

Types = immediate over-denture; transitional over-denture; remote over-denture.

Immediate denture = which are constructed before all the remaining teeth have been removed and is inserted immediately after removal of remaining teeth.

Obturator = which is used to close a congenital or acquired opening in palate.

Types = feeding Obturator/surgical Obturator/interior Obturator/hollow Obturator/metal base Obturator/palatal Obturator/speech bulb type Obturator.

SPACE MANAGEMENT

- **Best space maintainer** = natural tooth.
- Loss of space may lead to = malocclusions; impaction of the erupting tooth, etc.
- Maximum amount of space loss occurs = during first 6 months after extractions.
- Untreated proximal caries may also cause space loss due to drifting of the teeth.
- Premature loss of primary tooth may cause impaction/retarded eruption of its counterpart permanent tooth; so use the space maintainer.
- At an average, 4–5 months are required to move through 1 mm of bone. If more bone is present, a tooth will take more time to erupt through it.
- Arch length decreases during eruption of permanent teeth due to loss of E-space/leeway space.
- If deep COS is present; a 1 mm linear space is required per side for every mm of depth of COS to level it.
- Space m/m is imp in posterior area of deciduous dentition than in anterior area.
- Early loss of mandibular E may lead to mesial drifting of mandibular 6, and thus loss of space. So guiding appliances are used, i.e. distal shoe/Roche's/Willet's appliance is inserted.

- If bilateral loss of teeth is to be prevented then use lingual holding arch or Nance palatal arch.
- If natural spacing is present in primary incisor area, then no space maintainer is required.
- Loss of first permanent molar before eruption of 2nd permanent molar at the age of 8–9 yrs causes bodily shift of 7 in place of 6.
- But if 6 is lost at a later age, i.e. during eruption of 7 or after eruption of 7 then mesial tipping of 7 occurs.
- Loss of primary canine can lead to distal tipping of incisors in the space. It may hamper with the intercanine width increase in U/L arches. It may lead to midline shift.

Space analysis: (Refer to section of orthodontics for cast/space analyses.)

Appraisal	Mm	Clinical significance
Large space excess	+ 3 mm	Long term planning
Space excess	< + 3–0	Wait and watch; do nothing
Equivalency	0	Watch carefully
Deficiency	< 0 to –2 mm	Use mandibular lingual holding arch
Deficiency	– 3 to – 6 mm	Space regain/expansion
Large deficiency	> – 6 mm extractions	Space regain/expansion/

Different methods of space analysis

- Nance's method
- Carey's analysis
- Johnston-Tanaka analysis
- Profitt's analysis
- Tweed's method
- Moyer's analysis

Classification of space maintainers

- Fixed/removable/semi-fixed
- Active/passive
- Functional/nonfunctional
- Banded/bonded
- Unilateral/bilateral
- Maxillary/mandibular
- e.g. band and loop, band and bar, trans-Palatal Arch, Lingual Holding Arch, Lingual Holding Arch with U-loops in premolar regions, Nance Palatal Arch, RPD, distal loop appliance, lip bumper, etc.

HYPOTHYROIDISM: Delayed eruption of teeth.

Cretinism = i.e. congenital hyperthyroidism. It is present at birth; short arms and legs; i.e. dwarf. Jaws are smaller and so crowding is there. Delayed primary/pmt dentition; MACROGLOSSIA is there and so anterior openbite is there.

HYPOPITUITARISM : It does not appear before 4 yrs age; there is delayed dentition. Decreased or retarded growth; due to decreased GH; prolonged reunion of primary teeth.

ACHONDROPLASIA : Growth of limbs is limited due to lack of calcifications in cartilages of long bones. Head size is large; nasal bridge and maxilla are deficient; skeletal class III m.o. here is deficient growth of cranial base due to early closure of synchondroses; it is related to increased father age.

DELAYED ERUPTION: Is also seen in fibromatosis gingiva; rickets; Gardener syndrome; chondro–ectodermal dysplasia; Ellis-van Creveld syndrome.

SUGAR SUBSTITUTES

1. Caloric sweeteners = sugars and sugar alcohols.
2. Non-caloric sweeteners = e.g. aspartame; acesulfamate potassium; saccharin; sucrolose; neotame.

Glucose / dextrose, fructose / levulose and invert sugars are caloric sweeteners.

Sorbitol is less cariogenic than sucrose.

Xylitol has antimicrobial, antiplaque properties and is a sugar substitute for diabetics.

Sucrose, maltose, fructose are cariogenic sugars.

Cane sugar contains which carbohydrate.

DENTAL CARIES

3 THEORIES of caries:

1. Proteolysis theory by Gottlieb and Frisbie.
2. Proteolytic–chelation theory.
3. Acidogenic/chemico-parasitic theory by Miller.

Proteolytic chelation theory

- According to this concept, first organic component of enamel is attacked and then, the breakdown products chelates with the tooth minerals.

Acidogenic theory = it is the most popular theory.

- The acid produced from carbohydrate first causes the **decalcification of inorganic** part and then the **disintegration of organic** part of the tooth.
- Main bacteria = are *Strept. mutans; Strept sanguis; Strept salivarius.*
- Sucrose is the main cariogenic sugar.
- *S. mutans* is not present in oral cavity of infants at birth and is detected only after primary teeth begin to erupt.
- pH of acid produced = 5.5–5.2.
- 0.2% Chlorhexidine gluconate si antiplaque agent. Details from article.
- Acids diffuse in enamel surface through organic inter-prismatic material and start demineralising outer edges of HA crystals.
- Outer surface of enamel is more resistant to demineralization, so the greatest amount of demineralization is seen 10–15 microns below the enamel surface. It forms the INCIPIENT subsurface CARIES lesion and is seen as the white spot.

- Remineralisation of subsurface lesion is possible only if the surface is intact, with the help of saliva. Fluoride is also helpful.
- 3 peaks of new caries lesions are seen at = 4–8 yrs; 11–19 yrs; 55–65 yrs.
- Since the enamel calcification at the time of eruption is incomplete, and it requires 2 yrs for its completion under saliva, so the teeth are more susceptible to caries during 1st 2 yrs of eruption. The pits and fissures are deeper in immature teeth.
- Environmental factors have greater influence on caries than the genetic factors.

Definitions

1. Incipient caries = it is the early lesion, seen as the white spot on the enamel surface, without continuity defect. There is subsurface demineralization. It can undergo remineralization.
2. Occult caries / hidden caries; these cannot be identified clinically but detected on R/G only, e.g. bite wing, OPG. Latest methods, e.g. FOTI (fibre optic transillumination) and ERM (electrical resistance method). It is associated with low caries rate due to

GRADING OF ROOT CARIES (According to Billings 1986)

Property	**Grade 1**	**Grade 2**	**Grade 3**	**Grade 4**
Surface texture	Soft	Soft, irregular	Soft	Deeply penetrated
Dental explorer	Penetrable	Penetrable	Penetrable	Deeply penetrated
Surface defects	No	< 0.5 mm deep	> 0.5 mm deep	Deeply penetrated
Pigmentation	Light tan to brown	Tan to dark brown	Light brown to dark brown	Brown to dark brown
Synonyms	Initial	Shallow	Cavitation	Pulpal

fluoride exposure; the hidden lesions as known as FLUORIDE BOMBS / FLUORIDE SYNDROME.

3. Arrested caries = i.e. progress of lesion is stopped; it is as known as eburnation of dentin.
4. In rampant caries= lower incisors are attacked.
5. In nursing caries = upper incisors are attacked, because milk gets pooled around these teeth.
6. Linear enamel caries = as known as odontoclasia; it occurs in neonatal line of max anterior primary teeth.

First national oral health survey conducted by IDA = was in 1984

About IDA.

CARIES PROCESS

- Demineralization = it occurs at a critical pH of 5.2–5.5 or below.
- Remineralization = can occur if pH is neutral by buffering and Ca and PO_4 ions in saliva can inhibit the process of dissolution by COMMON ION EFFECT.
- Buffer action of saliva is due to = PO_4 and CO_3 ions.
- 3 Primary factors for caries (given by KEYS, 1960) are susceptible host, i.e. tooth; microflora and local substrate.
- 4th factor, i.e. TIME was added by newborn 1982.
- Irradiations, enamel hypoplasia; vitamin deficiency; diabetes; protein deficiency during the dental development increase the chances of caries.
- Ions, e.g. Se, Cd, Pb, Mn, Ba = increase caries.
- Caries susceptibility of deci teeth is = EDCBA.
- Caries susceptibility of pmt teeth is = 6 are most susceptible and lower 1, 2, 3 are least susceptible teeth.
- Sequence of caries attack in deci teeth is = mand molars; max molars; max anteriors.
- D are less susceptible to caries than E.
- Mand 6 are more susceptible to caries than max 6.

CARIES ACTIVITY TESTS: Amina's seminar also:

1. Lactobacillus count = by dentocult test, i.e.

   if count > 10,000 cfu /ml = high activity.

   if count < 1,000 cfu /ml = low (CFU = colony forming units).

2. *Strept. mutans* count: It is not a very reliable test. It is based on the fact that bacitracin inhibits growth of all other strept except *S mutans*.

3. Cariogram = There are 5 sectors of pie diagram, i.e.

Green	Chance to avoid caries
Dark blue	Diet
Red	Bacteria
Light blue	Susceptibility
Yellow	Circumstances

4. Snyder test = bromocresol dye is used.
5. Salivary reductase test = diazoresorcinol dye is used.
6. Enamel solubility test.
7. Alban test.
8. *S. mutans* adherence test.
9. *S. mutans* screening test.
10. Buffer capacity test.
11. Dewar's test.
12. Fosdick calcium dissolution test.
13. Viscosity measurement.

DIAGNOSIS OF CARIES: Exploration; R/G

Among the latest methods are:

1. FOTI = decayed part of tooth has a lower index of light transmission than the sound tooth part, it appears as darker shadow; it is good esp for anterior teeth.

2. Fluorescence = in carious teeth, the emission spectra shift towards red range, i.e. more than 540 nm under UV light. With argon laser light, carious tissue appears dark, fiery, orange-red. DIAGNODENT is based on fluorescence.
3. Electronic resistance measurements/ERM = increased conductance or decreased resistance shows the p.o. hypo- or demineralization. It occurs due to increased pore volume in the enamel.
4. Ultrasonic = i.e. using sound waves for caries detection; a higher amplitude echo is produced at the cavity site.
5. Dyes = for enamel caries = calcein; zyglo ZL–22. For dentin caries, fuschin, acid red system, 9–aminoacridine.

NURSING AND RAMPANT CARIES

Nursing caries = max anterior teeth are carious due to milk pooling there.

Mand anterior teeth are spared due to tongue covering and salivary pooling there.

s/s = neck of the tooth is involved in a ring–like pattern, along the gumline.

Rampant caries = is an acute, widespread caries with early pulpal involvement of teeth which are usually immune to decay, e.g. mand incisors, cusp–tips, etc. are affected most. Here rapid appearance of new lesions occurs.

Massler defined rampant caries as: Suddenly-appearing, rapidly burrowing, wide spread and uncontrollable caries causing early involvement of pulp and involves those teeth/surfaces regarded as immune to caries.

Caries rate is = 10 or more lesions/yr.

Proximal surfaces of lower anteriors involved.

Reader's Notes

3

Oral Surgery

Electrosurgery = it involves the use of electric current in performing various surgical procedures.

Principal = passing of an alternating current through the body using 2 electrodes. The large electrode is dispersive and small is active.

- Effects of the current = dehydration; warming of the area; coagulation; tissue destruction.

Types of electrosurgery

Electro-fulguration/ electro-dessication	High frequency High voltage Low amperage	One electrode used
Electro-coagulation	High frequency Low voltage Low amperage	2 electrodes
Electro-cutting	High frequency	2 electrodes
Electrocautery	Low voltage High amperage	One electrode

Principles of surgery

1. Asepsis/sterilization
2. Atraumatic procedure
3. Infection control
4. Haemostasis

- Increased susceptibility to infections occurs in:
  - D. Mellitus
  - Leukemia
  - Pt. on corticosteroid treatment
  - Uraemia, etc.
  - Quinidine can cause thrombocytopenia

Response of the patient to an operation is divided in **4 phases of convalescence:**

1. Acute injury; **catabolic state**; for 2–5 days; negative N_2 balance; increased production of catecholamines and corticosteroids.
2. Patient's appetite increases; diuresis begins.
3. **Anabolic phase**—increased appetite; gains strength; positive N_2-balance; for 2–3 weeks; lean muscle mass is restored.
4. Gain in fat.
   - For approx 2 days after operation, there is Na and H_2O retention and so less Na and H_2O should be given I/V.
   - Increased production of corticosteroid occurs after injury especially free 17-hydroxycorticosteroids esp CORTISOL.
   - If patient was on a prolonged steroid therapy, his adrenal-pituitary axis gets suppressed and so he is not able to respond to trauma. These patients require **replacement therapy** with steroids to avoid PROFOUND shock, etc. during extractions/surgery, etc.

STERILIZATION (Also refer to the section of microbiology for details.)

- Moist heat is most reliable and least expensive method.
- Sterilization = means the total destruction of microbes, virus and spores.
- Bactericide = destroys the bacteria.
- Bacteriostatic = inhibits the bacterial growth.
- Autoclaving = 121°C × 15 psi × 15 min or 134°C × 30 psi × 3 min.
- 3 min FLASH CYCLE is best for unwrapped instruments.

Dry heat	120°C
Boiling water	100°C
Autoclaving	121°C
Oil bath	175°C
Gas	10.8°C
Irradiations	
Filteration	

Antisepsis and disinfection

- Alcohol 70%
- Hexachlorophene 3%
- Iodine$_2$ and its compounds 2–5%
- Aq. Quat. Ammonium compounds
- H_2O_2 3%
- Sodium hypochlorite
- Phenols
- Formaldehyde and glutraldehyde
- Chlorhexidine 20%
- Cetrimide 0.5%

Boiling water sterilization

- Cannot remove spores.
- At 100°C × 30 min.

DRY HEAT STERILIZATION/HOT AIR OVEN

- For disinfection of dental handpieces, oils, powders, papers, clothes, etc.
- Slow method
- 121°C × 6 hrs.
- 160°C × 2 hrs.

- Dry heat will not attack glass and will not rust instruments.
- Less expensive.

Chemical or cold sterilization: SLOW = 18–24 hrs required.

- Most widely used for DISINFECTION.

1. 70–90% solution by wt. of ***ISOPROPYL ALCOHOL***
   - Poorly effective vs all micro organism.
   - NOT AT ALL effective vs spore formers.
   - Expensive.
   - Does not work in p.o. body fluids.
   - Can rust the instruments.
2. ***Benzalkonium chloride*** (a quaternary ammonium compound.)
   - Used for general sanitation and housekeeping.
3. ***2% glutraldehyde*** = best; bactericidal.
4. ***2–5 % Hexachlorophene.***
   - Bacteriostatic
5. ***8% formaldehyde***
   - ***20% formalin***
   - ***I_2 and iodophores***
   - ***Chlorinated bis-phenols***

GAS STERILIZATION

- For heat-sensitive and water-sensitive instruments.
- **Ethylene oxide** gas is used = bactericidal.
- Use ethylene oxide at room temperature and a 30% HUMIDITY for 12 hrs.
- Used for dental handpieces, etc.
- Gas is expensive.
- Gas > 3% of room air can be EXPLOSIVE.
- Items should be aerated after sterilization for 24 hrs.
- Used for INDUSTRIAL use.

CHEMICAL VAPOUR STERILIZATION (CHEMICLAVE)

- Formaldehyde + Alcohol + water vapours.
- 132°C (270°F) × 20–40 psi × 20–25 min.

Adv. SHORT cycle; No rusting of instruments; No aeration required; But high cost.

For industrial sterilization

- ***Ionizing radiations.***
- **Gamma** and accelerated beta rays.
- **e.g.** for the mass sterilization of syringes, etc.

RADIATION SOURCES

1. Electron accelerators
2. Radioisotopes
   - Co 60 and Cerium 137 = give gamma–rays

Important points

- Oils and grease should be removed before sterilisation.
- Instruments should be completely immersed in water to prevent RUSTING.
- Hypodermic needles and syringes should be sterilized by AUTOCLAVING.
- Instruments should be stored in AUTOCLAVED MUSLIN or paper packs.

Conversion data

1. To change F to C = subtract 32 from F and divide by 1.8. (F = Fahrenheit; C = celsius).
2. To change C to F = multiply C by 1.8 and add 32.
3. 1" = 2.54 cm.
4. 1 oz = 28.35 gm.
5. 1lb = 453.5 gm.
6. 1kg = 2.2 lbs.
7. 1 gallon = 3.78 liters.

For **hand-scrubbing**

- ♦ Soaps containing HEXACHLOROPHENE or Iodophors are used.
- ♦ 10 minutes scrubbing is required.

Other principles

- ♦ Surgeon's back and the gown **below the level of waist** is UNSTERILE.
- ♦ ONLY the interior of glove should be touched with hands. Exterior of the glove is considered STERILE.
- ♦ Surgeons and nurse/assistant **should pass BACK-TO-BACK** in the OT.
- ♦ In OT—the **level of surgical table** is the line of demarcation for asepsis.
- ♦ In dental clinics—**level of ARM–REST** of the dental chair is line of demarcation of asepsis.
- ♦ Gloved hands may be scrubbed between patients, using a 2 min. scrub with HEXACHLOROPHENE SOAPS.
- ♦ O_2 cylinder = black cylinder with white collars.
- ♦ N_2O cylinder = blue cylinder.

INCISIONS

1. Pen-grasp method.
2. Table knife method.
   - Skin is more difficult to incise than mucosa.
   - Incision on skin should be placed into the creases of skin relaxation. It helps in wide exposure as they are the cleavage lines of superficial tissue planes.

- ♦ Cleavage Dissection = here, the tissue layers are exposed by accurate clipping of tissues with a sharp scissors or scalpel; it produces a LESS BLIND TRAUMA than blunt dissection.
- ♦ If incision is placed in LINE OF TENSION = sutures will be under maximum stress and so more SCAR.
- ♦ Gentle handling of tissues; aseptic conditions.

- Incision should be clean, atraumatic, perpendicular to skin.
- During suturing on skin—a slight EVERSION of skin edges is preferred.
- Avoid infections.

Principles of skin incisions

- Incision can be placed in a relatively hidden area.
- Incision can follow LANGER'S lines. These lines are the direction of collagen fibres, i.e. lines of tension in the collagen fibres of dermis. Incision parallel to them does not gape and a thin scar is formed after suturing.
- Incision should not be placed in a direction so that muscles may pull the edges of wound and widen the scar.
- Best place of incision is skin crease, these are the areas where muscle pull is absent.
- Incision in growing children tend to heal with a broad scar, it is due to stretch of scar due to somatic growth.
- Always mark the incision on skin with pen, etc. before incision.
- Skin is incised at right angles to the surface except within the eyebrow, where the cut should be angled along the line of the eyebrow hairs.
- Skin edges of neck and facial wounds should not be grasped with dissecting forceps, etc. or they will get crushed and damaged.
- Stitch should enter not more than 2 mm from the wound edges and pass to a depth of 4 mm, embracing a greater width of s/c tissues.
- There should be no dead spaces.
- Cut edges at the surface should be slightly raised in order to produce a final scar, which is flat and level with the rest of the surface.

SUTURE TECHNIQUES–classification

1. Interrupted sutures.
2. Continuous sutures.

3. Continuous locked or blanket sutures.
4. Subcuticular sutures.
5. Continuous mattress or horizontal sutures.
6. Vertical mattress sutures.
7. Square knot sutures.
8. Halsted interrupted mattress sutures.

Bandages

1. Stockinette bandage.
2. Barton's bandage.
3. Towel bandage.
4. Barrel bandage.
5. 4-tailed bandage.

Poor wound healing—why?

- Diabetes.
- Poor nutritional status especially Vitamin C deficiency.
- Protein deficiency.
- Poor amino acid metabolism.

Suture materials—classification

(a) absorbable/non-absorbable.
(b) braided/non-braided.
(c) monofilament/multifilament.
(d) metallic/nonmetallic.

1. Absorbable

e.g. Catgut = made from serosa of sheep intestine; chromic gut.

- Must be wet to be manageable.
- Absorbed by metabolic activity.
- Highly tissue reactive.

- Polyglycolic acid sutures—easy to handle; less tissue reactive; less expensive.
- Polyglactin 910 and collagen.

(a) **Natural fibre** (enzymatic absorption)

- **monofilament**—catgut/collagen.
- **multifilament**—none.

(b) **Synthetic fibre** (hydrolytic absorption)

- **Monofilament**—glycolide/caprolactone (monoacryl).
  - Glycolide/dioxanone/trimethylene carbonate (biosyn).
  - Polydioxanone (PDS).
  - Polyglycolide/trimethylene carbonate (maxon).
- **Multifilament**—glycolide/lactide (vicryl, polysorb, dexon).

2. Non-absorbable material

(a) Natural fibres = silk, cotton, linen.

(b) Synthetic fibres = Dacron, nylon, polyester, polypropylene.

- Have superior tensile strength
- **Minimum capillary action**
- Less inflammatory reaction
- But difficult to handle and **hard to tie**.

Natural fibre

- **monofilament**–none
- **multifilament**–cotton; silk

Synthetic

- **monofilament**
  - Polyamide (nylon)
  - Polybutester (novafil)
  - Polypropylene (prolene, surgipro, surgilene)
  - Polytetra fluoroethylene (PTFE)
  - Steel
- **multifilament** = polyamide (nylon); polyester (e.g. dacron); steel

Ideal properties

1. It should have adequate strength.
2. It should be sterilisable.
3. It should evoke little tissue reaction.
4. It should have a contrasting colour.
5. It should have good handling and knot tying characteristics.

Sutures are sized such that **No. 3 is the largest and 7–0 is the smallest** in general use. The more zeros in the number, the smaller the diameter of the strand. 3–0 and 4–0 are used intraorally.

A. Absorbable sutures

1. Gut
2. Collagen
3. Polyglycolic acid and polyglactin 910.

GUT: It is derived from sheep's intestinal submucosa or bovine intestinal serosa. It is of 2 types:

- **Plain gut** = this is stiff and has **insecure knot handling** characteristics.
- **Chromic gut** = this is plain gut, which has been **tanned with a solution of chromium salts** prior to being spun, ground and polished.

Gut suture is **absorbed by proteolytic degradation** and phagocytosis. This is accompanied by considerable inflammation and tissue reaction.

COLLAGEN: Is obtained by grinding the native collagen of deep flexor tendons of cattle.

POLYGLYCOLIC ACID and POLYGLACTIN 910: They are resorbed by hydrolysis. They are synthetic polymers, and produce very little tissue reaction. When braided, they are the **strongest of the absorbable materials**.

B. Non-absorbable materials

1. Silk
2. Nylon
3. Cotton and linen

4. Metal
5. Dacron polyester, teflon coated polyethylene, polypropylene.

SILK

- **Most popular suture material** for intraoral use.
- Excellent handling characteristics.
- Produces a moderate tissue reaction.
- It is inexpensive.
- Does not irritate the adjacent mucous membrane.
- If retained for a long time, produces a **rail-track scar.**
- Its complications are suture abscess, inclusion cyst (the epithelium invades down into the connective tissue).
- Remove silk in 5–10 days.

NYLON

- Can be obtained in braided or monofilament forms.
- Because of its stiffness, a **large knot is required.**
- It has a tendency to tear through the non-keratinized tissue, therefore **nylon is not frequently used intraorally.**

COTTON and LINEN

- Cotton suture is made from non-continuous natural fibres of cotton, which are combined into yarns and then twisted into piles.

METAL

- Stainless steel or tantalum sutures, either monofilament or braided.

Multifilament sutures = source of infections as cp to monofilament sutures due to capillary actions; monofilament sutures get loose more often.

Suture needles—1/2–5/8″ length; types are:

1/2 circle round edge

1/2 circle cutting edge

Swaged needle

Eyed/non-eyed needles

- Lateral cutting edge helps easy suturing through ligamentous tissues.
- 18" length of suture material.
- Wire is strongest of all suture materials.
- Wire mesh = used to fill in the bony defects and lost bone contours. TANTALUM mesh is best, but expensive.
- Sutures should be placed at > 5 mm intervals; helps in proper seepage of exudate.
- Chromic gut resorbs more slowly than the plain gut.
- Interrupted sutures are preferable to continuous sutures on skin.
- Slightly EVERT the line of skin incision during closure. It permits some subdermal contractures without separation in the line of incision.

Consistency of swellings/growth

Soft	In lipoma
Firm	Fibroma
Cartilage hard	Pleomorphic adenoma
Bony hard	Osteoma
Rock hard	Malignant lymphatic nodes
Rubbery hard	Affected nodes in Hodgkin's disease

Edges of ulcers

Undermined	Tuberculous
Punched-out	Gummatous ulcer
Rolled	Rodent ulcer
Rolled, raised and everted	Malignant ulcer

Different cells

PMN cells	Increase in **acute infections** and after trauma; trauma; blood loss and cardiac infarction, etc.
Lymphocytes	Increased in pertusis, **glandular fever** and lymphocytic leukemia.
Monocytes	Increases in **protozoal infections;** in monocytic leukemia; in glandular fever.
Eosinophils	Increased in **parasitic disease;** intestinal worm infestations; **allergies,** e.g. asthma, urticaria.
Punctate basophilia	In **lead poisoning**.

Eye signs seen in toxic goiter

Von-Graefe's sign	Lid lag sign.
Joffroy's sign	Absence of wrinkling of forehead, when head is bent down and patient looks up.
Moebius's sign **Exophalthmos** **Anxious looks**	Difficulty in convergence.

Sub mandibular approach

- Cut placed 2 cm below the inferior borders of mandible; in the line of skin tension; it avoids cutting of the mandibular branch of 7th N.
- Incision should rest on solid bone/firm base.
- Major facial vessels lie deep to superficial ms of expression and PLATYSMA.
- Md Br of 7th N lies just deep to platysma, directly over the facial A; superficial to anterior border of masseter.
- STYLOMANDIBULAR lig separates parotid and submandibular glands.

Surgical approach to TMJ

- Danger of damage to 7th N.
- Blair = inverted-L or reverse question-mark incision.
- Wakely = T-incision; horizontal bar of T is placed over the zygomatic arch.
- Lampert's ENDAURAL approach.

Hypertension

Essential HT = increased BP for which definite aetiology is unknown.

Mild or moderate HT =	systolic BP	< 200 mm Hg
	Diastolic BP	< 110 mm Hg
Severe HT =	SBP	> 200 mm Hg
	DBP	> 110 mm Hg

Avoid Na-containing I/V solutions.

Cyclosporine-A = may cause gingival hyperplasia.

Vitamin K deficiency–2, 7, 9, 10 clotting factors depressed.

B.P.	mild	if	DBP 90–104 mm Hg
	moderate		105–114 mm Hg
	severe		> 115–125 mm Hg
	malignant		> 125 mm Hg

Adrenal insufficiency

S/s—Weakness; wt loss; fatigue and hyper-pigmentation of skin and mucosa.

Secondary adrenal insufficiency

- Due to chronic therapeutic steroid administration.
- S/s of patient are moon facies, buffalo hump and thin translucent skin.

Thyrotoxicosis: Only thyroid disease, in which an acute crisis may occur. It is due to raised circulating levels of T_3 and T_4 hormones.

S/s of excessive thyroid H

- Fine brittle hair
- Hyper-pigmentation of skin
- Increased sweating
- ↑ BMR; ↑ HR
- **Wt. Loss**
- Palpitation
- Exophthalmos

Thyroid gland **should not be palpated** as it can also trigger crisis.

Atropine and Adr should be avoided in these cases.

PREGNANCY

- Elective procedures should be avoided in 1st and 3rd trimesters.
- Best time for elective procedures–2nd trimester.
- Position of the patient during the Rx.
- Maximum time of procedure allowed.
- How much LA can be given.
- What are the C/I during pregnancy.

Dental medicines to be avoided in pregnancy

- Aspirin and other NSAIDS
- Carbamazepine
- Chloral hydrate
- Corticosteroids
- Diazepam, etc.
- Diphenhydramine hydrochloride
- Morphine
- Nitrous oxide
- Pentazocine HCl
- Phenobarbital
- Promethazine HCl
- Propoxyphene

- Tetracyclines
- If N_2O gas is to be used, at least 50% O_2 should be used with it.
- N_2O should not be used during first trimester.
- Drugs least likely to cause fetal harm are: lidocaine/bupiva caine/ acetaminophen/codeine/penicillin/erythromycin.
- Aspirin should not be given in late 3rd trimester = due to its ANTICOAGULANT property.
- Pt. should not be in SUPINE position, to avoid compression of IVC (inferior vena cava).
- Should be placed slightly to one side during surgery.

Drugs to be avoided in LACTATION

- Ampicillin
- Aspirin
- Atropine
- Barbiturate
- Chloral hydrate
- Corticosteroids
- Diazepam
- Metronidazole
- Penicillin
- Propoxyphene
- Tetracycline

Safer drugs in lactation

- Acetaminophen
- Antihistamines
- Cephlaxin
- Codeine
- Erythromycin
- Fluoride
- Meperidine

- Oxacillin
- Pentazocine

ASA classification of physical status

ASA I	A normal healthy patient.
II	A patient with mild systemic disease, or significant health risk factor.
III	A patient with severe systemic disease which is not incapacitating.
IV	A patient with severe systemic disease, which is a constant threat to life.
V	A moribund patient, who is not expected to survive without operation.
VI	A declared brain-dead patient, whose organs are being removed for donor purposes.

Instruments (details/classification)

- Most commonly used scalpel blade for intraoral surgery = No. 15 blade.
- **Hemostat** = for controlling bleeding from incised Vs and As.
- **Halsted's mosquito/Artery forceps** = used as haemostats.
- **Adson forceps** = to grasp the soft tissues, to stabilize the flaps during suturing.
- **Allies tissue forceps** = has locking handles and teeth to grip the soft tissues firmly, during removal of soft tissues/fibrous/ granulation tissues.
- **Russian tissue forceps** = large, round-ended, tissue forceps for removal of tooth fragment from their socket.
- **Rongeur forceps** = for removing the bone.
- **Blumenthal rongeur** = side cutting/end cutting forceps–can be inserted into the sockets for remaining inter-radicular bone also.
- **Chisel and mallet** = for bone removal.

- **Monobevel chisel** = used for bone removal.
- **Bibevel chisel** = used for tooth splitting.
- **Difference b/w chisel and osteotome** = chisel is monobevel instrument and osteotome is bibeveled.
- **Bone files** = for final smoothening of bone before suturing; used with PULL motion only.
- **Needle holder** = its beak is shorter and stronger than that of hemostat; face of the beak is crosshatched for a positive grasp of needle and suture.
- **Needle** = is held approx at 2/3rd of the distance between the tip and end of needle.
- **Suture** = size most commonly used to suture oral mucose is 3–0, black silk, poly-filament (which is easy to tie).
- Most commonly used suture scissor is the **DEAN scissors.**
- **Austin retractors** = are cheek and soft tissue retractors; has a right angle.
- **Minnesota retractor** = is an offset broad retraction.
- **Rubber bite blocks** = to help hold the mouth open, e.g. in Rx of ankylosis, hypomobility, etc.
- **Molt mouth prop** or side action mouth prop for opening the mouth wider.
- **CO_2 laser** = latest method of cutting; efficient cutting; good hemostasis; better healing.

Dental elevators = its 3 parts are handle + Shank + Blade

3 types of elevators
- Straight/gouge type = Most common used.
- Triangle/penant shape type = CRYER.
- Pick type = CRANE pick; apex elevator.

Principle of elevators

Lever principle = mechanical advantage is 3.

- **Most commonly used principle.**
- Here the elevator is a lever of first class.
- Effort arm is longer than resistance arm.

- Mechanical advantage = output force/input force = 3 for each pound of pressure.

Wedge principle = Mech. Adv. is 2.5 for each pound of pressure.

- e.g. apexo-elevators.
- Is like a movable inclined plane.
- Used to remove the apices of roots from the sockets.

Wheel and Axle principle = Mech. Adv. is 4.6 for each pound of pressure.

- Should be used carefully as it applies maximum pressure.
- May cause fracture of bone if used improperly.

EXODONTIA

Definition: The ideal tooth extraction is the painless removal of whole tooth or root with minimal trauma to the investing tissues, so that the wound heals uneventfully and no postoperative prosthetic problems are created.

METHODS: There are 2 methods of extraction:

1. Forceps extraction = also known as intra-alveolar extraction.
2. Surgical method = also known as trans-alveolar extraction or open method.

MECHANICAL PRINCIPLES OF EXTRACTIONS

1. Expansion of bony socket.
2. Use of a lever and fulcrum to remove a tooth.
3. Insertion of wedge or wedges–to help the tooth/root to rise in the socket.

Analgesia = loss of pain sensation; without loss of other forms of sensations (e.g. pressure; temperature, etc.).

Anaesthesia = loss of all forms of consciousness and also a loss of motor functions.

EXTRACTIONS

- For md teeth = chair should be as low as possible.

- For Mx teeth = upper jaw of patient should be at the height of operator's shoulder.
- Patient should be in SEMI-RECUMBENT POSITION.
- Autoclaving = best way for sterilization.
- Molt's curet is used to check the anaesthesia for severing the soft tissues.
- Palatal/lingual beak of the forceps is placed first on the tooth.
- Long axis of forceps should be parallel to the long axis of tooth.
- First pressure is placed towards the apex of the tooth to set the forceps at CEJ.
- No more than 4 ml of LA solution with 1:1 lac conc. of adrenaline for a total dose of 0.04 mg in any 30 min. interval should be injected in a patient having angina.

Contra indications of extractions

- Irradiated jaws may develop an acute radio-osteomyelitis after extraction due to lack of BLOOD SUPPLY.
- Uncontrolled DM = wound infection and healing problems.
- Cardiac problems = a post-infection patient is not subjected to surgery within 6 MONTHS of his infarction.
- Hemophilia, leukemia.
- ADDISON'S Disease (i.e. STEROID deficiency) is an absolute CI. They cannot withstand the STRESS of an extraction without taking any steroids. (Read Pts. on STEROID TREATMENT).
- PUO (pyrexia of unknown origin), SABE.
- **Pregnancy** = 2nd trimester is SAFEST.
- Senility is a relative C/I = patient may have a negative N_2 balance.

Relative contra-indications to extractions

1. Uncontrolled diabetes.
2. Acute blood dyscrasias.
3. Untreated coagulopathies.
4. Adrenal insufficiency.

5. Teeth should be removed only 6 mos after myocardial infarction.
6. In previously irradiated jaws, at least 1 year is allowed for maximum recovery of circulation. It helps in proper healing.
7. Acute infections in the floor of mouth is a C/I to any form of anaesthesia (GA/LA) in an outdoor patient.
8. Mimp C/I to LA is the po acute infection at the site of operation. It may lead to spread of infections and LA is not effective due to acidic nature of pus.
9. PO of haemangioma is C/I for LA.
10. Disease which impairs patency of airway or respiratory efficiency is C/I for GA.
11. Adr/N Adr should not be injected in patients taking tricyclic antidepressant drugs; as then hypertension or cardiac arrhythmia may occur. The effects of Adr and N Adr get potentiated with them.
12. In such patients, prilocaine with felypressin, i.e. a no-amine vasoconstrictor should be used.
13. Patients with H/O hypersensitivity to sulphonamides should not receive LA with PABA rings.

ABSOLUTE C/I of EXODONTICS

1. Arteriovenous or sinusoidal aneurysms.
2. Central haemangiomas.

DEFINITIONS

- **ODONTOTOMY** = i.e. cutting of the tooth apart.
- **Odontectomy** = removal for partly erupted/unerupted tooth by surgical excision.
- **Replantation** = replacing the tooth after extraction and RCT; it is known as elective/intentional replantation.
- **Ankylosis** = i.e. bone fuses directly to the root surface.
- **Replacement resorption** = i.e. after replantation, ankylosis occurs and progressive replacement of root occurs by bone.
- **Autotransplantation** = also known as **tooth autograft**. It is the transplantation from one position to another position within the same mouth.

- **Allogenic tooth transplant** = also known as **tooth allograft**; is a tooth transplanted from one patient to another.
- **Curettage** = is the removal of pathologic tissues from around the root.
- **Hemisection/odontosection** = is the cutting of the tooth in half and removal of root with overlying crown part.
- **Amputation/radisectomy** = is the root removal with the coronal tooth structure remaining intact.
- **Gingival curettage** = is the scrapping of soft tissues walls of the pocket.
- **Gingivectomy** = is the removal of soft tissue wall of the pocket to the point at which the tissue is attached.
- **Gingivoplasty** = is the contouring of gingival tissues.
- **Osteoplasty** = is the reshaping of alveolar process, without removal of the supporting bone.
- **Ostectomy** = is the removal of supporting bone.
- **Apicoectomy** = is the removal of a part of the root end.

Principles of apicoectomy (Refer to the section on endodontics Vol. I.)

- While cutting the apical part of the root, the cut should be placed in an oblique direction to maintain the length of the root, rather than in the horizontal direction, which then reduces the length of the root.
- Retrograde filling material should be biocompatible.
- A hermetic seal is a must with obturation.

Important points

- PA granulation tissue should be removed with a small curet. But it is not done in MAXILLARY INCISOR AREA, because the veins here have no valves and so the infected material and thrombi may ascend into the cranial cavity to form CAVERNOUS SINUS THROMBOSIS.
- Socket must be compressed after extraction
  - To re-establish the normal width of the alveolar ridge.

- Brings gingival margins near to each other.
- Helps maintain the clot in position.

♦ In uncomplicated cases, the remaining posterior teeth in maxilla and mandible on ONE side can be removed in one visit.

♦ If maxillary tuberosity fractures during extractions; every effort should be made to retain it, as it is important for denture retention.

♦ **Mechanism of action of cold** at surgical site = cold acts by producing vasoconstriction and so decreases the exudation of fluid and blood into tissue spaces.

♦ **Mechanism of heat** = leads to vasodilation and increases circulation, more rapid removal of tissue breakdown products and greater influx of defensive cells and antibodies.

♦ **Mechanism of action of saline rinses** = since the saline water is hypertonic, and the exudate is having less conc. of salts but more water, there exists an osmotic gradient to expel out the excess fluids from the inflammed tissues under the influence of hypertonic saline rinses.

♦ **Prophylactic odontectomy of 3rd molars** = best time is when the R/G shows the roots of 3rd molars to be half to 2/3rd formed. It is generally at 16–17 yrs of age.

♦ Mesioangular impaction is easiest and distoangular impaction is most difficult to remove.

Other points

♦ While removing the apical 3rd of root/tip, the tip of apexoelevator is placed between the socket well and the highest side of the fragment (which is closest to the rim of alveolar socket).

♦ Long **Winter's elevators** are used for removing mand. molar roots and are never used elsewhere.

♦ A **root apex** = is defined as a root fragment < 5 mm in its greatest dimension.

♦ If 2, 3, 4 no. of teeth are to be removed at one visit, the chances of fracture of labial plate are reduced if canine is removed first.

♦ Root displaced in max antrum is mainly of max premolars and molars and most often the palatal root.

- **Tannic acid** powder placed on a pack adj to the bleeding socket helps to arrest the bleeding.

Position of the operator

- For extraction of right mand 3 –8 teeth, the operator should stand behind the patient.
- For rest of the teeth, he stands on right side of the patient.
- For removal of maxillary teeth, the chair is adjusted s.t the site of operation is **8 cm, i.e. 3 inches below the shoulder** level of the operator.
- For mand teeth, the chair is adjusted s.t the tooth to be removed is **16 cm/6 inches below** the level of operator's **elbow**.
- **Hearing** is the **last sense lost** under GA and first to be regained as the consciousness returns.
- When average extractions are being done, limit the extractions to the **equivalent of 12 roots** on one occasion.
- If patient is allergic to procaine, then lidocaine may be given
- Vasoconstrictor action of LA with adrenaline is useful to control bleeding.
- In GA–more bleeding occurs, as it has no vasoconstriction property.
- Extraction of teeth should be done from posterior to anterior, if multiple extractions are to be done.

Forceps principles

1. Beaks should be placed as far apically as possible.
2. Beaks should be placed as parallel as possible to the long axis of the tooth.
3. Applications of excessive forces should be avoided.
4. First direction of placement of forceps is in apical direction.

Order of extraction

Teeth should be removed in a systematic fashion, i.e.

1. Very loose and painful teeth are extracted first.
2. Roots are extracted before whole tooth.

3. Lower teeth are removed before the upper teeth.
4. Posterior teeth are removed before the anterior teeth, so that the vision is not obstructed by bleeding.
5. All extractions of one side should be completed before starting on other side.
   - Since anaesthesia becomes effective in maxilla first, so the maxillary teeth are extracted first.
   - Most posterior teeth are removed first for better vision.
   - First molars and canine are removed after their adjacent teeth are removed, so that better purchase can be obtained and also advantage of earlier alveolar plate expansion is gained.
   - **8 7 5 6 4 2 3** is the order of removal.
   - More difficult and more posterior teeth should be removed first during multiple extractions because Haemorrhage from earlier extraction will not hamper the vision and field of work of these teeth.

Types of extraction

1. Trans-alveolar (open, surgical) extraction.
2. Intra-alveolar (closed) extraction.

Alveoloplasty—or alveolectomy is the surgical removal of a part of the alveolar process.

- Most of the initial resorption will be completed in 3 weeks after extractions.

Types

1. **Simple alveoloplasty.**
2. **Radical alveoloplasty** = e.g. in cases of extreme overjet, labial plates are removed for satisfactory prostheses replacements.
3. **Inter-radicular alveoloplasty** = no flap/periosteum is raised and so less resorption/postoperative pain occurs.

Complications of exodontics

- **Postoperative haemorrhage** is the **most common** complication of exodontia.

- **Oro-antral fistula;** mostly in case of palatal root.
- Buccal roots of M and PM are pushed laterally through the wall of maxilla and lie **above the attachment of the BUCCINATOR** ms.
- **Infratemporal space** lies directly posterior and superior to the tuberosity of maxilla, where lie the neurovascular structures. Avoid any dislodgement of tooth, root, etc. in this area.
- If haemorrhage is coming from a bone bleeder, the dull side curet is used to **burnish** the bone in the area of haemorrhage or socket may be packed with **"Gelfoam soaked in Thrombin".**

Dry socket/localized osteitis

- Also known as alveolar osteitis; localised osteitis.
- It is due to loss of blood clot form the sockets.
- Develops on 3–5th postoperative day and has severe, continuous pain and necrotic odour.
- Develops in mandible more frequently than maxilla. It is mainly due to less blood supply in mandible.
- Vasoconstrictor in LA may be a cause as they interfere with blood supply to the bone.
- No pus but foul odour and severe radiating pain is there.
- A septic alveolus is a denuded bone surface.
- Dry socket repair usually takes 2–3 weeks.
- Dry socket aka ALVEOLITIS SICCA DOLOROSA, i.e. (Inflammation of alveolus/Dryness/Pain).
- CURETTAGE is C/I in dry socket, as it leads to spread of infection.
- Treatment of dry socket is PALLIATIVE, i.e. packing with THYMOL IODINE POWDER and BENZOCAINE CRYSTALS dissolved in EUGENOL.
- **Trypsin** also applied = to stop bacterial growth.

Exodontia in children

- Bones are softer in children and more pliable.
- Maxillary sinus is small or absent.

- Mand canal is lower in respect to the teeth.
- Healing is more rapid; greater remodelling capacity.
- Greater porosity of bone in child, there is better penetration of LA and so infiltration anaesthesia can be used in molar region of mandible and in other parts of maxilla and mandible.
- Position of inferior alveolar foramen in respect to the OP varies in children, so the block should be given accordingly.
- **Inferior alveolar nerve block level** varies in children with age in very young patients, as related to the level of OP; the injection is to be given at or above the level of OP in young children; as cp to adults; in which it is given below the OP.
- With nerve block, patient should be instructed/cautioned against/about biting the numb lip/buccal mucosa/tongue, which is the **most common injury** to the child after LA.
- Bilateral inferior alveolar block is not C/I, but tongue may fall back posteriorly in the larynx and may cause problem in breathing.
- **Cowhorn forceps** should never be used to remove deciduous teeth as it may lead to avulsion of premolars.
- **Cryers elevators** should never be used in children to remove deciduous roots as it may lead to the damage to tooth buds.

Surgical Flaps (Refer to section of perio also.)

Principles of flap designing

- **Base of flap should be broader** than the free end, to maintain the BLOOD SUPPLY.
- Should be sufficiently large for **adequate vision** and area of operation.
- Incision should be made over the bone not to be removed, i.e. flap should be well supported by bone on repositioning. Flap margins should **rest on the sound bone**.
- Incision should not be started at the tip of interdental papilla but at the proximal line angle of the tooth. Integrity of I/D papilla should be maintained.

- Avoid tearing of periosteum.
- Should be no sharp angles in the flap.
- Vertical/oblique incisions should not be placed over a root eminence.

Types of incisions

Types of flaps: e.g. envelop flap; 2 sided triangular flap; 3 sided rhomboid flap; semilunar flap; pedicle flap.

- **horizontal**
- **semilunar/elliptical/curved** = helps to maintain the attached gingival.
- **vertical** = most desirable to be used; it may be single, i.e. triangular flap or double, i.e. trapezoidal flap has vertical incision extending from the mucobuccal fold to horizontal gingival incision–around the neck of the teeth, incision should be directed away at 45 degrees from the tooth to be removed.
- **Ochsenbein–Luebke flap** = is a combination of semilunar and vertical incisions.
- **Envelop flap** = has no vertical releasing incision; used for posterior mandibular and palatal surgery; also known as **Bayonet shaped flap**.

Premedication/relaxation of patient pre-surgically.

- 0.1 gm of pento barbital sodium oral.
- 2 ml of pento barbital sodium oral.
- 20 mg of diazepam I/V to achieve Verrill's sign, which may be supplemented with meperidine (Demorol) or N_2O–O_2.

IMPACTED TEETH

- **Impacted tooth** = A tooth which is completely or partially unerupted and is inhibited by bone/tooth/soft tissue s.t. its further eruption is unlikely.
- **Malposed tooth** = A tooth, erupted or unerupted, which is in an abnormal position.

- **Unerupted tooth** = A tooth which has not perforated the oral mucosa.
- **Oxycephaly** = known as steeple head; top of head is pointed.
- **Chair position** = low enough so that the operator's right elbow is opposite the pt's (R) shoulder.
- An impacted tooth is more easily removed, if it is displaced to a buccal position (as cp to lingual) and if it is at a higher occlusal level.
- Distoangular impaction is more difficult to remove.
- **Cow-horn forceps** (No. 16) is **not used for extraction of lower deci**. molars because sharp beaks of this forceps can cause damage to the unerupted premolars.
- During extraction of Max. primary. Anterior teeth = No/little pressure should be placed lingually, because permanent teeth lie lingual to them.
- A very young patient is BEST managed under GA, usually of INHALATIONAL TYPE.
- In p.o. infection, LA is not always profound and is less effective.
- Nerve block is most effective and allows injection in a noninfected area. As it is given at a distant site other than the localised infection, it can be used to remove the tooth in p.o. of infection without the fear of spread of infection by injection. However, antibiotic coverage is necessary in such cases to avoid bacteremia/septicemia.
- Injection in an infected area may cause SPREAD OF INFECTION. So GA may be used in p.o. ACUTE INFECTION.
- **TRISMUS** = i.e. inability of patient to open his mouth. ETHYL CHLORIDE spray on the ms in spasm can help open the mouth.
- Oral procedures taking > 30 min. should be done under "LA with premedication". Premedication help in removing the anxiety and fear of the patient.

IOPA–**WAR lines/Winter's lines**: For mandibular 3rd molar impactions.

Line	Details
White line	• Joins the buccal cusps of erupted molars and extended posteriorly. • Indicates the **relative depth** of 3rd molars.
Amber line	• Runs at the level of the crest of interdental septum b/w the molars. • Represents the **bone level covering** the impacted tooth.
Red line	• Is a **perpendicular** drawn on the amber line from an imaginary point, where the elevator will be applied. • Indicates the **amount of resistance** and difficulty encountered during extraction.

Difficulty index for removal of impacted mandibular third molars:

Classification spatial relationship	Value
Mesioangular	1
Horizontal/transverse	2
Vertical	3
Distoangular	4
Depth	
Level A	1
Level B	2
Level C	3

Ramus relationship/space available	
Class I	1
Class II	2
Class III	3

Difficulty index

- Very difficult 7–10
- Moderately difficult 5–7
- Minimally difficult 3–4

CLASSIFICATION OF IMPACTED Mandibular third Molars: By Pell and Gregory.

(A) According to the relation of tooth to ramus of mandibular and 2nd molars

Class I	There is sufficient amount of space between ramus and distal of M_2 for accommodation of MD crown diameter of M_3.
Class II	Space between ramus and M_2 is less than MD diameter of M_3.
Class III	All or most of the M_3 is located within the ramus.

(B) Relative depth of M_3 in bone

Position A	Highest position of tooth is on a level with or above the O.P.
Position B	Highest position of tooth is below OP, but above the cervical line of M_2.
Position C	Highest position of tooth is below the cervical line of M_2.

(C) Position of long axis of impacted M_3 in respect to. the long axis of M_2 (Winter's classification)

- Vertical; Horizontal; Inverted;
- Mesio angular
- Disto angular
- Bucco angular
- Linguo angular
- Buccal version
- Lingual version
- Torso version

Relationship of impacted maxillary M_3 to the maxillary sinus

1. Sinus approximation (SA)—no bone or a thin portion of bone between the impacted maxillary 3rd molar and maxillary sinus.
2. No sinus approximation (NSA)—2 mm or more of bone between M_3 and maxillary sinus.

Classification of impacted maxillary canines

Class I	Impacted canines located in palate (1) Horizontal (2) Vertical (3) Semivertical
Class II	Canines located on labial /buccal surface of maxillary (1) Horizontal (2) Vertical (3) Semivertical
Class III	Impacted canines located in both the palatal process and labial or buccal maxillary bone.
Class IV	Canines located in alveolar process, usually vertically between incisor and first PM.
Class V	Canine located in an edentulous maxillary.

Haemorrhage

- Definition = it is an acute loss of circulating blood.
- Total blood is = 7% of the body wt.
- Most effective method of control haemorrhage for almost all intraoral wounds = PRESSURE.

Hypotensive anaesthesia—i.e. during GA, the patient's BP is decreased with hypotensive agents to decrease the bleeding.

- Adr. (in LA, etc.) can produce cardiac-arrhythmias if used with Halogenated GA and may also cause postoperative reactive hyperaemia.
- But felypressin (0.03 IU/ml) with Prilocaine 3% used during HALOTHANE GA does not cause reactive hyperaemia.

Classification

1. **Primary** = occurs as a normal part of surgery.
2. **Reactionary** = i.e. after few hours post-operatively.
3. **Secondary** = i.e. after 7–10 days of extraction.

Types of haemorrhage

1. **Arterial Hg** = pulsating nature; vigorous flow of blood; bright red colour of blood.
2. **Venous Hg** = no pulsating nature; flow is slow; dark red colour.
3. **Capillary Hg** = oozing, non-pulsating; intermediate, red in colour.

- **Intravascular Hg** = i.e. due to deficiency of clotting factors.
- **Extravascular Hg** = i.e. there is a normal clotting system.
- **Stick ties** = it is the suture placed in the soft tissues lateral to the free end of vessels, which has been clamped, to prevent the Hg. The knot is tightened to occlude the vessels by compression of the adj. tissues, after removal of hemostat.

Methods to control extravascular Hg

- Pressure.
- Direct occlusion with haemostats.
- Coagulation by precipitation of proteins.
- Production of artificial clots.

Class I haemorrhage	Loss of upto 15% blood
Class II haemorrhage	Loss of upto 16–30% blood
Class III haemorrhage	Loss of upto 30–40% blood
Class IV haemorrhage	Loss of > 40% blood

Feature	**Class I**	**Class II**	**Class III**	**Class IV**
Blood loss	< 750 ml	750–1500	1500–2000	> 2000 ml
Blood loss	< 15 %	15–30 %	30–40	> 40 %
Pulse rate	< 100	> 100	> 120	> 140
B.P.	Normal	Normal	Decrease	Decrease
Pulse pressure	Normal/ increased	Decreased	Decreased	Decreased
Respiratory rate	14–20	20–30	30–40	> 35
Urine output	> 30 ml/hr.	20–30	5–15	Negligible

- Provision of an artificial fibrin network.
- Hastening coagulation to produce vasoconstriction.
- Production of an adherent.
- Administration of systemic agents.

Coagulation of proteins can be done by:

- Electrocoagulation.
- Cryotherapy
- Styptic and astringents = e.g. ferric subsulfate; Monsel's solution; tannic acid; tea-bags.
- Thrombin and absorbable gelatin sponge.

Haemostatic agents—e.g.

- Gelfoam.
- Topical thrombin.
- Oxidized cellulose.
- Avitene.
- Local pressure.
- Adrenaline pack.
- Turpentine or tannic acid; but cause skin burns.
- Thrombin; it is expensive.
- Russel-viper venom; it is very expensive.
- Oxidized regenerated cellulose (**Surgicel**) = is absorbable; **acts as a fibrin trap**.
- Horsley's bone wax (Bees wax + olive oil + phenol in the ratio of 7:2:1).

  - **Bone wax** (Bees wax + salicylic acid).
  - Artificial clot may be produced by OXIDIZED = cellulose and regenerated **oxidized cellulose (surgicel).** It attracts RBCs and produces artificial clot.
  - **Absorbable gelatin sponge** (gelfoam) = forms artificial fibrin network by disrupting platelets.

- **Thrombin** = topical use, clots fibrinogen to produce rapid hemostasis.
- **Epinephrin** = causes vasoconstriction; topical solution is 1:1000; or Inj. 1.8 ml of 1:100,000 Adr can also control primary Hg.
- **Cyanoacrylate** Adhesive Monomers = it bonds to oral tissues and coagulum, and so produces a protective dressing on the surgical site.

Hemophilia (Also refer to the oral patho/pedodontics section.)

- Due to deficiency of factor VIII (AHG) in plasma.
- Defective gene is on X-chromosome; it is sex-linked inheritance.
- At levels of 25–50% of AHG in blood = no trouble to patient unless major trauma occurs.
- At 10–25% = bleeding even on minor cuts.
- At < 10% = **bleeding occurs in joints** and Ms esp. **knee joint.**
- Blood CT is normal with factor 8 levels above 1–2 %.
- CT is not prolonged until the level of AHG falls below 1%.

Hemophilia

1. Most common bleeding problem in hemophilics = spontaneous bleeding in the joints.
2. Most frequently affected joint = elbow/knee.
3. In cases of haemarthrosis, the factor VIII levels should be raised up to = 30–50%
4. In cases of haematoma, the factor VIII levels should be raised up to = 50%.
5. In cases of GI bleeding, the factor VIII levels should be raised up to = > 50%.
6. In cases of lacerations, the factor VIII levels should be raised up to = 30–50 % and supplemented by eACA or transemic acid.
7. In cases of head injury, the factor VIII levels should be raised up to = 100 %.

8. In cases of infilteration anaesthesia in the maxillary jaw, the factor VIII levels should be raised upto = 30 %.
9. In cases of extraction, deep scaling, IAN block, the factor VIII levels should be raised upto = 50%.
10. In cases of surgical extractions, the factor VIII levels should be raised upto = 100 %.
11. For major elective surgeries = 50–70 % level for 2–7 days.
12. For normal hemostasis = 70–100 % level + EACA or Tranexamic acid should be given.
13. Prophylactic Rx is = gene therapy.
14. 4 things can be given to such patients = FFP (fresh frozen plasma), cryoprecipitates, DDAVP, and factor 8 concentrates. The Rx can be started with FFP.
15. Relative specific activity of factor 8 as compared to other plasma proteins is = 1 in FFP; 30 in cryoprecipitates; 3 lac in highly purified factor 8 preparations.
16. BEST is = purified factor 8 concentrate as it does not cause LOADING.
17. Development of recombinant factor 8 represents one of the milestones in biotechnology.
18. DDAVP = has vasopressin like action; should not be given to < 1 yr old child; not useful in head trauma and intra cranial bleeding; helps release of VWF (von willebrand factor), which is a carrier of factor 8. It can be given if factor 8 levels in blood is > 10%.

Preparations which contains factor 8 are:

1. Fresh whole blood = 5–7% level.
2. Fresh/frozen plasma = 15–20% level.
3. Cryoprecipitates prepared from frozen plasma.
4. Freeze-dried animal AHG = 60–100% level.
5. Freeze-dried human AHG = 50–60% level.
   - Cryoprecipitates and fresh frozen plasma are mainly used during exodontia.
   - Cryoprecipitates is 5–15 times more concentrated.

- For minor injuries and single tooth extractions 5–20 % of AHG levels required.
- For multiple extractions = 10–40% levels AHG required.
- For major trauma or surgery = 100% AHG is required.
- **Endotracheal intubation should not be done**, as it may lead to bleeding in the region of glottis.
- **Mandibular block injections (of LA) are absolutely C/I**– because it may cause persistent Haemorrhage into the parapharyngeal tissues.
- **Only absolute safe site for injection is PDL**. (Not even infiltration).
- **Socket should not be sutured** after extraction because otherwise blood collected in the socket may seep down the fascial planes of the neck.
- **Aspirin is absolutely C/I**, as it impairs platelet functions. Paracetamol/dihydrocodeine may be given.
- **EACA**—is anti-fibrinolytic substance; used for treatment during hemophilia.
- **Tranexamic acid** = decreased plasminogen activity by **competitive inhibition** and also decrease activity of plasmin; safer than EACA.

Christmas disease: deficiency of factor IX.

Cryoprecipitates does not contain factor IX and so is not used for Rx of Christmas disease.

- Vitamin K is required for production of 2, 7, 9, 10–factors in LIVER.
- **Von-Willebrand's dis** = also known as pseudo-hemophilia; increased BT

Ehlers Danlos syndrome

1. Fragile skin = hyper–elastic; **difficult to suture;** gaping wounds.
2. Scarring = scar instead of contracting, **tend to spread.**
3. Hyper-mobile joints = also in Marfan's syndrome.
4. Excessive bruising.

Hereditary Haemorrhagic Telangiectasia

Also known as **Osler-Weber-Rendu** disease.

- Triad of Telangiectatic lesions
- Hereditary
- Haemorrhagic diathesis
  - Is due to **purely mechanical defect** in vessels.
  - **Fragile vessels** are liable to RUPTURE.

Haemorrhagic lesions

- Astero-venous (AV) or sinusoidal aneurysms and central haemangiomas are absolute C/I for exodontics/surgical procedures.
- Aspirate any radiolucent lesion before surgery.
- If undiagnosed central venous lesion is exposed by extraction immediately REPLACE the tooth to act as stopper.
- Management of central aneurysm and haemangiomas includes surgical excision, irradiation, curettage and embolization.
- Haemorrhages from soft tissue lesions, e.g. ranula and mucocele can also occurs.
- Treatment of soft tissue haemangiomas and aneurysms is CRYOTHERAPY; **Fibrosing solutions** like sodium morrhuate; resection, etc.
- LYMPHANGIOMAS usually **do not cause a haemorrhagic threat**. It may be treated by surgical excision or by cryotherapy.
- **Bone bleeding** = controlled by Burnishing the bleeding bone; crushing the areas with hemostat; using bone wax; gelatin sponge pack with thrombin.

SHOCK

Definition = it is an abnormality of circulatory system, which results in inadequate organ perfusion, e.g. skin, kidneys, CNS.

Compensatory mechanisms may prevent a measurable fall in systolic pressure until 30% of blood volume is lost.

Types

- Hypovolaemic
- Cardiogenic
- Septic
- Neurogenic
- Vasovagal
  - Septic and neurogenic shocks are due to peripheral pooling and decreased venous return and decreased cellular uptake.
  - Shock is mainly due to either **poor oxygen delivery** or poor oxygen use at cellular level. So due to anaerobic metabolism, **lactic acid is produced** leading to increased serum lactate level. So **primary metabolic acidosis** and compensatory **respiratory alkalosis.**
  - There occurs passing of Na and H_2O into the cells and K^+ into the serum.
  - Fluid from extracellular compartment shifts to the vascular compartment.
  - So use **CRYSTALOID SOLUTIONS as primary treatment** of shock to restore homoeostasis.
  - Vascular space = 5% of total body weight.
  - Extracellular space = 20% of total body weight = (5% intravascular/plasma + 15 % of extravascular/interstitial).

S/S of hypovolaemic shock

1. **Decreased cardiac output** = is due to decreased various returns in hypovolaemic shock.
2. **Cool, clammy extremities** = due to vasoconstriction.
3. **Tachycardia and Tachypnoea** = both are EARLY symptoms of shock, and represent a compensatory increase in O_2 delivery.
4. **Arterial BP = postural hypotension** is the most sensitive sign of early hypovolaemic shock.
5. **Central venous pressure decreased** due to poor venous return.
6. **Arterial blood gases.**

- PO_2 should not be allowed to drop below 60.
- Fair reserves exist with PO_2 = 60–90.

7. **Renal function:** normal GFR = 125 ml/min.
   - Renal blood flow decreases with fall in GFR and urine output.
8. **Haematocrit** = to monitor continuous blood loss and progress of shock.

Treatment

- ♦ O_2
- ♦ Replenish vascular volume, e.g. Ringer's lactate.
  - No place for glucose, so water and artificial plasma expanders, e.g. dextran.
  - **Position of the patient** – Body supine
    – Legs elevated
    – Head down
  - Monitoring.

  1. BP; HR, Resp. rate, temperature.
  2. Renal flow should be more than 20 ml/hr.
  3. Arterial blood gases-PO_2 > 60.
  4. CVP.
  5. Haematocrit.

8 measurements for the follow up of shock

1. Arterial BP = (120/80 mm Hg)
2. Pulse rate = (80/min)
3. CVP = (5 cm H_2O)
4. Urine flow = (50 ml/hr).
5. Cardiac index = (3.2 liters/min/m^2).
6. Arterial blood - PO_2 = 100 mg Hg
   PCO_2 = 40 mg Hg
   PH = 7.4
7. Arterial blood lactate = 12 mg/100 ml.
8. Haematocrit = 35–45%.

TISSUE TRANSPLANTATION

Autogenous grafts = tissue taken from same individual.

Allogeneic graft/allograft: tissue taken from an individual of same species, who is not genetically related to the recipient.

Isograft/syngenesio plastic graft = taken from an individual of same species genetically related to recipient.

Xerograft = tissue taken from donor of other species, e.g. animal.

Graft = is the true transplantation of living tissue.

Implant = transplantation of nonviable tissue, e.g. freeze–dried allogenic bone; xenogenic implants of animal bone.

Alloplasts = are synthetic materials of non-animal origin, e.g. Hydroxyapatite, POP, etc.

Antigen = invading agent causing initiation of immune response.

Antibody = specific protein developed in the body in response to the Ag.

Humoral immunity = plasma cells, large lymphocytes and reticulum cells produce Abs and release them in circulatory body fluids. It lasts for as long as the specific Ab persists in body fluids.

Cells mediated immunity/tissue immunity = certain cells do not release Abs, but react with foreign materials. It may last indefinitely.

Allograft response = is rejection of tissue graft between unrelated members of same species. It occurs due to cellular reaction of host to the graft.

White grafts = high resistance gets developed in a donor after rejection of first allograft. Now if a 2nd allograft is placed from same donor, it gets destroyed even more RAPIDLY. These 2nd grafts are known as White grafts.

Autogenous grafts = also known as autografts; self-grafts.

- Obtained from the same individual.
- Only type of graft which provides living and immunocompetent cells.
- **Block** grafts = are solid pieces of both cortical and cancellous bone, e.g. iliac crest; and ribs.

- **Particulate marrow-cancellous bone**/PMCB grafts = are obtained by harvesting the medullary bone and associated endosteum and haematopoietic marrow. It provides greatest concentration of osteogenic cells; obtained mostly from ilium.
- **Composite grafts** = they contain both soft tissues and osseous elements, e.g. pedicle grafts, i.e. some blood supply to graft is maintained with the original site.
- **Free graft** = graft is totally removed from its site and immediately replaced. The blood supply is restored by reconnection of blood vessels.

Allogenic grafts

- Aka allografts/homografts.
- Are taken from another individual of same species.
- e.g. freeze dried.
- Cannot participate in phase I of osteogenesis, because osteogenic cells get destroyed by freeze drying, etc.
- Offers a hard tissue matrix for phase II induction of osteogenesis.

Xenogenic graft

- Aka heterograft/xenograft.
- Taken from a different species.
- Antigenic dissimilarity of these grafts are greater than allogenic grafts.
- It is rarely used.
- Does not provide viable cells for osteogenesis.

3 methods to attenuate immune response

1. Modify host's immune mechanism
   - Thymectomy
   - Irradiation
   - Immuno suppressive drugs = it is generally used in major organ transplant.

2. Alter the inherent graft ANTIGENIC properties
   - Irradiation
   - Freezing
   - Freeze drying

   It is mostly used is ORAL SURGERY.
3. By storing transplant organ in INTERMEDIARY HOST

Storage of allergenic bone for transplantation

- Best = Cryobiological, i.e. by cooling, freezing or freeze–drying.
- Grafts are more completely REVASCULARIZED and remodelled.

Bone and cartilage have less cellular content, but a LARGE amounts of calcified/uncalcified matrix which is NONVIABLE.

- During cryogeny–**only cellular death occurs**, without altering the remaining osseous structure of graft, which is the essential part for the development of an effective graft substance.
- **Osteogenic process** is purely PASSIVE.
- Extracellular matrix of the graft acts as a system of ABSORBABLE surface on which new bone can grow.
- **Sterilization** can be done by ETHYLENE OXIDE and Beta propiolactone.
- **Autogenous bone graft** is MATERIAL of choice in most orthognathic surgical sites.
- Autogenous **iliac crest bone** is recommended for rebuilding the HEIGHT of deficient alveolar ridge.

Purpose of decalcification of allogenic bone is to release more BONE–MORPHOGENETIC–Proteins (BMP) as a stimulator of osteo-induction in appropriate progenitor cell substrates.

Other graft materials are

- Partially decalcified allogenic bone.
- Completely decalcified allogenic bone.
- Allogenic banked cartilage.
- Xenogenic bone graft = it

- Stimulates an immune response.
- Major antigenic component of animal bone is contained within the organic fraction of the tissues; e.g. calf bone.

Autogenous grafts

- Usually used to restore large areas of lost mandibular bone.
- Costochondral RIB graft is employed to reconstruct the disarticulated mandible, as the cartilage part stimulates the TMJ and condyle.
- RIB graft.
- Iliac graft.

Autogenous particulate marrow cancellous bone graft (PMCB)

- Autogenous haematopoietic marrow and cancellous bone containing marrow are the only type of bone graft materials capable of ACTIVELY inducting osteogenesis.
- Particulate marrow graft are better than the solid grafts in RAPID regeneration of large defects. It is easy to obtain through a small opening.

In Cleft Lip and Palate

- Autogenous cancellous bone grafts are most effective.
- Grafting is done between 5–12 yrs age.
- Canine is moved in occlusion between 8–12 wks after grafting (at 9–11 yrs age).

COMPOSITE GRAFTS

- They contain both hard tissue and soft tissue.
- Obtained from chest wall or iliac crest (with superior iliac circumflex A attached).

WOUNDS AND INJURIES

Soft tissues injuries: e.g. abrasion; contusion; laceration.

Contusion

- Is also known as bruise.
- Produced by an impact **from blunt object.**
- Without breaking the skin or mucous membrane.
- Submucosal or s/c haemorrhage occurs.
- Ecchymosis is seen after 48 hrs.
- Skin continuity is usually not broken.

Abrasion

- Painful due to involvement of nerve terminals.
- Is produced by rubbing or **scraping off** of the covering surface; exposes NERVE endings.
- It results **from friction.**
- Wound is superficial and produces RAW BLEEDING surface.
- Bleeding is capillary in nature.

Laceration

- It is a tear in the epithelial and subepithelial tissues.
- It is most frequent type of injury.
- Wound **resulting from tear**, with sharp margin.
- Produced **by SHARP object.**

BURNS–"RULE of 9"

- **First degree** = which produces **erythema** of skin.
- **Second degree** = which produces **vesicle formation.**
- **Third degree** = which causes **complete destruction** of epidermis and dermis, extending into or beyond the S/C tissue.
- Major **systemic problem** with burns = shock esp OLIGEMIC/ HYPOVOLEMIC shock, due to fluid/colloid loss.

Estimated **need for replacement** in first 24 hrs is

1. Colloid = % of body burned × Body weight × 0.25.
2. Electrolyte = % of body burned × body weight × 0.50.

3. Glucose in water = 2000 ml.
   - Requirements for second 24 hrs. = half the amount required for first 24 hrs. + 2000 ml. of glucose in water.

Closure of wound

1. **Objective = accurate co-adaptation/**approximation of layers of tissues with elimination of all dead spaces.
2. Handle the tissue **Gently**.
3. Suture to form watertight seal.
4. Deeper ms and S/C tissue should be **closed by inverted buried interrupted sutures** with absorbable (plain gut/PGA) sutures.
5. Under tension should not be placed.
6. Sutures should be **placed at equal distance** and **equal depth** on either side of the wound.
7. Slight **eversion of skin margins** should be produced to avoid contracture scars.

Prophylaxis against Tetanus

- Caused by *Clostridium tetani*.
- Active immunization is long tasting.
- Given as 0.5 ml in 3 doses.
  - First dose = zero day
  - Second dose = 6 wks.
  - Third dose = 6–12 mos.
  - Booster dose = every year.

Passive Immunity—By I/M inj. 250 units of Human Anti-tetanus globulin (ATG).

Traumatic injuries to teeth and associated structures: Please refer to the section on pedodontics for details.

Repair of displaced tooth

1. **Hematoma phase** = upto 24–72 hrs.
   - Blood clot formed.
   - Early organization.

2. **Fibrous repair phase**
   - 3rd day–3 weeks.
   - Prevent additional injury to blood clot.
3. **Final bone forming phase**
   - For 4–6 weeks.
   - Bone formation completed.
   - Undesirable movement/traumatic stress leads to surgical failure. So avoid it.
   - Most traumatic wounds of oral cavity are OPEN and all such injuries should be treated as infected wounds.

FRACTURE OF JAWS

Classifications and definitions

Pathological fracture = bone gets weakened by some underlying pathology and get fractured under very less stresses than it can bear normally.

Simple fracture = is in which the overlying integument is intact; bone is broken completely but not exposed to air.

Greenstick fracture

- One side of bone/cortical plate is broken and other is bent.
- Seen often in children as their bones are soft.
- Time required for healing is minimal.

Compound fracture

- Here an external wound is associated with break in the bone.
- Fracture is open to outside air.
- Almost all jaw fractures in the teeth region are compounded through PDL.

Comminuted fracture = is one in which the bone is splintered or crushed.

Displaced/undisplaced fracture

Favourable/unfavourable fracture

FACTORS

Bones get easily fractured due to weakening under certain systemic conditions

1. Endocrine disorders
   - Hyper parathyroidism
   - Post menopausal osteoporosis.
2. Developmental disorders
   - Osteopetrosis
3. Systemic disorders
   - Reticuloendothelial diseases
   - Paget's disease
   - Osteomalacia
   - Mediterranean anemia
4. Local disorders
   - Fibrous dysplasia
   - Tumours and cysts

Healing of BONE

3 phases

1. Haemorrhage = clot organization and proliferation of blood vessels; lasts upto 10 days.
2. Callus formation
   - Woven bone/**primary callus** formed.
   - Lasts from 10–20 days.
   - **Secondary callus** = haversian systems formed.
   - From 20–60 days.
3. FUNCTIONAL/Reconstruction phase
   - Mechanical forces are required.
   - Haversian systems line up according to STRESS–LINES, as according to **Wolff's law of trabeculation.**
   - Bony shape moulded with functional use.
   - Runs for 2–3 yrs.

Healing of fracture-studied by Weinmann and Sicher, occurs in 6 phases

1. Clotting of blood of hematoma = 6–8 hrs.
2. Organisation of blood of hematoma
   - Capillaries invade = 24–48 hrs.
   - Fibroblasts invade = 24–48 hrs.
   - Proliferation of blood vessels.
3. Formation of fibrous callus–10 days
   - Fibroblasts are most important cells.
   - Decreased number of white cells.
   - Partial obliteration of capillaries.
   - End of hyperemic phase.
4. Formation of primary bony callus
   - 10–30 days.
   - Very low calcium content.
   - Woven bone is formed.
   - Can't be seen on R/G.

PRIMARY CALLUS– 4 types

(a) Anchoring callus

- Develops on outer surface of bone near periosteum.
- Spongy bone, produced by OSTEOBLASTS.
- Extends some distance away from fracture.

(b) Sealing callus

- Develops on INSIDE surface across the fractured ends.
- Fills the marrow spaces.
- Forms from ENDOSTEAL PROLIFERATION.

(c) Bridging callus

- Develops on outer surface between the anchoring callus on the 2 #ed ends.
- It is the ONLY one, which is **primarily CARTILAGINOUS.**

(d) Uniting callus

- Between the ends of bones and between the areas of other primary calluses.
- It forms only after the development of other calluses.

5. **Secondary Callus** = is the MATURE bone, which replaces the immature bone of primary callus.
   - More **heavily calcified.**
   - **Can be seen on R/G.**
   - Haversian system not formed UNIFORMLY.
   - HAS LAMINATED bone, which can withstand the active force.
   - 20–60 days.
6. **FUNCTIONAL reconstruction of fractured bone**
   - Bone subjected to functional stresses.
   - Haversian systems get uniformly oriented.

MAXILLARY FRACTURES

Le Fort's Classification

Le Fort I	– Horizontal fracture/Floating Jaw/Low level fracture/Guerin fracture.
Le Fort II	– Pyramidal fracture/Sub-zygomatic fracture.
Le Fort III	– Transverse fracture/Craniofacial dysjunction/High level fracture/Supra-zygomatic fracture.

Modified Le Fort classification

Le Fort I		Low Mx fracture
	Ia	Low Mx II/multiple segment
Le Fort II		Pyramidal fracture
	IIa	Pyramidal and nasal fracture
	IIb	Pyramidal and Naso-orbito-ethmoidal (NOE) fracture

Le Fort III	Craniofacial dysjunction
IIIa	Craniofacial + nasal fracture
IIIb	Craniofacial + NOE
Le Fort IV	Le Fort II or III fracture and cranial base fracture
IVa	Supra orbital rim fracture
IVb	Ant. Cranial fossa + SOR fracture
IVc	Ant. Cranial fossa + orbital wall fracture

Orbital blow-out fracture

- When an object of slightly greater diameter than the orbital rim strikes protruding eyeball,
- The rapid rise in the intra-orbital pressure fractures the orbital floor.
- The contents get displaced in the antral cavity like a trap-door.
- It is seen as **hanging-drop sign** in the Water's view R/G.
- It interferes with the IO/IR ms and so diplopia occurs in the vertical/upward gaze.
- It causes enophthalmos.

Blow-in fracture

- i.e. an inward buckling of the orbital floor and so decrease in volume of orbit occurs.

CSF Rhinorrhoea

- It occurs with the fracture of cribriform plate of ethmoid bone.
- Mucus associated with cold will dry with the starching of the handkerchief.
- But **CSF dries without starching.**
- CSF produces **TRAM LINE pattern** on face and **a halo–effect** on the sheet and pillow.
- CSF has **much higher glucose content.**

- Associated with Le Fort II, and III; ethmoid bone fracture; cribriform plate and severe nasal fractures.
- Patient with head injury **should not be given MORPHINE,** as it may depress the respiratory centre.

Various s/s associated with fractures

CSF rhinorrhoea	Le Fort II, and III; ethmoid bone fracture; cribriform plate and severe nasal fractures.
Damage to infra-orbital and zygomatic nerves	Le Fort II and zygomatic fractures.
Cranial N damage in orbit	In Le Fort II and III; zygomatic fracture.
Hooding of eye	In zygomatic fracture; in Le Fort III fracture. Level of globe drops and upper eyelid comes down. Occurs when fracture **passes above** the Whitnall's tubercle.
Diplopia	Mainly due to interference in the activity of ocular ms especially IO/IR/LR; it should be recorded in all the nine gauges.
Epiphora	Increased lacrimation; occurs in Le Fort II and III fractures.
Telecanthus	Increased distance b/w canthi of eyes; due to severe naso-ethmoidal fractures.
Circum-orbital ecchymosis	Seen in zygomatic fractures; Le Fort II and III fracture
Sub-conjunctival hacmorrhage	
Black eye	

Neurological evaluation after trauma

Battle's sign	Area of ecchymosis behind the ear in mastoid area, e.g. in basilar skull fracture esp. middle cranial fossa.
Raccoon eye	Area of ecchymosis around the eye, e.g. in anterior cranial fossa fracture.
Marcus–Gunn pupil	It is an afferent pupillary defect due to optic N damage; the involved eye constricts to the light in the opposite eye and dilates as the light is brought into the involved eye.
3rd nerve palsy	Unilaterally dilated pupil, which does not react to the light and appears displaced laterally due to paresis of Medial Rectus ms.
Epidural hematoma	Haemorrhage b/w dura and inner table of skull; caused by tear of middle meningeal A by fracture in the temporal area, pressure on 3rd n and so dilated pupils Lucid interval is present.

Difference between epidural and subdural hematoma

- Lucid interval
- **Subdural hematoma** = occurs when veins bridging the cortex to the venous sinuses are torn.
- **Concussion** = is the temporary loss of consciousness with no permanent organic brain damage.
- **Contusion** = is a bruising of the brain.
- **Jafferson fracture** = is a comminuted fracture of the ring of vertebra C–1.
- **Hangman's fracture** = is a fracture through the pedicles and laminae of C–2.
- **Most frequently damaged**/injured cranial n in fractures = 6th N.

- **Optic N** is protected by a ring of compact bone. The fracture line involving orbit goes around that foramen rather than through it.
- **Crow's foot** skin creases are present on the outer corner of the eyes; the incision should be given in these creases to avoid significant scar formation.
- If the fractured zygomatic arch impinges on coronoid process of mandible, then it interferes with normal range of excursion of mandible.
- Do not use morphine in patients of fracture and head injury as it:
  - Depresses the cough reflex.
  - Causes pupil constriction.
  - Depresses level of consciousness.
  - Depresses respiration.
  - Drug of choice here is diazepam (sedative) and pentazocine (analgesic).
- Haemorrhage anterior to orbital septum causes lid–ecchymosis.
- Haemorrhage posterior to orbital septum includes subconjunctival haemorrhage; it is sharply limited by septum and tarsal plate.
- **Retrobulbar haemorrhage** = if decompression is not done, it may lead to blindness by ischemia of optic N due to occlusion of **short posterior ciliary As.**

Suspensory ligament of lockwood

- Maintains the level of eye globe.
- Passes from medial attachment of lacrimal bone to Whitnall's tubercle, which is present on inner aspect of zygomatic bone just below fronto-zygomatic suture.
- If fracture occurs below Whitnall's tubercle, there is no alteration in the level of eye globe.

Signs and symptoms of Le Fort I fractures

- **Ecchymosis** in the buccal sulcus below zygomatic arch.
- Disturbed occlusion.

- Mobility of teeth bearing segment is ascertained by = grasping the teeth and applying slight and firm movement.
- **Cracked–pot sound** = occurs on percussion of upper teeth.

Signs and symptoms of Le Fort II and III fractures

- Massive oedema of face is a characteristic feature = **moon–face appearance.**
- Bilateral circum-orbital ecchymosis.
- Subconjunctival ecchymosis.
- Maxilla is displaced down and backward = **dish-face deformity.**
- Gagging of occlusion and anterior open bite.
- Floating maxilla.
- Cracked pot sound on teeth percussion.

Signs and symptoms peculiar of Le Fort II fractures

- Step deformity and mobility at infra-orbital margin.
- No change in the pupil level because line of fracture passes below the lateral attachment of suspensory ligament.
- Hematoma in upper buccal sulcus in first and second molar region = as the fracture line passes across the zygomatic buttress.
- CSF rhinorrhoea is not a constant finding.
- **Subconjunctival Haemorrhage.**
- **Black eyes.**
- CSF rhinorrhoea if cribriform plate of ethmoid bone gets fractured.
- H/O unconsciousness
- Lesions of cranial Ns **(esp 6, 7th).**
- **Battle's sign** (ecchymosis in line of the posterior auricular A in MASTOID area) after 24 hrs of fracture.

Signs and symptoms peculiar of Le Fort III fractures

- **Also known as High level fracture.**
- Tenderness and separation at fronto-zygomatic suture.

- Fracture line passes above the Whitnall's tubercle and so ocular level is lowered and **hooding of eye** occurs.
- Profuse CSF rhinorrhoea.
- Results in depressed posterior end due to pterygoid ms attachment and so Ant open bite.
- Dish face/transverse fracture.
- Orbit separated at zygomatico–frontal suture.
- Bleeding from ear (shows middle cranial fossa fracture).

Diplopia: i.e. double vision

- due to injury to **inferior oblique ms** or due to depressed orbital fracture.
- In NOE fracture.
- In zygomatic complex fracture.
- In orbital blowout fracture.

Zygomatic arch fracture

- Seen best by **JUG HANDLE/Water's view.**
- Treatment by **Gillies approach.**

Ophthalmoplegia and ptosis = due to involvement of **3, 4, 6th Ns.**

Fixed and dilated pupils = due to **disturbances in p-sympathetic** Ns.

Proptosis = by paresis of **extra-occular ms**, which normally exert a retracting influence on the globe.

Sensory disturbance = due to **ophthalmic div of 5th N.**

McGregor and Campbell's lines: Seen in OMV/ PNS view.

- **First line** = path from zygomatico-frontal suture to superior orbital margin across the glabella region to superior orbital margin and zygomatico-frontal suture of the other side.

  Second line = from zygomatic tubercle to continuous line of zygomatic arch till it blends into zygomatic bone and the line continues along inferior orbital margin, across the frontal process of maxilla and lateral wall of nose through septum and then same course on the opposite side.

- **Third line** = from condyle across the mandibular notch, coronoid process of the mandible to lateral wall of antrum and continuous through the medial wall of antrum or lateral wall of nose at the nasal floor level and the same course on the opposite side.
- **Fourth line** = occlusal curve of the U/L arches.
- **Fifth line** = lower border of mandible from one angle to other side angle.

TREATMENT

- If maxillary tuberosity is attached to the periosteum = it can be left alone with or without splinting.
- Rx of zygomatic arch and/or complex fracture = by **Gillies temporal approach; Bristow's elevator** is use.
- Fixation of zygomatic arch fracture is not required because temporalis fascia attached along the superior aspect of the arch effectively immobilizes the segments.
- For reducing nasal complex fracture—**Walsham's and Asch's forceps** are used.
- Delayed Rx of zygomatic complex fracture may lead to interference of mandibular movements. So coronoidectomy should be done.
- Delayed Rx of nasal complex fracture and dish face deformity may require osteotomy and alloplastic implants.
- Damage to nasolacrimal duct may occur in Le Fort II and nasal complex fracture. So epiphora may develop.
- Improperly reduced Le Fort 1, 2, 3, fractures may cause posterior gagging of occlusion and anterior open bite.

Steps of treatment of a fracture

1. Reduction
2. Fixation and immobilization

Immobilization

Internal fixation		**External fixation**
	By	
• direct osteosynthesis		• craniomandibular
• suspension		• craniomaxillary
• support		• suspension from cranial vault

Direct osteosynthesis:	Suspension from cranial vault
• trans-osseous wiring	• circumzygomatic
• bone plate and screws	• zygomatico-mandibular
• Kirschner wire	• inferior orbital border–mandibular
• Steinmann pins	• fronto-mandibular
	• pyriform fossa-mandibular

WHAT ARE THE ABC'S OF PATIENT MANAGEMENT?

A	Airway maintenance with cervical spine control
B	Breathing and ventilation
C	Circulation and control of haemorrhage
D	Disability and neurological status
E	Exposure

AVPU method of patient's level of consciousness

A	Alert
V	Responds to verbal stimuli
P	Responds to pain
U	Unresponsive

Glasgow coma scale

- Evaluated for a patient of head injury.
- It has 3 areas of assessment, i.e. eye response, verbal response and motor response (EVM).
- Maximum GCS index = 15.
- Minimum GCS index = 3.

Grade response	Motor response	Verbal response	Eye
6	Obeys command	–	–
5	Localizes pain	Oriented	–
4	Withdraws from pain	Confused conversation	Spontaneous opening
3	Abnormal flexion	Inappropriate words	Opens to speech
2	Extensor response	Incomprehensible words	Opens to pain
1	No response	None	None
Mnemonic	OLWFEN	OCIIN	SSPN

MANDIBULAR FRACTURES

- Mandible is the strongest and most rigid component of the facial skeleton.
- Are the most common fractures of the facial skeleton, followed by maxilla, zygoma and nasal bones.
- Fracture of mandible requires high forces (425 lbs); while fracture of maxilla requires low forces (140 lbs).
- Fracture of neck of condyle acts as a safety mechanism and prevents the middle cranial fossa fracture.
- Relative lines of weakness in mandible are = 3rd molar region and canine regions due to its long root.

- **Civilian type fracture** = mandibular fracture with no gross comminution of bone.
- **Gun shot type fracture** = mandibular fracture with gross comminution of bone and with extensive loss of hard and soft tissues.

Types of fracture

- **Simple** = not associated with outside atmosphere but in oral cavity, the fracture is associated through PDL to outer environment and so becomes compound.
- **Greenstick type** = mostly found in children; bones are very slender and elastic; one cortex is bent and other is intact.
- **Compound** = fracture associated with outer atmosphere through PDL in tooth bearing segment.
- **Comminuted** = multiple fragments of bone at the same fracture site.
- Displaced and undisplaced fracture.
- Favourable and unfavourable fractures.
- Horizontal and vertical fractures.
- **Pathological** = bone weakened by pathological conditions, e.g. neoplasm, osteomyelitis.
- **Complicated** = severe fracture involving vessels, nerves, etc.
- **Impacted** = 2 segments of fractures are interdigitated and cannot be dislodged.
- **Atrophic** = thickness or size of bone gets decreased very much.
- **Multiple fracture** = involving more than one bone or at multiple sites of the same bone.
- Most common fracture of mandible = **angle.**

Guardsman fracture

- Is a multiple fracture.
- Is due to fall on the midpoint of chin with fracture of both condyles and the symphysis, e.g. in epileptics, soldiers, elderly patients.

Displaced fracture = Due to **muscular sling of the mandible,** i.e. masseter and medial pterygoid ms. It displaces posterior fragment of jaw UPWARD, aided by TEMPORALIS.

- Anterior segment is displaced DOWNWARD by suprahyoid ms.
- Posterior segment also displaced MEDIALLY, by especially medial pterygoid m. and aided of SUPERIOR constrictor m.

Symphysis fracture = displaced by the bilateral POSTERIOR and SLIGHT LATERAL pull of SUPRAHYOID and DG ms.

Condyle fracture = displaced by the pull of lateral pterygoid m in an upward, anterior and medial direction.

Direction of fracture line

- **Horizontal favourable** = line of fracture **extends in a distal direction** towards the alveolar ridge while the fracture at inferior border is located ANTERIORLY.
- **Horizontal unfavourable** = fracture extends **forward towards the alveolar ridge** from a posterior point on the inferior border.
- **Vertical unfavourable** = line extends **from a posterolateral point to an antero-medial** point.
- **Vertical favourable** = fracture line extends **from an anterolateral to the posteromedial** point.

Condyle fracture: Shift of midline occurs towards the fractured side.

- Premature posterior occlusion (open-bite).
- Condyle dislocated forward/medially due to LATERAL PTERYGOID Ms.

M/m of condylar fracture SHOULD BE CONSERVATIVE, i.e. closed treatment especially in unilateral case.

- Main growth centre of mandible is located in the CONDYLAR region.
- Main mandibular growth occurs between 1–5 years of age in human; followed by a period of quiescence at 5–10 years age and then active mandibular growth from 10–15 years age.

- Growth during 10–15 years age is mainly due to muscular functions more than the growth centre. (functional matrix theory of growth by MOSS).
- So the most **critical period** for condylar fracture is 1–5 years.
- So the most **critical situation** is a fracture dislocation in a child of 2 ½ years old or less.
- **Wolff's law** = i.e. the shape of the bone conforms to the stresses placed on it during function.
- In children
  1. Condylar fractures are Rxed CONSERVATIVELY mostly.
  2. IMF is placed for 2 weeks.

Time for repair

- Most md. fractures heal well enough to allow removal of fixation in 6 weeks.
- Young adults = 4–4½ weeks.
- Children = 3–4 weeks.

Classification of the fractures based on the presence of dentition by Kazanjian and Converse

Class	Teeth present/absent
I	If teeth are present on both sides of the fracture line.
II	If one tooth is missing on one side of the fracture line.
III	If no tooth is present on either side of the fracture line, e.g. edentulous mandible.

Fracture at the angle

- Influenced by the medial pterygoid-masseter sling.
- Can be vertically and horizontally–favourable or unfavourable.
- Medial pterygoid is stronger m than the masseter.

- Pull of masseter is in upward and forward direction.
- Pull of MT is in U, F, medial/lingual direction.
- In vertically unfavourable fracture—the fracture line runs in U and F directions, i.e. site of fracture line at lower border is distal and on alveolar border it is mesial. The posterior fragment is pulled U, F and lingually.
- If fracture line runs U and B towards the alveolar border—it is vertically favourable fracture.
- In horizontally unfavourable fracture = the fracture line runs in bucco-lingual direction, parallel to the pull of ms. The line starts distally on buccal surface and comes mesially on the lingual surface.
- In horizontal favourable fracture—the line starts mesially on buccal surface and comes distally on the lingual surface.

Fracture at symphysis and parasymphysis

- Mylohyoid and geniohyoid ms form a diaphragm at the floor of mouth.
- Transverse midline fracture of symphysis are not displaced.
- Oblique fracture tends to overlap. The fracture part with genial tubercle is displaced lingually by ms pull.
- Bilateral parasymphyseal fracture gets displaced posteriorly under the influence of genioglossus mainly.
- Tongue falls in oropharynx only if patient's level of consciousness is depressed in bilateral parasymphysis, e.g. in head injury.
- In severe cases, detachment of genioglossus m. may lead to loss of tongue control and airway obstruction.
- Displacement of condyle occurs mainly in the antero-medial direction, i.e. upward; forward and medially, under the influence of lateral pterygoid m.
- Fracture of coronoid process occurs by reflex contraction of temporalis m; displacement occurs upwards; a rare fracture; limited mandibular movements especially on protrusion occurs.

Fracture of edentulous mandible

- Bilateral fracture occurs mostly near the posterior attachment of mylohyoid m.
- Anterior fragment gets extreme displacement (because there is no dental interference/interlocking) in D and B direction; which is due to digastric and myloyoid ms. It is known as **bucket-handle displacement**. It may cause respiratory distress.
- Mandible is weak due to bony resorption.
- With ageing —the periosteal blood supply becomes increasingly important. So the periosteum should be preserved as much as possible as it helps in healing. Healing problems occur due to decreased blood supply.
- No precise reduction of fracture is required.
- Modified Gunning splint is used mainly.
- Primary bone graft, e.g. ribs, iliac crest, etc. used in ultrathin mandible. 5 cm long rib graft is sufficient.
- Open reduction of fracture in aged patients may lead to loss of periosteum.
- Clinical examination = ecchymosis/hematoma in lingual sulcus is pathognomonic. It is because on the lingual side, the mucosa of the floor of mouth overlies the periosteum of mandible.

CONDYLAR FRACTURES

1. Intracapsular and extra capsular.
2. Unilateral and bilateral.
3. Displaced and undisplaced.
4. Intracapsular are rare; extracapsular are most common.
5. Displacement is due to pull of lateral pterygoid m, which is attached at antero-medial aspect of condyle.
6. Bleeding from the middle ear may due to the fracture of petrous temporal bone and with CSF otorrhoea. It is a significant finding and should be immediately dealt with.
7. **Battle's sign** = ecchymosis of skin just below the mastoid process; especially seen with fracture of base of the skull.

8. Gagging of molars on the same side of fracture.
9. Mandibular deviation on opening towards the side of the fracture.
10. If bilateral displaced fracture is there, then anterior open bite develops.

Treatment

- Immobilization is must for adequate healing.
- Malunion is more common than nonunion.
- Minimum period = for 3 weeks, i.e.

If in a **young adult** with fracture of **angle of mandible** taking **early** treatment, in which the **tooth is removed** from the fracture line.

- It requires **3 weeks** for treatment.
- If tooth is retained in the fracture line = add 1 week.
- If fracture is at symphysis = add 1 week.
- If age is > 40 yrs = add 1–2 weeks.
- If child/adolescent = subtract 1 week.
- Active movements are must for intracapsular fracture in children; immobilization is contraindicated, to avoid analysis.

SUMMARY	**Intracapsular**		**Extracapsular**	
	Unilateral	**Bilateral**	**Unilateral**	**Bilateral**
Children	Zero	Zero	7–10 days	7–10 days
Adults	2 weeks	2–3 weeks; elastics for 4 weeks	4 weeks	4–6 weeks

Intracapsular fracture in children

1. Disturbance of growth occurs because condylar cartilage which is growth site in mandible gets involved.
2. Fibrous/bony ankylosis may occur.
3. It should be Rxed by active movements only to avoid the ankylosis, no immobilization is recommended.

Extracapsular fracture in children

1. Should be Rxed conservatively.
2. Risk of ankylosis is less.
3. Early movement is done.
4. But if painful, then 7–10 days of immobilization can be done.

Unilateral intracapsular fracture in adults

1. Occlusion is undisturbed.
2. No immobilization of mandible done.
3. If painful, then IMF done for upto 2 wks only.

Unilateral extracapsular fracture in adults

1. IMF is done for 4 wks if occlusion is disturbed due to fracture-dislocation.
2. If not displaced, then no active Rx required.

Bilateral intracapsular fracture in adults

1. IMF should not be done for more than 2 weeks/2–3 weeks, otherwise ankylosis or stiffness may occur.
2. Intermaxillary elastic forces used at night for 6 weeks after removing IMF.

Bilateral extracapsular fracture in adults

1. Dislocation is anteromedially by lateral pterygoid ms.
2. Occlusal gagging and anterior open bite.
3. IMF done for 4–6 weeks.
4. Open reduction may be required.

Fracture of mandible in children

- May interfere with growth.
- Difficulty in IMF because of loose deciduous teeth and young permanent teeth.
- Morphology of deciduous molars is also troublesome during IMF.
- Gunning splint may be required.

- Unerupted teeth may get damaged if trans-osseous wires, bone plates and pins are used. So these are contraindicated in children.
- Healing is very rapid.
- Slight imperfections in reduction get compensated by growth and remodelling.
- Prolonged follow up is required.

TREATMENT OF MANDIBULAR FRACTURES

- Different methods of immobilization can be used depending on demand.
- Fractures must always be tested clinically before releasing the IMF.

Methods	**Details**
Dental wiring	Direct wiring done by Gilmer; 0.45 mm/ 26 gauge soft s.s wire is used; wire should be stretched by 10% before use.
Eye lets	Ivy Hearley 5 eyelets used in each arch.
Arch bars	e.g. a Winter's; Jelenko; Erich bars best if the patient has insufficient no. of teeth for effective inter-dental eyelets. Mostly, Erich arch bar is used. Upper and lower bars are fixed and then tied with wires to close the mouth in occlusion. It is known as inter-maxillary fixation (IMF).
Cap splints	Especially used when there are multiple loose/damaged teeth, which have to be retained, e.g. Gunning splint for edentulous mandible.
Trans-osseous wiring	
Circumferential wiring	
Fig-of-8 wiring	

(*Contd.*)

Methods	Details
Bone plating	Simple bone plates, compression bone plates/EDCP/2-hole/4-hole plates, etc. • The screws should engage the inner cortical plate of mandible. • The holes in compression plates are such that their widest diameter lies nearest the fracture line.
External pin fixation	• Pins of s.s. or Ti are used. • Are approx 3 mm or 1/8 inches in diameter. • Are not parallel to each other but diverge. • Are attached by cross bars.
Bone clamps	• e.g. Brenthrust splints.
Kirschner wires	• For transfixation; are of 2 mm diameter.

ACUTE INFECTIONS OF ORAL CAVITY

Pus producing bacteria = **Staphylococcus**

Deep cervical fascia has 4 part

- Investing layer/superficial layer
- Carotid sheath
- Pre-tracheal layer
- Pre-vertebral layer

1. Superficial/**investing layer** splits and encloses
   - 2 ms = SCM m and trapezius
   - 2 glands = Parotid and submandibular
   - Forms suprasternal space.

Associated with 3 fascial compartments, i.e. submandibular, submental and parotid.

2. **Carotid sheath** = contains CCA/ICA/IJV/Vagus N.

3. **Pre-tracheal layer** forms investment for THYROID GLAND.
4. **Visceral space** = lies between pre-tracheal and pre-vertebral layers; is continuous with mediastinum of thorax.

Masticator Space

- Formed by splitting of investing layer of deep cervical fascia at lower border of mandible, which runs both medially and laterally to ramus enclosing masseter, temporalis, ramus, medial and lateral pterygoid ms.
- Continuous with space of body of mandible subperiosteally.
- Involved after dental extractions especially of **third Molars.**
- **Subperiosteal abscess** occurs, so incision should be given till bone.
- **Trismus** = due to masseter-medial pterygoid sling irritation.

Temporal pouches

- 2 = superficial and deep.
- Superficial pouch lies between temporal fascia and temporalis m.
- Deep pouch lies deep to temporalis m between the muscle and skull.
- Communicate with infratemporal and pterygopalatine fossae.

Submental space = contains **Submental lymph nodes,** which drain median part of lower lip, tip to tongue and floor of mouth.

- Floor formed by **mylohyoid m.**

Submandibular/Digastric space

- Floor formed by **MH and hyoglossus M.**
- Contains **superficial part of submandibular gland.**
- **Deep part of SMG** continues posterior to mylohyoid m. **into sublingual space.**

Sublingual space = lies **above the mylohyoid** and laterally bound by inner surface of body of mandible **above the MH line.**

- Floor is formed **by MH m.**
- Contains **sublingual gland**, SM duct, **deep part of SMG**, lingual N, 12th N. and terminal branch of lingual A.

Lateral pharyngeal space–aka parapharyngeal space

- Extends from BASE of skull to level of HYOID bone.
- Subdivided into **2 parts by STYLOID process**—Anterior and Posterior.
- Carotid sheath is in **posterior compartment** (containing ICA/IJV/9, 10, 11, 12 Ns and cervical sympathetic TRUNK).
- Posterior compartment has NO LYMPH NODES.
- Most often involved by spread of infection from masticator space; palatine tonsil, parotid gland; etc.
- Especially by infection of **max. 3rd molar.**

PAROTID SPACE

- Formed by splitting of investing layer of deep fascia.
- **Stylomandibular ligament** separates parotid from the submandibular space.
- Stylomandibular ligament is formed by Investing Fascia.
- Br. of 7th N lies **deep to the superficial part** of parotid gland.
- Not involved directly by dental infections.

Pterygopalatine/and Infratemporal Fossae

- Involved by **infections of upper molars especially M_3.**
- PPF fossa communicates with **infratemporal Fossa** through pterygo-maxillary fissure (PMF).
- PMF is continuous with inferior orbital fissure (IOF).
- IOF has infra orbital N (which is a continuation of Mx N).
- ION gives br. = Ant. and middle superior Alveolar N, which supply Mx 1–5 and upper gums).
- PPF also communicates with pterygoid canal.

- Pterygoid canal has VIDIAN N. (made of gr. Petrosal br. of 7th N). + Deep petrosal N.
- Gr. Petrosal N = gives preganglionic para-sympathetic fibres to pterygopalatine ganglion.
- Deep petrosal n = has posterior ganglionic sympathetic fibres from superior cervical sympathetic ganglion.
- Foramen ovale and F. Spinosum are in Greater Wing of sphenoid bone.

Ludwig's Angina

- From mandibular Molars infection.
- **Roots of mand. Molars lie BELOW the attachment of MYLOHYOID** m.
  - 3 fascial spaces are involved bilaterally = submand + sublingual + submental.
  - Bilateral involvement.
  - **Open-mouth appearance** of patient—due to elevated floor of mouth and tongue is protruded and elevated.
  - Cause = **Haemolytic streptococci.**

Cavernous sinus thrombosis

- **STAPHYLOCOCCAL** infection.
- Due to extraction of **acute infected maxillary anteriors** and curettage of the sockets.
- Infected thrombus ascends in the veins **due to absence of valves in angular/facial and ophthalmic vs.**
- Paresis of **3, 4, 6th Ns.**
- Venous obstruction in retina; conjunctiva or eyelid occurs.
- Meningeal irritation occurs.

Miscellaneous points

- Osteolytic lesions in cancellous bone can't be detected on R/G. It is only seen if a part of cortical bone is destroyed.

- Attachment of buccinator and mylohyoid ms determine the path of pus eruption, i.e. intraoral or through the skin.
- To search for broken needle in the tissues, it should be searched in a direction perpendicular to the direction of insertion.

CYSTS (Also refer to the sections of oral pathology Vol. 1.)

Congenital cysts	**Others**	**Developmental cysts (Inclusion type)**		**Odontogenic cysts**
		Retention	**Fissural**	
Thyroglossal duct cyst	Haemorrhagic	Mucocele	Nasoalveolar cyst	Dentigerous
Branchiogenic cyst	Traumatic	Ranula	Median cyst	Periodontal
Dermoid cyst			Incisive canal/ nasopalatine cyst Globulo-maxillary cyst	Primordial/ fissural Keratocyst; OKC

Important points

- If protein level in aspirated fluid of cyst is less than 4 mg %, its is OKC.

Aspiration of fluid and its inference

Light straw coloured fluid with cholesterol crystals	Cyst
Creamy white fluid with keratin suspensions	OKC
Brick red fluid No fluid	Haemorrhagic cyst Solid growth

Congenital cysts: or branchial cleft type.

1. **Thyroglossal duct cysts**
   - Are in MIDLINE.
   - Lie between thyroid gland and foramen cecum.
   - Move upward with swallowing.
2. **Branchiogenic cyst**
   - Arise from persistancies of 2nd branchial cleft.
   - Present along the **anterior border of SCM m.**
3. **Dermoid cyst**
   - Occurs along the **natural lines of union.**
   - Causes **Bony Erosion** beneath them.
   - Contains hair, sebaceous glands, sweat glands and tooth structure.
   - In floor of mouth–cause swelling in the same location as RANULA but it has a **yellow** colour.
   - More superficial to branchiogenic cleft cysts and not attached to lateral pharyngeal wall.

Developmental cysts–(Inclusion cysts)

(a) Fissural type

1. **Nasoalveolar**
   - At the junction of globular, lateral nasal and maxillary processes.
   - Swelling at the attachment of ALA of nose.
   - They are not central bony lesions.
   - R/G = negative findings.
2. **Median cysts**
   - Forms in median fissure of palate from embryonic remnants.
   - Occurs more posteriorly in the palate as cp. To INCISIVE CANAL CYST.
3. **Incisive canal/Nasopalatine cysts**
   - Located **in the centre** of the bone.

4. **Globulomaxillary cyst**
   - At the junction of globular and maxillary process.
   - Between L.I. and canine teeth.
   - Cause divergence of roots of these teeth.
   - **Pear - shaped radiolucency in R/G**.
   - Teeth are VITAL.

(b) Retention cysts

Mucocele

- Due to obstruction of ducts of minor salivary glands.
- Lie just **below the oral mucosa**.
- Present especially on lips/buccal mucosa, etc.
- Treatment = **complete excision with involved gland** and duct.

Ranula

- ♦ Arise from sublingual gland.
- ♦ Bluish colour due to thinning of mucosa. Seen as the belly of the frog, and hence is the name.
- ♦ Larger size than mucocele.
- ♦ Tongue may be raised.
- ♦ Does not pit on pressure.
- ♦ Contain stringy–mucoid material.
- ♦ Best treatment is MARSUPIALIZATION.
- ♦ **Partsch operation** is also known as MARSUPIALIZATION.
- ♦ **Waldron's operation** = is a 2-stage operation, which consists of marsupialization first and then the ENUCLEATION of cyst membrane at a later stage.

CRYOSURGERY

It involves the application of cold solutions to tissue to freeze and destroy it. *ROBERT BOYLE* observed that the freezing of tissues produced necrosis.

EFFECTS OF FREEZING

- The events that are involved in cellular necrosis during freezing are as follows.
- Formation of extracellular ice.
- Concentration of extracellular solutes.
- Decrease in intracellular water.
- Cell shrinkage.
- Concentration of intracellular solutes.
- Cell membrane damage.
- Formation of intracellular, ice.
- The most expensive type utilizes **liquid nitrogen** to freeze the surgical site through an insulated probe. Liquid nitrogen can be used to achieve temperatures of **–196°C.**
- Other refrigerant media are **carbon dioxide, nitrous oxide** and **freon.** This may reach temperatures of **– 20°C to – 89°C.**
- Generally **4-5 minutes** of freezing at –80°C will result in sufficient tissue necrosis to eradicate most intraoral mucosal lesions.

MAXILLARY SINUS

- Also known as **Antrum of Highmore.**
- It is the first paranasal sinus to develop; it grows laterally from middle meatus of nasal cavity at approx 17th day IU; start developing at 3 mo IU.
- Expands by pneumatization into developing alveolar process.
- It Vol. is 10–15 ml is the capacity of adult sinus; size is 34 × 33 × 23 mm (L, H, W).
- It is largest of all the 4 PNS.
- **Pyramidal** in shape = **apex in root of the zygoma/zygomatic process of maxilla.**
- Grows during 7–15 years age.
- It is lined by respiratory epithelium, i.e. pseudostratified ciliated columnar epithelium and periosteum.

- It opens at OSTIUM MAXILLAE in the **middle meatus of nasal** wall.
- Opening/ostium lies 2/3rd of the distance up from the inferior part of the medial wall and drains into nasal cavity; is at a higher level than the floor and so there is drainage problem.
- It opens in the posterior end of hiatus semilunaris in middle meatus of nasal cavity b/w middle and inferior nasal conchae.
- Covered inside by **ciliated** epithelium known as **Schnedrian membrane.**
- In infants and children = floor of sinus is always higher than the floor of nose and so better drainage due to gravity is possible from window operation.
- In adults = the floor of sinus is lower than nasal floor.
- **Nasal antrostomy** = opening is made in the **inferior meatus**, where bone is very thin.
- Posterosuperior alveolar br of Mx nerve (br of **5th N)** supply the lining of membrane.
- **Blood supply** = from infra orbital A (br of Mx A).
- Lymph drainage = submandibular LN.
- Best r/g view for diagnosis = water's view; OPG.
- If acute sinusitis = r/g shows air filled levels.
- In chronic sinusitis = r/g shows opacifications, polyps and mucosal thickenings.
- Normal flora of sinus = aerobic streptococci; anearobic G (–ve) rods, e.g. bacteroides and fusobacterium.
- Sinusitis of non-odontogenic origin = mainly aerobes especially *Strept pneumonial*, *H. influenzae* and *Staph. aureus*. The anaerobes are bacteroides, peptococcus, fusobacterium.
- Sinusitis of odontogenic origin = main anaerobes, e.g. peptococcus; peptostrept; bacteroides and eubacterium and aerobic strept.
- Penicillin, erythromycin and clindamycin are effective vs odontogenic sinusitis.

Functions

- Gives resonance of the voice.
- Warms the air.
- Lightens the skull
  - **Water's view** (PNS view) of R/G shows all sinuses.
  - During acute sinusitis, teeth may be painful, as their roots approximate the lining of sinus.
  - Lining becomes thick due to cellular proliferation in chronic Mx sinusitis.
  - Fractured root of molars may enter the sinus.
  - Mx 3rd molar may slip in INFRATEMPORAL FOSSA during extraction.

Caldwell–Luc operation

- Cuspid–2nd molar area is exposed.
- **Opening** is made in the facial wall of antrum ABOVE THE BICUSPID ROOTS.

ORO-ANTRAL FISTULA = an opening communicating between the sinus and the oral cavity. It may get formed by entry of roots of the maxillary molars due to improper extractions.

DANKER'S OPERATION = i.e. joining the anterolateral nasal opening with canine fossa opening (piriform aperture).

Salivary glands (Also refer to the section on anatomy; oral pathology.)

- Minor salivary glands are mucus type.
- Parotid = largest; serous.
- 7th n lies deep to parotid's superficial lobe and passes between the lobes rather than within the parotid substance.
- Parotid duct passes anteriorly and medially; open at the level of mx 2nd molar in buccal vestibule.
- Submandibular gland is mucoserous/mixed.
- At the post border of mylohyoid m–SMG enters the sublingual space and gives off its excretory duct, i.e. Wharton's duct. The

duct opens at the caruncle lateral to lingual frenum. It crosses beneath the lingual N at the level of 3rd molar and above the lingual N at the level of 2nd molar.

- Sublingual gland = is mucus; lies above the mylohyoid m; its landmark is plica sublingualis; has got multiple ducts; it has **simple ductal system.**
- Minor glands = are mucous in nature; has got **simple ductal system.**
- Ductal pattern of SMG and parotid glands resembles the **leafless tree.**

Anatomical weaknesses

- SMG lies in dependant position; may cause retrograde infections.
- Lumen of the duct of SMG and parotid glands are broader than their opening and may get blocked by the obstructions formed by the setting of epithelial cells and salivary fluid contents.
- Duct of SMG and parotid glands take a radical turn along their course, which acts as favourite point for lodgement of obstructions.
- Retention cysts develop due to rupture of a duct into the gland parenchyma and then filling with salivary secretions. It does not fill with radiopaque solutions in sialography.
- **Branchial cleft cyst** = It arises from the epithelium between the branchial arches, occurs as the swelling on the lateral aspect of the neck or in the floor of the mouth.
- **Mixed tumour** = Also known as **pleomorphic adenoma**; most commonly occurs in parotid and minor glands, ball-in-hand appearance in sialogram, does not respond to radiations; so surgical excision with the normal part of gland supporting it has to be done, recurrence is possible.
- **Muco-epidermoid tumours** = Are malignant, occur most frequently in parotid gland; involve ductal and acinar structures of the gland.
- **Stones/sialolithiasis = Most common in submandibular** glands and ducts (83%), parotid (10%), sublingual (7%), best Rx for stone is **trans-oral sialo-lithotomy** for SMG, save lingual N.

- Secretions of SMG contains more calcium.
- Relation of 7th ns and it s branches with parotid gland.

Consistency

Abscess	Fluctuant
Dermoid cyst	Doughy
Stones	Dense/stellate
Infected/obstructed gland	Firm/tense
Tumor	Fixed/painless

Definitions

- **Sialodochitis** = i.e. inflammation of salivary duct; it is the dilation of salivary duct secondary to epithelial atrophy with irregular narrowing caused by reparative fibrosis.
- **Sialadenitis** = inflammation of salivary gland.
- **Sialolithiasis** = stone in salivary gland.
- **Sialo-angiectasis** = gland and duct system is vastly dilated by stasis of the salivary secretions.
- **Sialogogues** = agents which increase the salivary flow.

SIALOGRAMS

- **Sialography** = radiographic study after injecting radiopaque oil in the ductal system. The r/g obtained is known as **sialogram.**
- **Lipiodol** as the radiopaque solution is used. Iodised oil has antiseptic action also.
- **Water-based** contrast medium is better than the oil based media; why, because oil irritates the soft tissues; and its clearance is slow as compared to water based medium.
- Sialadenitis = **leafy-tree appearance.**
- Sialolith = **link sausage appearance.**
- Mixed tumour of parotid = **ball-in-hand** deformity in many cases.
- Sjogren's syndrome = **branchless-fruit- laden tree/cherry–blossom** appearance.

Leafless tree	Normal acinar structure of parotid
Leafy tree	Sialadenitis; terminal acini of parotid gland are dilated
Link-sausage dilation	Sialolith; blocking collecting ducts; sialodochitis
Ball in hand deformity	Mixed tumor of parotid

Summary

Parotid	Serous	Stenson's duct; opens near max 2nd molar	Lies superficial to masseter ms
Submandibular	Mixed	Wharton's duct; opens in floor of mouth	Posterior border of mylohyoid m
Sublingual	Mucus has 8–20	Bartholin's duct; small ducts of Rivinus	Lies on superior surface of mylohyoid ms

TEMPOROMANDIBULAR JOINT (Also refer to the sections of anatomy; orthodontics, oral pathology.)

It is a type of Ginglymo-arthroidal joint.

- Condylar type of synovial joint (complex).
- Articulating surfaces covered with AVASCULAR fibrous tissues rather than HYALINE cartilage.
- Articular surface of condyle faces U and F. Neck of condyle appears to be bent anteriorly.
- Articular disc has concavo–convex upper surface and concave lower surface. It divides TMJ in superior and inferior compartments.
- Disc is very thin and **avascular in centre**, so healing is a problem in disc.
- Lateral pterygoid M attached to disc and pterygoid fovea at the anterior of the condyle of mandible.

Capsule

- Superior portion of capsule is loose and permits anterior gliding movement.
- Inferior portion is TIGHTER and allows HINGE movement.

Temporomandibular ligament = runs D and B from zygomatic arch to condylar neck.

- It gives DIRECT SUPPORT TO THE CAPSULE. It is the main ligament of the joint.
- Nerve supply: Auriculotemporal and masseteric br. of 5th N; prioprioceptive.
- Blood supply: superficial temporal br of ECA.
- Movement in upper compartment = GLIDING.
- Movement in lower compartment = Rotation + Gliding.

TMJ pain = Jaw deviates to the affected side during normal opening motion.

- **Injection therapy** of TMJ pain by **Hydrocortisone** helps in reducing the inflammation. Drug is deposited **in superior compartment**.

Sclerosing solutions

- For treatment of hypermobility/subluxation/luxation.
- Injection is given **in capsule** overlying the upper condylar neck only to aid in fibrosis and tightening of that structure.
- Solutions should not be injected into JOINT.

- High condylectomy/**condylar shaving** is done in cases of extensive proliferative changes or erosion of condylar head.
- **Costo chondral graft** are useful in children with agenesis of condyle, as they can help during growth spurt for growth of mandible.
- Treatment of luxated condyle-downward and backward pressure on the mandibular posterior teeth and the mandible is then moved in a downward/backward and upward direction to place it in condylar fossa.

- **Ankylosis** = most common cause is trauma; it may lead to micrognathia/**bird-facies** due to lack of condylar growth in children.
- Ankylosis can be bony/fibrous; unilateral/bilateral; intra-articular/extra-articular; complete/partial.

Movement	Muscles
Depression	Lateral pterygoid.
Elevation	Masseter medial pterygoid temporalis.
Protrusion	Lateral and medial pterygoid ms.
Retrusion	Posterior fibers of temporalis.
Lateral	Medial and lateral pterygoids of each side acting alternately.

Arthrosis

- Initial stage of arthritis.
- No R/g findings seen.

NEUROLOGICAL DISORDERS

Definitions

Paralysis	• Loss of or impairment of motor function in a body part.
Paresis	• Is incomplete paralysis.
Anesthesia	• Is the loss of any and all sensations.
Ageusia	• Loss of specific sensations of taste.
Analgesia	• Loss of sensitivity to painful stimuli.
Hyperesthesia	• Excessive sensitivity.
Hypoesthesia	• Decreased sensitivity especially to touch.

Definitions (*Contd.*)

Hyperalgesia	• An increased sensitivity to pain.
Hypoalgesia	• Decreased sensitivity to pain.
Pain detection threshold	• Is the lowest level, at which a given stimulus is considered painful.
Pain tolerance threshold	• Is the level of maximally tolerated stimulus and is highly variable; it is altered by pharmacological and hypnotic techniques.
Sensory dissociation	• Loss of certain senses with simultaneous maintenance of other senses.
Paresthesia	• Any altered sensation.
Dysesthesia	• Is a painful paresthesia, e.g. burning, boring, stabbing or phantom pain.
Referred pain	• In which symptoms are felt in distant tissues and are unrelated to the true pathological site.
Phantom pain	• Is the awareness of a previously extracted tooth or a burning tongue after glossectomy, why?

- **Phantom bite syndrome** = it is the situation where a patient cannot find a position of comfort despite having worn dentures for many years.
- **Components of pain** = 3, perception; affect/emotion; and reaction.
- **Nociceptors** = 1–5 micron nerve fibres; are unmyelinated/thinly myelinated; are A–delta and C–type fibres; activated by serotonin, prostaglandins AG.
- **Gate-control theory** = given by **Melzack and Wall;** the gate is located in the **caudal portion of the brain stem trigeminal**

synaptic regions especially in subnucleus caudalis of the descending trigeminal tract.

- **Somatic sensations** = trigeminal nerve; max and mand divisions; 5th n. contains the largest proportion of myelinated axons and smallest proportions of unmyelinated axons on the entire somatic sensory system.
- **Multiple sclerosis** = is a demyelinating disease (Also refer to section on oral pathology).
- In *D mellitus*, polynephropathy of 5th nerve may occur, which is symptomatic degeneration of many nerves.
- Sympathetic nerve supply to maxillofacial region arises in cervical spinal cord and after synapse in the superior cervical chain ganglion, it is distributed along the arteries to glands and smooth ms.
- Para-sympathetic neurons arise in brain stem cells columns of 3, 7, 9th cranial ns , which then synapse in ciliary, sphenopalatine otic and submandibular ganglia and is distributed to smooth ms, salivary glands and lacrimal glands.
- **Gustatory sweating/auriculotemporal nerve syndrome** = is due to severance of auriculotemporal n and its associated autonomic fibres; and then the inappropriate regrowth of 9th n parasympathetic fibres along the vacant sympathetic paths, which then terminate in sweat glands rather than salivary acini.
- **Motor supply** = originate in upper motor neurons; comes to lower motor neurons; from LMN the peripheral extracranial processes go to skeletal ms and form the cranial nerves.
- All the lower motor cranial ns except 4th nerve are completely UNCROSSED in their courses to skeletal ms, so any lesion of LMN produces a deficit in all the ms supplied by that nerve.
- Lesions of UMN of 7th n cause a deficit in lower facial ms only; it is due to some crossing of UMNs, which cause double innervation to some parts of facial motor nucleus.
- Lesions of LMNs of 7th n produce a deficit in all the ms supplied by this nerve, i.e. upper and lower facial ms.
- **Diagnostic nerve blocks** = it is a simple and most revealing technique for locating and characterizing neurological lesions.

Tests of cranial N functions

3, 4, 6 ns 5 7 9, 10 11 12	Extraocular ms functions Masticaroty ms functions Facial ms functions Palatal; pharyngeal; laryngeal functions Sternomastoid; trapezius ms Tongue functions
Somatosensory functions	.5, 7, 9 ns
Special functions	
1 2 7, 9 8	Smell Vision Taste Hearing
Autonomic functions	
Sympathetic	Pupillary dilation, eye lid tone; sweating; vaso-constriction; salivation
Para-sympathetic	Pupillary constriction; serous salivation

Idiopathic trigeminal neuralgia

- Also known as tic douloureus, because of ms spasm.
- Unilateral; does not cross the midline.
- Commonest mainly on RHS; in females; in 6th decade age.
- There are trigger zones.
- Fibres of 5th n does not cross the midline of face; so it is unilateral.
- Expression less face known as starey face.
- Segmental demyelination of the sensory root of 5th nerve, may occur due to the anomaly of superior cerebellar A may be the cause.

- Rx = carbamazepine; phenytoin; decompression and complete resection of ganglionic posterior root fibres; peripheral neurectomy, etc.

Different neurological diseases

Vago-glossopharyngeal neuralgia	9, 10th nerves; sensory, autonomic and motor fibers involved more on LHS pain in the base of tongue, tonsillar pillars, soft palate and external auditory canal syncope, hypotension; bradycardia = are due to effect on N of HERING, which is responsible for initiating carotid sinus reflex activity.
Eagle's syndrome	Due to elongated, ossified stylohyoid ligament, which causes pressure on the nerves in the area of F spinosum Rx = intracranial rhizotomy of posterior roots of 9th and 10th nerves; no use of peripheral neurectomy.
Geniculated neuralgia; nerve; aka intermedius neuralgia	Due to sensory/intermedius part of 7th N. Unilateral entity is known as Ramsey-Hunt syndrome. Pain in deep external auditory meatus; auricle and soft palate.
Migraine	Unilateral pain in temporal area, appears before 16 yrs of age, is due to excess vasodilation of extracranial vessels, e.g. maxillary A and dural part of (MMA), middle meningeal A. Rapid pain relief by digital pressure of CCA/ ECARx = ergotamine tartarate (a vasoconstrictor agent)
Cluster headache	Also known as periodic migrainous, neuralgia, histamine, cephalgia.

Different neurological diseases (*Contd.*)

	Invloves ciliary neuralgia, vidian neuralgia and sphenopalatine (sluder's neuralgia). No trigger points; problem is along the course of greater superficial petrosal n. Rx = ergotamine tartarate, methysergide (serotonin antagonist).
Atypical facial neuralgia	Pain does not follow the distribution of somatic sensory trigeminal nerves. Palpable tenderness at the carotid bifurcation and along the ECA branches. 5, 7, 9, 10 and cervical afferent fibers are involved distribution of pain is along the maxillary A and its terminal branches, i.e. middle meningeal; deep temporal; and sphenopalatine division.
Bell's palsy	Due to neuritis of 7th nerve within the facial canal. If chorda tympani n is involved, then impaired taste sensation over anterior 2/3rd tongue occurs. If nerve to stapedius ms involved = then loud noise intensification occurs. If upper motor neuron lesions = the upper facial ms are spared lower facial ms are involved. In lower motor neuron lesions = whole face is involved.
Orbital edema	3rd, 4th and 6th nerves get involved, 1. 3rd n neuritis = Horner's syndrome, i.e. ptosis, anhidrosis and pupillary constriction; deficient upward gaze.

Different neurological diseases (*Contd.*)

	2. 4th n neuritis = inability to rotate the eye ball down and out ward. 3. 6th n paralysis = impaired lateral gaze.
Causalgia	Is due to injury to mixed peripheral nerves; is a deep burning pain of post-traumatic nature. It is caused by the excitation of demyelinated sensory nerve segments by adjacent unmyelinated sympathetic fibers, i.e. artificial synapsing of efferent sympathetic fibers with somatic sensory fibers. In regenerated fibers—the distance between nodes of Ranvier is shorter and conduction velocity is decreased; they are poorly myelinated.
Phantom pain	Patient who have got amputation of a body part often experience a sense of awareness of the missing part known as phantom phenomenon; complain of phantom teeth is a usual phenomenon.

- **Pulpal ns** are poorly myelinated.
- **Leprosy** is the only known direct infection of peripheral fibres.
- H. zoster is the only definite viral infection of peripheral nervous system. It occurs in sensory N distribution of 5, 7, 9, 10 nerves; mostly involves ophthalmic div of 5th n; it occurs due to VZ virus latent in the larger neuron cell bodies of sensory ganglia.
- **Raynaud's phenomenon** = fingers and toes respond to cold and emotional stress with pallor, cyanosis, and trophic skin changes due to vasospasm.
- Most common disease associated with connective tissue disease neuropathies = diabetes mellitus.

- **Nutritional neuropathy** = mainly occurs in branches of nerves most acutely affecting vibratory and position senses.
- **Wernicke's encephalopathy** = occurs by thiamin deficiency in chronic alcoholism.
- **TENS** = i.e. transcutaneous electronic nerve stimulation = it is based on the gate control theory, where stimulation of large cutaneous fibres through transcutaneous electronic stimulation may be responsible for overriding the pain input from structures, e.g. TMJ and ms.
- **Syringobulbia** = degenerative disease of medulla oblongata; there is dissociated sensory loss of pain and temperature but not of touch; occurs due to cavitation and gliosis.

Traumatic nerve injuries

Inferior alveolar N	With fracture of mandibular body; ostectomy, etc.
Infraorbital N	Zygomatico-maxillary complex fracture.
Lingual N	Mandibular 3rd molar surgery.
Long buccal N	By raising the buccal flap for 3rd molar surgery, mandibular osteotomy, etc.
Nasopalatine N	Impacted maxillary canine surgery.
Mental N	Skin graft, vestibuloplasty of mandible, periapical surgery of mandibular premolar region.

Degeneration

1. **Segmental demyelination** = is selective dissolution of the myelin sheath segments; slowing of conduction velocity occurs.
2. **Wallerian degeneration** = it is the disintegration of peripheral nerve fibres and myelin sheaths, which spreads distally from the point of injury.
3. **Dying back neuropathy** = degeneration begins in the most peripheral nerve tissues and progresses centrally from that point.

It occurs due to metabolic intoxications; anaesthesia and paraesthesia appear peripherally and progresses centrally.

CLEFT LIP AND PALATE (Also refer to orthodontics and pedodontics.)

Classifications and causes: hereditary/congenital.

- **Cleft lip CL.**
- **Cleft lip and alveolus CLA.**
- **Cleft lip and palate CLP = unilateral/bilateral; partial/ complete.**
- **Midline CL** are rare.
- **Soft palate cleft.**
- **Incomplete cleft palate** = i.e. only secondary plate is involved.
- **Complete cleft** = involves alveolar ridge and hard and soft palates.
- **Occult cleft palate** = are submucosal clefts, i.e. muscle slings of soft palate are not united. No cleft is seen intraorally.
    - Cleft lip is known as **cheiloschisis.**
    - Cleft plate is known as **palatoschisis.**
    - CLP are congenital.
    - Incidence = 1:800 live births.
    - CL are more frequent in males.
    - Isolated CP more frequent in females.
    - Cleft develops b/w 6–10th weeks of IUL.
    - CL are more common on LHS than RHS.
    - Lip forms by fusion of fronto-nasal and lateral maxillary processes.
    - Palatine shelves contact at the MIDLINE and fuse from anterior to posterior forming the palate.
    - Point of fusion of future hard palate with septum is the site of ossification of future VOMER.
    - Cleft occurs due to lack of mesodermal proliferation along the lines of fusion of embryonic processes.
    - With increased maternal age–there are increased chances of cleft.

- **Cheilorrhaphy** = cleft lip repair; done at 3 weeks to 3 months age.
  - Lip is corrected as early as is medically possible.
  - **Millard's rule of ten = wt** = 10 lbs; **age** 10 wks; **Hb** 10 gm%; **WBCs** 10,000.
- **Staphylorrhaphy** = aka soft palate closure. Soft palate cleft is closed b/w 18–24 mos, leaving the hard palate open.
- **Palatorrhaphy** = i.e. palate repair.
  - For normal speech and swallowing.
  - Bony union of hard palate area is not achieved and the hard palate defect is covered with obturator till 5–6 yrs age **for proper maxillary growth to occur.**
  - At 2 yrs age = soft palate is repaired for proper velo-pharyngeal function.
- **Uranorrhaphy** = is the hard palate closure.
- **Alveolar bone grafting**
  - Provides support for the teeth.
  - Helps to improve arch contour.
  - Stabilises mobile premaxilla in bilateral clefts.

Early alveolar grafting has adverse influences on maxillary growth and development.

In bilateral clefts = the premaxilla is excessively thrust forward due to septal-premaxillary ligament, which influences the amount of anterior and upward rotation and due to the influences of septum and vomer.

In bilateral complete clefts = the blood supply to premaxilla is from the vomer and septal midline source only. So there are no collateral anastomosis and there may be interference in blood supply and growth after surgical setback.

- 70% of adult premaxilla is the alveolar bone, so if teeth are lost, there is alveolar atrophy and lip support is lost. So save the teeth.
- 9–12 yrs of age is the BEST time for the graft, when the canines root is 1/4th to 1/2 formed.

- Bone graft used is of **cancellous particulate** type and helps to form a bridge, which will unite maxilla.
- Grafting is done after orthodontic expansion of maxillary arch, coordinating with the mandibular arch.
- For Rx of malposed premaxilla–the surgical correction to normal position and bone grafts are best done between 8–14 yrs age.

Speech AID appliances, e.g. obturator.

- To cover the velopharyngeal insufficiency.
- Help in developing the muscle action.

Speech difficulties in CLP cases

- Retardation of consonant sounds = B, D, K, P, T, G.
- Hypernasality.
- Articulation problems.
- Hearing problems.
- Velopharyngeal mechanism is disturbed due to discontinuity of ms from one side to the other side, i.e. velopharyngeal insufficiency.
- Compensatory mechanism occurs by development of Passavant's ridge.

ACQUIRED DEFECTS

Grafts

Graft = a tissue which is transplanted and expected to become a part of the host to which it is transplanted.

Type of response the immune system of the body mounts against the foreign grafts is primarily a **cell mediated response by T- lymphocytes.**

Free/pedicled.

Spilt thickness/full thickness.

Spilt thickness graft

- Good assurances of a "take".
- But have marked tendency to contract.

- Also known as **Thiersch's graft.**

  Best for the defects oral/nasal cavity and orbits.

Full thickness graft

- Also known as **Wolfe's Graft.**
- Less tendency to contract.
- Superior to spilt thickness graft as far as matching the face colour is concerned.
- Decreased chances of graft survival as cp to split thickness graft.

Local flaps

- Use the contiguous tissues and include advancement, rotation and transposition.
- Also known as **French flap.**

Rotation flap

Transposition flap = is one that is rotated at an angle, jumping an area of normal tissue to reach the defect.

Inturned flap = here, the margins of a defect are inside, undermined, and turned in to form the back side of the defect if a double lining is required.

Pedicle flaps: Has s/c tissue and skin both.

- **Z-plasty** is a double rotation flap; most effective method for releasing tension on a tissue contracture.

  Rotation of flap allows the direction of tension to be changed.
- **V-Y flap**
  - Is a type of advancement flap.
  - Acts as a lengthening procedure.
- **Y-V Flap** = acts as a shortening procedure.
- **Abbe or Estlander flap** = is used for repairs of full thickness losses of lip; achieved by rotation of flap from one lip to the other.
- **Musculocutaneous flap** = for extensive defects of head and neck.

- **Distant or pedicle flaps** = are those carried over an area of normal skin on a pedicle, which later sectioned and returned to the donor site.
- **Bone grafts.**
  - Fresh autogenous bone, e.g. iliac bone.
  - Large spaces within the substances of cancellous iliac bone allow rapid revascularisation with survival of many of the graft cells.
  - Dense bone has low osteogenic power, because of the increased need for its resorption and replacement, e.g. tibia; rib.
  - Spilt rib graft are better as they have open specs present for revascularisation.
  - Iliac bone is much more resistant in PO infection.
  - Greater the area of graft-recipient bone contact, the more certain and more rapid regeneration.

ARTIFICIAL IMPLANTS

1. **Alloplasts** are inert foreign body implants.

Metals

1. Vitalum = Co + Cr + Mo
2. Tantalum
3. 18–8—SMO steel = 18 Cr + 8 Ni + 4 Mo.

Titanium

- Is RADIOLUCENT.
- Extreme light.
- High degree of strength.
- Resistant to corrosion.
- Tantalum and vitallium—both are RADIOPAQUE.

Synthetic resins = e.g.

- Methyl methacrylate MMA.
- Polyethylene.

- Polyvinyl alcohol.
- Telon/PTFE = most chemically-inert and least irritating to tissue autoclavable.

Rubber silicones/silastics

- Autoclavable.
- Contourable.
- Non-irritating to the tissues.

Proplast = is a composite of PTFE and carbon fibres.

- **Microprosity** = pore vol. 70–90 vol%, pore size 80–400 nm; helps in tissue-ingrowth.
- Used for contour correction.
- Autoclavable.

PROPLAST-II

- Composite of PTFE and **aluminium oxide**; white colour.
- Used below thin skin, e.g. nasal bridge.

Reconstruction of mandible

- Plates for correction of continuity defect for adequate functions and esthetics.
- Also maintain the position of bone fragments till grafting is done.
- Autogenous bone graft is the material of choice (osteogenic effect).
- Grafts may be in the form of Block/chips/osteo-periosteal/pedicle.
- Osteo-periosteal graft contains all the elements required for osteogenesis of bone.
- Sliding bone graft for Rx of defects is also a method.

Advantage of Iliac bone GRAFTS

- Cancellous.
- Allows rapid transmission of tissue fluids and nutritive elements.
- Provide pathway for the ingrowth of cells.

- Readily contoured to desired shape.
- Resistant to infection.
- Rapid vascularization and consolidation.
- **Composite graft** of autogenous iliac cancellous bone marrow and frozen lyophilized cortical allogenic bank bone can be used for larger bone defects.
- **Costochondral graft is best** for the reposition of mandibular joint in both the growth period and later in life.

Tumours (Refer to the section of oral pathology for details.)

- **Block resection** = of the involved bone should extend into and include 10 mm of the normal peripheral bone surroundings the tumour mass.
- **Enostoses** = i.e. osteomas arising from the INNER surface of bone cortex also known as **central osteomas**.
- **Exostoses** = i.e. locally circumscribed bony growths developing outside the cortical plates. Also known as **peripheral osteomas**.
- **Myxoma** = honeycomb appearance in R/G.
- **Osteogenic sarcoma** arise from bone forming cells, generally occur in children **during periods of active growth.**
- **Sunray appearance** of osteoblastic sarcoma is due to the radiating spicules of bone extending outward from the cortex.
- All types of **sarcomas metastasise to LUNGS** through the bloodstream.

Fibro osteoma

- Occurs mainly in females and in maxilla.
- Tumour may obliterate the maxillary sinus.
- Does not invade nasal structures.
- In hyper osteosis and Paget's disease, the nasal meati are obliterated.

Ewing's tumour

- Arises from endothelial lining of the blood or lymph vessels.
- Growth is radiosensitive, so treated by x-rays.
- s/s = elevation of body temperature pain; swelling.

Multiple myeloma

- Arise from bone marrow cells.
- **"Pain of wandering type"** is an outstanding symptom.
- **Bence-Jones proteinuria.**
- Alk Pase level is normal.
- R/G = **multiple punched out round lesions** in multiple bones, which are the sites of bone marrow.

Central giant cell tumour

- Arise in bone of cartilaginous origin.
- e.g. symphysis, angle of mandible, canine fossa of maxilla.
- Root resorption of teeth.
- Perforation of cortices.
- Highly vascular and haemorrhagic.

Peripheral giant cell tumour

- Also known as giant cell epulid.
- Arise from connective tissue of dental periodontium.

Biopsy

- It is the removal of tissues form a living individual for diagnosis by microscopic and histopathologic examination.
- It has got the **most diagnostic value.**
- It is of following **types** = excisional; incisional; aspiration; punch; exfoliative cytology; fine needle aspiration cytology.
- Specimen should be immediately placed in **10% formalin** or 4% formaldehyde solution, which is **20 times the volume of the surgical specimen.**
- **Oral cytology** = used for monitoring of dysplastic changes in mucosa; unreliable method; lesion is scraped and placed in fixing solution.
- **Aspiration biopsy** = i.e. to aspirate fluid/air from the lesion for examination; e.g. straw coloured fluid (cyst); pus (inflammatory/

infectious lesion); air (traumatic bone cavity); blood (hemangioma, aneurysmal bone cyst, central giant cell granuloma).

- **Incisional biopsy** = is done if lesion is of bigger size, e.g. larger than 1 cm; a part of normal tissue is also included in the sample for comparison purpose; a deep/narrow biopsy should be taken.
- **Excisional biopsy** = removal of entire lesion is done; normal tissue is also involved for comparison and to ensure total removal; done for smaller lesions < 1 cm diameter.

Procedure for removal of jaw tumours

- **Enucleation/curettage** = local removal of tumour by instrumentation in direct contact with lesion. It is used for very benign lesions.
- **Resection** = also known as **en-bloc resection**; it is the removal of a tumour by incising through uninvolved tissue around the tumour, thus removing the tumour without direct contact during instrumentation.
- **Marginal/segmental resection** = resection of a tumour without disruption of the continuity of bone.
- **Partial resection** = resection of tumour by removing a full–thickness part of the jaw; here jaw continuity is disrupted.
- **Total resection** = resection of a tumour by removal of the involved bone, e.g. maxillectomy; manidbulectomy.
- **Composite resection** = resection of a tumour with bone, adjacent soft tissues and contiguous lymph node channels.

ODONTOGENIC INFECTIONS

- Normal flora of oral cavity are = aerobic G (+) cocci; anaerobic G (+) cocci; anaerobic G (–) rods.
- Most common aerobic bacteria are G (+) strept and staph.
- Anaerobic G (+) cocci are strept; peptostrept; and peptococci.
- G (+) rods are eubacterium and lactobacilli.
- G (–) anaerobic rods are bacteroides and fusobacterium.
- Most of infections are mixed, i.e. aerobic–anaerobic 60%.

- Most common odontogenic infections is a vestibular abscess.
- Infections spreads along the line of least resistance in the bone.

Maxillary spaces	**Mandibular spaces**
Canine spaces	Submental space
Buccal spaces	Sublingual and submandibular space
Infratemporal spaces	Masseteric Temporal Pterygo-mandibular

SITE OF LOCALIZATION OF ACUTE DENTAL INFECTIONS

Tooth	**Usual exit from bone**	**Relation of exit to ms attachment**	**Which m/ms involved**	**Site of localisation**
Max CI	Labial	Below	**Orbicularis oris**	Oral vestibule
Max LI	Labial Palatal	Below –	**Orbicularis oris** –	Oral vestibule Palate
Max 3	Labial	Below **Above**	**Levator anguli oris** –do–	Oral vestibule **Canine space**
Max 4, 5	Buccal Palatal	Below –	**Buccinator/ Zygomaticus major/minor ms; levator labii superioris** –	Oral vestibule Palate
Max 6–8	Buccal Buccal Palatal	Below **Above** –	**Buccinator** **Buccinator** –	Oral vestibule **Buccal space** Palate

EXTENSION OF LOCALIZED MAXILLARY ABSCESSES

1. Mx 1, 2 = Labial cortical plate; upper lip swells.
2. Mx 3, 4, 5, 6, 7 = Swelling of cheek upto eye. Infection can spread to pterygoid plexus, cavenous sinus or IJV.
3. Md 1, 2, 3 = **Apices lie above the origin of inferior incisive and mental ms.**
   - If it spreads on lingual side = it involves **SUBLINGUAL space ABOVE the mylohyoid ms**, which has its origin close to lower border of mandible.
4. Md 4, 5 = depressor anguli oris, the triangularis and quadrate m, arise near the lower border of mandible, BELOW the apices of PM. PA abscess localizes first into the VESTIBULE, on labial side.
   - Lingual perforation will infect **SUBLINGUAL SPACE above mylohyoid m.**
5. Md 6, 7.

If buccal perforation

- Swelling in SULCUS if roots are short.
- If roots are LONG = below the buccinator m insertion and so S/C tissue is involved.

If lingual/perforation

- If below the mylohyoid m = abscess of submandibular space.
- If **above the mylohyoid m = abscess of sublingual space.**

6. Md 8.
   - Mostly perforates the LINGUAL Plate and so SUBMANDIBULAR space involved.
   - Origin of buccinator m at oblique line directs the spreading abscess D and F of M3 in the buccal vestibule.
   - Mand 1–5 teeth usually erode through labial–buccal plate and above the attached ms.

Tooth	Usual exit from bone	Relation of exit to ms	Which m/ms involved attachment	Site of localisation
Mand CI,	Labial	Below	**Mentalis**	**Submental space**
L!	Labial	Above	**Mentalis**	Oral vestibule
Mand 3	Labial	Above	**Depressor labii inferioris; depressor anguli oris; platysma**	Oral vestibule
Mand 4, 5	Buccal Above	Below **Buccinator**	**Depressor labii inferioris; depressor anguli oris; platysma** Buccal vestibule	Oral vestibule
Mand 6	Buccal Buccal Lingual	Above Below Above	**Buccinator** **Buccinator** **Mylohyoid**	Oral vestibule **Buccal space** **Sublingual space**
Mand 7	Buccal Buccal Lingual Lingual	Above Below Above Below	**Buccinator** **Buccinator** **Mylohyoid** **Mylohyoid**	Oral vestibule **Buccal space** **Sublingual space** **Submandibular space**
Mand 8	Lingual	Below	**Mylohyoid**	**Submandibular/ pterygopalatine spaces**

- Molar infections erode through lingual plate more frequently than the anterior teeth.
- 3rd molars infections almost always erode lingually.
- If the root apices of mand first molar are above the origin of buccinator, then infections is in oral vestibule.
- If apices are below the buccinator, then buccal space abscess occurs.
- Apices of 4, 5, 6 are almost always above the attachment of mylohyoid and so result in sublingual space abscess.
- Mand 7, 8 infections give rise to submandibular space infections as it perforates below mylohyoid ms.

Differences b/w cellulitis and abscess

Characteristic	**Cellulitis**	**Abscess**
Duration	Acute	Chronic
Pain	Severe and generalized	Localised
Size	Large	Small
Localisation	Diffuse borders	Well circumscribed
Palpation	Doughy to induration; board like	Fluctuant
po pus	No	Yes
Bacteria	Aerobic	Anaerobic

CANINE SPACE

- Lies **between levator anguli oris and levator labii superioris** ms.
- Involved due to **maxillary canine infections.**
- Canine is the only tooth with long root to allow bony **erosion superior to ms** of facial expression.
- Infection erodes superior to origin of levator anguli oris and below levator labii superioris ms.

- Swelling obliterates nasolabial folds.
- Spontaneous drainage occurs just inferior to medial canthus of eye.

Buccal space

- Involved when infection **erodes superior to buccinator m.**
- Due to infections of maxillary molars and premolars and mandibular molars.
- Swelling below zygomatic arch and above the inferior border of mandible.

Infratemporal space

- Involved by infections of **maxillary 3rd molars.**

Cavernous sinus thrombosis

- Infections spreads through pterygoid plexus and emissary vs or via angular veins and inferior or superior ophthalmic vs to cavernous sinus.
- These vains **do not have valves.**

Submental space

- Infected by the **infections of mandibular incisors.**
- Infection erodes **apical to mentalis m** and spreads under the inferior border of mandible.

Sublingual and submandibular spaces

- Involved by **lingual perforation** of infection of molars and premolars.
- Location of infected space is **determined by mylohyoid m attachment.**
- If **infections is above MH m, then sublingual space** is involved and occurs with premolars and first molars; intraoral swelling and raised tongue.
- If infection is **below MH m, then submandibular space** is involved; mainly involved by infections of 3rd molars.

- Mand 2nd molar may involve either of the space depending on its root length.
- **Sublingual space lies above MH m and submandibular space lies below MHm.**

Ludwig's angina

- **Bilateral** involvement of **submental; sublingual and submandibular** spaces.
- Due to streptococcal odontogenic infections.
- Breathing problems, trismus, elevated tongue, difficulty in swallowing.

Masseteric space

- Involved by the spread of **infections from buccal space.**
- Mand 3rd molar infections may spread.
- Severe trismus.
- Swelling over the angle and ramus of jaw.

Pterygomandibular space

- Lies **lateral to medial pterygoid** ms.
- **LA solution is injected** in this space during inferior alveolar block.
- **Little or *no facial swelling* seen, but significant trismus.**
- Significant diagnostic feature = *trismus without swelling.*

Temporal space

- Divided in 2 parts by temporalis m.
- Swelling occurs in temporal area **superior to zygomatic arch** and posterior to the lateral orbital rim.

Masticator space: Has 3 spaces, i.e. **masseteric, pterygomandibular and temporal** spaces; bounded by the ms of mastications.

Lateral pharyngeal space

- Involved **by infections of pterygomandibular space.**
- Medial to medial pterygoid ms and lateral to superior pharyngeal constrictor ms.
- Severe trismus; difficulty in swallowing.
- Swelling of lateral neck especially inferior to the angle of mandible.
- May lead to **thrombosis of IJV; erosion of carotid A;** interference with the functions of 9–12th Ns.

Retro-pharyngeal space

- Extends from the base of skull to C7 or T1 vertebra.
- Infections can spread to mediastinum.

Pre-vertebral space

- Extends from pharyngeal tubercle on the base of skull to the diaphragm.
- Involved by retro-pharyngeal space infections.

FASCIAL SPACES

Masticatory spaces: 3 SPACES.

1. **Buccal space:** Is between buccinator and masseter m. Connected posteriorly to PTERYGOMANDIBULAR Space and connected superiorly to zygomaticotemporal space.

2. **Pterygomandibular space**
   - Lateral boundary = medial surface of mandibular Ramus.
   - Medial boundary = medial pterygoid m.
   - Above = lateral pterygoid m.

- Its infection occurs most commonly ***by extraction of lower molars.***
- Abscess in this space points at the anterior aspect of masseter.

3. Zygomatico temporal/Retrozygomatic/Infratemporal space

- Space lies directly behind maxilla and zygomatic bones.
- Medial to insertion of temporal m.
- ***Infection of mx. Teeth*** drains through the cortical bone above the BUCCINATOR m. may spread to this space.

Parapharyngeal space (also known as lateral pharyngeal space) is continuous with RETRO-PHARYNGEAL space.

Pterygomandibular space communicates with the parapharyngeal space around the anterior and posterior borders of medial pterygoid m.

Submandibular space = is **divided by mylohyoid** m in sublingual (above the MH m) and submental (below the m.)

Submental space = lies between mylohyoid and platysma ms. It contains Ant. Belly of DG m; **PA infection of md. 1, 2, 3, 4, 5, perforate lingually below** the origin of mylohyoid m.

Sublingual space

- Lies below the mucosa (i.e. roof).
- Floor is mylohyoid m.
- Medially by = GH and genioglossus m.

- Sublingual cellulitis can spread across the midline.

Cavernous sinus thrombophlebitis: Infection can spread via 2 paths:

1. From anterior facial V to sup. ophthalmic V.
2. From posterior facial V to pterygoid venous plexus.
    - In first type–orbit is involved, danger signals are seen.
    - In 2nd type–intra-cranial/meningeal symptoms appear; no warning s/s seen. More dangerous.
    - Antibiotics may increase the chances of failure of birth control pills to prevent pregnancy.
    - Bactericidal antibiotics should be used than the bacteriostatic antibiotics.

Antibiotics for the odontogenic infections

Penicillin	Drug of choice; has a narrow spectrum and is bactericidal; only given "After Sensitivity Test" AST.
Erythromycin Clindamycin	If patient is allergic to penicillins.
Cephalexin Cefaclor	For broad spectrum.
Metronidazole; ornidazole, etc.	Only for anaerobes.
Tetracycline especially doxycycline	For gingival infections.
Clindamycin	May cause pseudomembranous colitis by Clostridium difficile.
Tetracycline	May cause photosensitivity and tooth discoloration.
Metronidazole	May cause disulfiram effect with alcohol.
Aminoglycoside	Kidney damage and 8th nerve damage antibiotics.
Chloramphenicol	Aplastic anemia.

- Bactericidal antibiotics interfere with cell wall formation of new bacteria, while bacteriostatic interfere with bacterial reproduction and growth.
- Usual recommended duration of antibiotics therapy is 2–3 days after the infection has resolved.

METASTATIC INFECTIONS

- Is the infection which occurs at a location physically separate from the portal of entry of bacteria, e.g. bacterial endocarditis.
- BE is mainly due to **alpha-haemolytic streptococci viridans.**

- Antibiotic prophylaxis should be given as = 3 gm of amoxicillin 1 hr before the procedure and 1.5 gm 6 hrs after the initial dose.
- Amoxicillin is the drug of choice than penicillin–V, because it is better absorbed from GIT; provides more sustained and higher plasma levels; and is effective killer of alpha–haemolytic viridans streptococci.
- Erythromycin and clindamycin are alternatives for patients allergic to penicillin.
- Erythromycin = 1 gm 2 hrs before and 500 mg 6 hrs after the surgery.
- Clindamycin = 300 mg 1 hrs before and 150 mg 6 hrs after the surgery.
- Clindamycin = is the alternative if patient cannot tolerate erythromycin.

OSTEOMYELITIS (Also refer to oral pathology.)

- Inflammation of bone marrow. It is the **infection of cancellous/ medullary part** of the bone.
- **Starts in medullary cavity**, involves cancellous bone, spreads to cortical bone and periosteum.
- It is due to compromise of blood supply and ischemia.
- **Mandible is more commonly involved** than maxilla, because blood supply of maxilla is much richer than mandible.
- Acute osteomyelitis occurs **most frequently in mandible** than in maxilla.
- **Bacteria** = streptococci; anaerobiccocci, e.g. peptostreptococci; G (–) rods fusobacterium and bacteroides.
- R/G = 10–12 days are required to be seen on it.
- Chronic osteomyelitis is seen as radiolucent **moth eaten appearance** on R/G.
- **Devitalised part of the bone is called as SEQUESTRUM.**
- Radiopaque areas are also seen in radiolucent areas known as **sequestra.**
- **Sequestra** are seen radiopaque due to osteitis–type reaction, in which bone production increases due to inflammatory reactions.

- Sequestrum becomes a site for **precipitation of ionized calcium,** which has been mobilized by the secondary osteolytic process and so it **appears more RADIOPAQUE** than the normal bone.
- **Involucrum** = is **radiolucent**, new bone.
- **Drug of choice** = penicillin; as it is effective veins strept and anaerobes.
- Drug of 2nd choice = clindamycin, if penicillin allergy is there.
- Surgical m/m = all tissue with compromised vascularity must be removed, i.e. sequestrectomy; decortication and saucerization.
- Mostly due to **M_3 infections.**
- R/G = early destruction of bone is not evident, until cortical bone is involved.
- Seen as **wormy appearance** on R/G.
- Curettage should not be done.
- **Saucerization** = after removal of sequestrum, the overhanging margins of bone are rongeured back to the cortical bone, which then rest on the intact medullary bone.
- Antibiotics should be given for 4–6 weeks.

Actinomycosis

- Is a bacterial infection; caused by *Actinomyces israelii; A. naeslundii; A viscosus;* G (+) branching rods; **anaerobic.**
- It does **not follow usual anatomic planes** as other infections, but burrows through them and becomes a lobular **pseudotumour.**
- **Multiple sinuses** on skin for drainage.
- **Sulfur granules** in exudate, which are **colonies of bacteria;** 1–2 mm in size.
- Multiple episodes of recurrent infections.
- Surgery = incision and drainage; excision of all sinuses.
- **Antibiotic** of choice = penicillin; 10 million units/day for 3–14 days I/V.
- And then long term **maintenance dose** = 500 mg qid for 3 mos.
- Drug of 2nd choice = tetracycline or doxycycline or minocycline as these can be given once/day.

HOST DEFENCE MECHANISMS OF THE BODY

Local defense	Humoral	Cellular defense
Anatomical barriers	Is a non-cellular type, e.g. by	It is cellular type, e.g.
• Skin	• Immunoglobulins	• Phagocytes; granulo – and monocytes
• Mucosa indigenous bacteria	• Complements	• Lymphocytes

Immunoglobulins (Also refer to the section of microbiology.)

- ♦ Are antibodies; help in phagocytosis of bacteria by leucocytes; produced by plasma cells/B-lymphocytes; are of 5 types:

IgG	75 %; defensive veins G + bacteria.
IgA	12 %; secretory Ig; prevents adhesion of bacteria to surface mucosa.
IgM	7 %; defends veins G (–) bacteria.
IgE	For delayed hypersensitivity reactions.
IgD	

- ♦ Primary phagocytes in early phase of infections are PMN leucocytes cells.
- ♦ Monocytes are seen in later stages and chronic infections
- ♦ T-lymphocytes play role in graft rejection and tumour surveillance.
- ♦ B-lymphocytes produce plasma cells and so the Ig antibodies.

RADIOTHERAPY (Also refer to the sections of oral pathology and radiology.)

- ♦ Used for the Rx of malignancies.
- ♦ Short wavelength x-rays or gamma rays of radium are used. Radioactive–Co is used to irradiate the tumour site. X-rays are used to sterilize the tumour from a distance.

- Rays destroy the neoplastic **cells by interfering with the nuclear** material required for reproduction, cell maintenance or both.
- Faster the cellular turnover, the more the susceptible is the tissue to the rays. (Which stage of mitosis is most vulnerable?)
- Tumour cells in stages of active growth are more susceptible.
- The more undifferentiated these cells appear, the more radiosensitive the tumour is.
- Normal cells, e.g. haematopoietic cells, epithelial cells and endothelial cells are also very susceptible.
- Salivary glands as such are radioresistant, but their **finer vasculature gets destroyed** by rays. It causes atrophy, fibrosis and degeneration and **xerostomia**.
- **Xerostomia** leads to rampant '**RADIATION CARIES'** of teeth; caries is seen around the entire circumference of the cervical part of tooth.
- OSTEORADIONECROSIS; ORN = is the devitalization of bone by radiations. It occurs **due to endarteritis; fibrosis of the blood vessels** and loss of fine vasculature. Turnover and repair rates of bone are slow. **Mandible is more affected than maxilla** due to higher density and poor blood supply.
- Irrigation with **dil hypochlorite solutions** help to oxygenate the areas of devital bone in Rx of ORN.
- **Hyperbaric O_2** gas increases the osteogenesis by **increasing the capillary proliferation** and leucocyte activity in irradiated bone. **150–750 mm Hg of O_2 is used for 2 hrs daily for 6–14 days.**
- Oral flora get altered; anaerobes and candida overgrow; 0.1% of Chlorhexidine and Nystatine are advised for Rx.
- All teeth with poor prognosis should be extracted before radiotherapy.
- Extractions should be done with removal of good portion of alveolar bone and atraumatic handling of flaps for better healing.
- Healing capacity greatly reduces with radiotherapy.
- Radiation dose = larger doses lead to more damage of normal tissues. If total dose is less than 5000 rads, the long term side effects are less.

- For squamous cell carcinoma, the most common tumour of oral cavity = > 6000 rads dose is required.
- Radiotherapy should be started 3 weeks after the extractions to give time for proper healing.
- RCT is difficult due to progressive sclerosis of pulp chambers in irradiated teeth.
- Hyperbaric O_2 = O_2 is given in the area before and after extractions under pressure. It increases local tissues oxygenation and vascular ingrowth in the hypoxic tissues and thus decreases the chances of ORN.
- Denture fabrication should be deferred for at least 6 months after the radiotherapy for those patients who were previously edentulous.

CHEMOTHERAPY

- Destroy or retards the division of rapidly growing/proliferating cells.
- Normal cells with high mitotic index are also affected, e.g. bone marrow, epithelium of GIT and oral cavity.
- Haematopoiesis system—myelosuppression occurs, i.e. leukopenia; neutropenic anemia; infections occur in oral cavity; spontaneous bleeding; gets corrected after 3 weeks of cessation of chemotherapy.
- Overgrowth of candida and G (–) bacilli occurs in oral cavity. It is Rxed with nystatine and chlorohexidine.
- 3 stages of chemotherapy.

IMPLANTS (Also refer to the section on prostho.)

Bone implant interface:

- Fibro-osseous integration = i.e. collagen fibres in between the interface.
- Osseo-integration = i.e. direct contact with bone occurs; bone ingrows through the implants.

Important points

- Bone temperature should be kept below 56°C during drilling to avoid bone damage.
- A low speed (1500–2000 rpm) should be used to drill the bone for implant placement.
- Areas of jaws with high % age of cortical bone, e.g. anterior mandible anchor the implant successfully.
- Areas of jaws with high % age of cancellous bone makes initial stability of implant more difficult.
- Minimum vertical dimension of bone for endosteal implant placement is 8 mm.
- Leave at least 2 mm bone between apical end of implant and inferior alveolar canal.
- Implant should have at least 1 mm of bone on buccal and lingual aspects.
- Maxilla has more cancellous bone, so a longer healing period is required.
- Peri-implant soft tissues environment and biomechanical overload of implant are the **2 most common factors** associated with breakdown of osseointegrations.
- Uncontaminated surface oxide layer of implant is necessary to obtain osseo-integrations of implant in the bone.
- Immediate placement of implant can be done after extraction if site is not infected. Implant is placed at least 4 mm apical to the apex of the tooth. It should be placed 2 mm below the alveolar crest to allow bone resorption after extractions.
- How to sterilize an implant, if it falls on floor from its container by infrared radiations?

Subperiosteal implants

- Fits on the top of supporting areas in maxilla and mandible under mucoperiosteum for support.
- Maxillary subperiosteal implants have **lower success rate** than mandible.

Transosteal implants

- Projections penetrate the mandible from its inferior border and rests on the inferior border.
- Can only be **used in anterior mandible.**
- Used in very atrophic mandible.

Endosteal implants

- Placed in alveolar and basal bone.
- Root form and blade form type of implants.
- **Root form implants** = cylindrical shape; 3–5 mm in diameter; and 7–20 mm long.
- **Blade implants** = wedge shape/rectangular; 2.5 mm wide; 8–15 mm depth; 15–30 mm length.
- **One stage implants** = placed in bone and projected immediately through oral mucosa.
- **2–stage implants** = first placed in bone to the level of cortical plate; healing period of 3–6–9 mos. for osseo-integration; then a second surgery is done to fit abutment, which projects in the oral cavity.
- **Threaded and non-threaded** implants.
- Implants are made of biocompatible materials, e.g. titanium; Ti-Al-V; with/without hydroxy-apatite coating.
- **Self–tapping implants** = used in maxilla where bone is soft.

COMPONENTS OF IMPLANTS

1. Implant
2. Sealing screw
3. Healing cap
4. Abutment
5. Impression post
6. Laboratory analogue
7. Waxing sleeve
8. Prosthesis retaining screw.

Implant	is placed in bone during first stage surgery.
Sealing screw	Placed in implant during healing phase after stage–one surgery. It is removed at stage–two surgery.
Healing cap	It is placed after stage–two surgery and before prosthesis placement to allow soft tissue healing.
Abutment	It screws directly into the implant. It supports the prosthesis.
Impression post	It helps the transfer of intra–oral location of fixture or abutment in the cast.
Laboratory analogue	It exactly represents implant or abutment in the lab cast. It is screwed into the impression post to be placed into impression before pouring.
Waxing sleeve	It is attached to abutment by prosthesis retaining screws on the cast and it becomes part of prosthesis upon the casting.
Prosthesis retaining screw	It penetrate the fixed restoration and secures it to the abutment.

Minimum distance b/w implant and anatomic structures

Buccal plate	0.5 mm
Lingual plate	1.0 mm
Max sinus floor	1.0 mm
Nasal cavity	1.0 mm
Incisive canal	Avoid midline; place away from the midline.

Minimum distance b/w implant and anatomic structures (*Contd.*)

Mental N	5.0 mm anterior to the mental foramen to avoid injury to the nerve.
Inferior alveolar canal	2.0 mm above the canal.
Adj. natural tooth	0.5 mm
Inter-implant distance	3.0 mm
Inferior border	1.0 mm

Minimum integration time

Anterior mandible	3 mos.
Posterior mandible	4 mos.
Anterior maxilla	6 mos; due to more cancellous bone.
Posterior maxilla	6 mos; due to more cancellous bone.
Into bone graft	6–9 mos.

Rehabilitation options

(A) For completely edentulous cases

1. ***Implant and tissue–supported overdenture***
   - Esp for mand denture.
   - **2 implants** are placed in mandibular symphysis area between mental foramina.
2. ***All–implant supported overdenture***
   - a minimum of **4 implants in lower jaw** and ***6 in upper jaw*** should be placed.
3. ***Fixed–detachable restoration***
   - **5 implants in mandible** and ***6 in maxilla*** are required.
   - Best for recently extracted cases with minimum bone loss.
   - Gives best psychological advantage to the patients.

(B) For partially edentulous patients: 2 main indications are:

- Free end–distal extension bases.
- Long edentulous span.

BIOMEDICAL WASTE/BMW MANAGEMENT

Categories of BMWs

Category	Type	Rx and disposal
1.	Human anatomical wastes	Incineration/deep burial
2.	Animal wastes	–do–
3.	Microbiology and biotechnology wastes	Local autoclave/ incineration.
4.	Waste sharps	Disinfection/autoclave, etc.
5.	Discarded medicines and cytotoxic drugs.	Incineration/destruction
6.	Soiled wastes	Incineration/autoclave.
7.	Solid wastes	Chemical disinfection, etc.
8.	Liquid wastes	Chemical disinfection/ discharge in drains, etc.
9.	Incineration ash	Dispose in municipal landfill
10.	Chemical wastes	Chemical Rx and discharge in drains.

Colour coding and type of container

Colour	Nature of waste	Category
Separately to be packed in **yellow** bags	Anatomical wastes like placenta, biopsies and all other human tissues including amputation material, surgical resection, etc.	1, 2, 3, 6
Yellow bags	Infectious wastes like waste from OT, emergency room, labor rooms, dressing of wounds, swabs, etc.	6

Colour coding and type of container (*Contd.*)

Colour	Nature of waste	Category
Red bags	Used syringes, I/V tubing, gloves, urine bags, catheters, etc. and all plastic materials.	3, 6, 7
Red bags separately.	All glass bottles.	7
Blue/white translucent puncture proof containers	All needles, sharps, scalpels, broken ampoules, etc.	4, 7
Black bags	All non-infectious BMW.	5, 9, 10

Note

1. **Plastic wastes** are not to be placed in yellow bags. They are to go **into red bags only**.
2. All bags shall be labelled as per **schedule IV (rule 6) of BMW (management and handling) rules 1998**.
3. General municipal wastes should not be packed in any of the yellow or red bags.

SCHEDULES OF DRUGS

Schedules	Properties
I.	• These drugs are not available for clinical use in US. • e.g. heroin, marijuana.
II.	• These drugs have high abuse liability. • Require written prescription and DEA no. • Prescription cannot be refilled without a new prescription. • e.g. morphine, meperidine, plain codeine, pentobarbital, oxycodone compounds.
III.	• These have lower abuse potential.

SCHEDULES OF DRUGS (*Contd.*)

Schedules	Properties
	• Prescription can be phoned in the pharmacy but require DEA no. • Prescription can be refilled upto 5 times in 6 months. • e.g. codeine and hydrocodone compounds; dihydrocodeine compounds; pentazocine.
IV.	Non-narcotic drugs with lower abuse potential DEA no. is required, e.g. chloral hydrate, diasepam etc.
V.	These are in low–dose preparation for OTC sales. primarily for cough syrup and anti-diarrheal purposes. NSAIDs are not scheduled drugs.

Stabilisation periods for dento-alveolar injuries

Injury	Duration
Mobile tooth	3–4 wks
Tooth displacement	3–4 wks
Root fracture	2–4 mos
Replanted tooth mature	7–10 days
Replanted tooth immature	3–4 wks

Physical types of lesions

Bulla	Loculated fluid in or under epithelium of skin/ mucosa; a large blister.
Crusts	Dried/clotted serum proteins on the surface of skin/mucosa.
Erosions	Superficial ulcer/excoriations.
Macule	Circumscribed area of colour change without elevation.
Nodule	Large palpable mass, elevated above the epithelium surface.

Physical types of lesions (*Contd.*)

Papule	Small palpable mass, elevated above the epithelium surface.
Plaque	Flat, elevated lesion; the confluence of papules.
Pustule	Cloudy/white vesicle, the colour of which results from the p.o. PMN cells/pus.
Scale	Macroscopic accumulation of keratin.
Ulcer	Loss of epithelium.
Vesicle	Small loculation of fluid in or under the epithelium; a small blister.

Characteristics of lesions that raise the suspicion of malignancy

Erythroplasia	Lesion is totally red or has a speckled red and white appearance.
Ulceration	Lesion is ulcerated or present as an ulcer.
Duration	Lesion has persisted for more than 2 wks.
Growth rate	Lesion exhibits rapid growth.
Bleeding	Lesion bleeds on gentle manipulation.
Induration	Lesion and adjacent tissues are firm to the touch.
Fixation	Lesion feels attached to adjacent structures.

COMPOSITIONS AND INDICATIONS OF FLUIDS

Isotonic saline, NS	NaCl = 0.9 gms, water for injection	Hyponatremia, hypochlorine, metabolic alkalosis, post-op maintenance
1/5 isotonic saline + 5 % dextrose	• Dextrose anhydrous = 5 gms • Dibasic K-phosphate = 0.13 g	Same as above

COMPOSITIONS AND INDICATIONS OF FLUIDS (*Contd.*)

	• Sodium chloride = 0.091 g • Na acetate = 0.28 g • Na metabisulphite = 0.021 g • K chloride = 0.15 g	
Dextrose 5%	Anhydrous dextrose = 5 g Water for injection	Early post-op period women Na excretion is less
DNS	Anhydrous dextrose = 5 g, Nacl = 0.9 g Water for injection	Intraoperative period; late post-op period
Darrow's solution	Anhydrous dextrose = 5 g KCl = 0.12 g Dibasic K phosphate = 0.12 g	Hypokalemia; started from 3rd post-op day toeplenish K loss Sod. Acetate = 0.026 g Sod metabisulphite = 0.021 g
Haemaccel	Polymer from degraded gelatin = 3.5 g Electrolytes and sterile distilled water to 100 ml Polypeptides are added for isotonicity.	Burns; extensive trauma.
Ringer's lactate/ hartmann's solution	Sod hydroxide; sod lactate; sod chloride, pot chloride; calcium chloride	GI losses, ECF volume deficit-hypovolumic shock; good results in intraoperative use.

R/G VIEWS (v) BEST FOR

Subcondylar fracture; condylar neck	Towne's view
Medially displaced condylar neck fracture	PA view

R/G VIEWS (v) BEST FOR (*Contd.*)

Ramus/body of mandible	LO at 15 degrees
Horizontal favorable/ unfavorable mand fracture	LO at 30 degrees
Frac. body mand, base of skull, zygomatic arch	SMV view
Max sinus	Water's/PNS view
Rim/floor of orbit	30 degree OMV
Coronoid	PA skull
Base of skull	Towne's and SMV
Zygoma; fracture of max-zygomatic complex	OMV
Sialolith of submand gland	Cross-sectional occlusal view
Impacted mand 3rd molar	Occlusal and IOPA
Zygomatic arch; base of skull	SMV/jug-handle view
Herniation and perforation of TMJ disk	Arthrography
Stenson's and wharton's duct sialoliths	OPG
Condyle neck fracture in TMJ view	Infracranial/ transpharyngeal view
Internal derangement of TMJ	MRI
Difference b/w CSF and blood	CT scan
Middle face fracture	Water's view
Fracture of mand condylar neck	Fronto-occipital; OPG
Medial wall, orbital roof	OM; lateral skull
Coronoid process	OM, PA view

R/G VIEWS BEST FOR (*Contd.*)

Palate	Oblique upper occlusal
Frontal sinus	Caldwell's view
Middle face fracture; BEST view	Water's view
TMJ space	Reverse towne's view; fronto-occipital

FRACTURES

- Le Fort I = guerin fracture/horizontal/floating palate/low-level fracture.
- Le Fort II = pyramidal/floating maxilla.
- Le Fort III = transverse; craniofacial dysjunction; high level fracture.
- **Panda facies** = in Le Fort fractures = it is bilateral black eyes due to circumorbital ecchymosis and facial oedema.
- **Blowout fracture** = hinged/trap door effect in R/G.
- Most common fracture of mid face = nasal bone.
- 2nd most common fracture of mid face = zygomatic bone.
- Most common fracture of face = nasal bone.
- 2nd most common fracture of face = mandible.
- Least common fracture of mandible = coronoid process; 1%.

SYNONYMS

1. JUG HANDLE V = oblique axial v/SMV = for zygoma.
2. Keyhole v = transpharyngeal/infracranial/Parma/McQueen projection v = TMJ.
3. Water's v = occipitomental view; OMV = PNS.
4. Caldwell luc v = PA v = frontal sinus.
5. Rheese v = oblique/optic foramen view.
6. Towne's v = occipitofrontal v = TMJ space.
7. Reverse Towne's = fronto-occipital view.

8. Transcranial v = posterior auricular approach of Lindblom = TMJ.
9. Transorbital v = zimmer projection = TMJ.
10. PA at–10 degrees = Caldwell view.

McGregor and Campbell's lines: Seen in OMV/ PNS view.

- **First line** = path from zygomatico-frontal suture to superior orbital margin across the glabella region to superior orbital margin and zygomatico-frontal suture of the other side.
- **Second line** = from zygomatic tubercle to continuous line of zygomatic arch till it blends into zygomatic bone and the line continues along inferior orbital margin, across the frontal process of maxilla and lateral wall of nose through septum and then same course on the opposite side.
- **Third line** = from condyle across the mandibular notch, coronoid process of the mandible to lateral wall of antrum and continuous through the medial wall of antrum or lateral wall of nose at the nasal floor level and the same course on the opposite side.
- **Fourth line** = occlusal curve of the U/L arches.
- **Fifth line** = lower border of mandible from one angle to other side angle.

R/G lines on IOPA for impacted teeth: known as Winter's lines/ WAR lines

- **White line** = line joining the buccal cusps of erupted molars and going posterior over the third molar region. A perpendicular line drawn to the occlusal plane of second molar represents the long axis of this tooth. It shows axial inclination of impacted molar in respect to the second molar. The relation to white line shows the relative depth of the third molar.
- **Amber line** = runs at the level of the crest of interdental septum between the molars and represents the bone level covering the impacted tooth.
- **Red line** = a line perpendicular from the amber line to an imaginary point where the elevator will be applied. It indicates the amount of the resistance and difficulty encountered during removal of third molars.

SIALOGRAMS

Sialodochitis = inflammation of salivary duct.

- Sialadenitis = leafy-tree appearance.
- Sialolith = link sausage appearance.
- Mixed tumor of parotid = ball-in-hand deformity in many cases.
- Sjogren's syndrome = branchless-fruit-laden tree/cherry-blossom appearance.

GRAFTS: Transplantation of LIVING tissues.

Autografts	From same patient.
Allografts/ homologus	Same species, i.e. from alleles.
Isografts	Same species, but genetically related to patient, e.g. monozygotic twin.
Xenografts	Another species, e.g. animals.
Alloplast	Synthetic material, non-animal origin, e.g. POP, hydroxyapatite.
Implant	Transplantation of NON-LIVING tissues, e.g. POP, HA.
Partial thickness	Aka Thiersch graft.
Full thickness	Aka Wolfe's graft.
Graft rejection	Occurs due to CMI; it leaves the reciepient in a condition of increased resistance. So when a second graft known as white graft is placed it is rejected much more rapidly than the first one.

DEFINE FOLLOWING

- Displaced fractures.
- Degloving injuries.
- Bucket handle displacement.
- Blow out and blow in fractures.
- Suspensory ligament of lockwood attachments.

Absolute C/I for using steroids

- Active/healed/incompletely healed TB.
- Ocular herpes simplex.
- Primary glaucoma.
- Acute psychosis.
- Allergy.

Relative C/I to steroids use

- Peptic ulcers.
- Cushing's syndrome.
- HT, DM.
- Osteoporosis.
- First trimester.
- Acute/chronic infections.
- Thromboembolic tendencies.

Only **3 emergency situations,** in which drug is administered before the oxygen are:

1. Acute allergy/anaphylaxis.
2. Insulin shock/hypoglycemia.
3. Narcotic overdose.

Others require prior oxygen therapy, i.e. ABCs and CPR.

Proper measure taken by the dentist if anaphylaxis reaction occurs = CPR immediately, Oxygen and Adrenaline.

Shock of adrenaline insufficiency is a problem= because it is not reversed by vasoconstrictors, e.g. adrenaline, etc.

Appropriate therapy for bronchospasm = I/V succinylcholine and oxygen by face mask.

Mechanical advantages

- Lever principle = 3.0.
- Wedge principle = 2.5.
- Wheel and axle principle = 4.6.

Stages of GA = details

- Stage I = stage of analgesia, conscious sedation.
- Stage II = stage of delirium.
- Stage III = stage of anaesthesia; surgical.
- Plane 1
- Plane 2
- Plane 3
- Plane 4
- Stage IV = stage of medullary depression; dangerous; death.

NERVE INJURIES

1. Neuritis = acute, reversible irritation of nerves.
2. **Neuropraxia/type I/first degree injury** = least severe injury; axonal conduction is interrupted; the nerve is intact; anatomic continuity of connective tissues sheaths and nerve axons is maintained; occurs due to blunt trauma, nerve manipulation/compression. Recovery is rapid, i.e. repaired within 4–8 weeks; no Wallerian degeneration occurs.
3. **Axonotmesis/type II/second degree injury** = occurs by tensile/crushing force; loss of axonal blood supply with potential demyelination; Wallerian degeneration occurs; necrosis and loss of nerve axons distal to the point of injury occurs; all layers of nerve are intact; gets repaired in 12–18 months.
4. **Neurotmesis/3rd, 4th, 5th degree injury** = loss of CT continuity to varying degrees; caused by blunt mechanical, e.g. stretch, contusion. The Wallerian degeneration occurs distal to the nerve trunk.
5. **Compression** is the most common mechanism of peripheral nerve injuries.
6. **Anaesthetic injury** = associated with sever stretch or disruptive injuries; prognosis is unfavourable; prognosis of extraosseous nerve repair is worse than intraosseous nerve injury.

7. **Paraesthesia** = nerve is intact clinically; best prognosis for spontaneous recovery.
8. **Dysaesthesia** = seen later in post–injury/post–surgical phases; may be seen with both divisions and incontinuity nerve injury; C/O pain in anatomic distribution of divided nerve and anaesthesia in that dermatome clinically (known as anaesthesia dolorosa). The pain should be controlled to prevent wide-range neuron sensitisation on priority basis.

Pattern of spread of odontogenic abscesses

Maxillary tooth	Potential spread sites
Molars/PMs	Swelling or sinus in buccal sulcus may spread to buccal space, i.e. lateral to buccinator.
Canine	Canine fossa-facial nasolabial fold area.
LI	May track to palate due to distal inclination of root, but usually labial.
CI	Labially, can give a swollen lip.

Mandibular tooth

3rd molars; (pericoronitis may track buccally along the inner aspect of buccinator to present in 5, 6 region), and 2nd molars.	Both have a potential to spread in many directions; submandibular space via lingual plate. Pterygomandibular space, lateral pharyngeal space and on down the neck. Spreading laterally, infection from the 3rd molar may give severe trismus with an extension in submasseteric space.

Mandibular tooth (*Contd.*)

First molar	Buccally, if lingual may be submental or submandibular depending on level of drainage and mylohyoid attachment.
PMs and Canines	Buccally.
Incisors	Labially.

Glasgow coma scale

Scale	Best motor response	Best verbal response	Eyes open
6	Obeys commands	—	—
5	Localises pain	Oriented	—
4	Normal flexion to pain	Confused conversation	Spontaneously
3	Abnormal flexion to pain	Inappropriate words	To speech
2	Extension to pain	Incomprehensible	To pain
1	None	None	Do not open

Score	CODE
15–15	5
11–13	4
8–10	3
5–7	2
5–5	1

Immunological features of vesiculo-bullous disorders

Disease	Direct immunofluorescence	Indirect immunofluorescence
Pemphigus	Intercellular IgG and C3	Titre correlates with disease severity
Mucous membrane pemphigoid	Linear IgG and C3 at basement membrane zone	Negative
Bullous pemphigoid	Linear IgG and C3 at basement membrane	Positive in 75% cases zone
Linear IgA disease	Linear IgA and C3 at basement membrane zone	Negative
Dermatitis herpetiformis	Granular deposits of IgA and C3 at the tips of dermal papillae	Negative

Classification of white patches

Genetic	• White sponge nevus • Darier's disease • Dyskeratosis congenita • Pachyonychia congenita • Hereditary intraepithelial dyskeratosis
Traumatic	• Chemical burns • Mechanical • Thermal burns = smoker's keratosis; nicotinic stomatitis
Infection	• Caniddosis/pseudomembranous and hyperplastic types; • Hairy leukoplakia • Syphilitic leukoplakia
Idiopathic	• Leukoplakia

Classification of white patches (*Contd.*)

Dermatological	• Lichen planusLupus erythematosus
Metabolic	• Associated with renal failure
Neoplastic	• Squamous cell carcinoma

Different types of nerve fibers

Fibre type	**Diameter, microns**	**Velocity; m/sec.**
A–alpha	13–22; **thickest**	70–120; **fastest**
A–beta	8–13	40–70
A–gamma	4–8	15–40
A–delta	1–4	5–15
B	1–3	3–14
C	0.51; **thinnest**	0.5–2; **slowest**

Nociceptors are unmyelinated or thinly myelinated fibers of slow conduction A–delta and C–type fibers.

Cranial nerve testings

Nerve	**Abnormal tests results**
1.	Unable to identify odours.
2.	Failure of pupil to constrict or presence of non-consensual gaze.
3.	Failure of pupil to constrict or presence of ptosis.
4.	Inability of eye to look to ipsilateral shoulder.
5.	Inability to feel light touch, i.e. sensory part; weakness of masseter ms, i.e. motor part.
6.	Inability of eye to look to ipsilateral side.
7.	Inability to raise eyebrows, hold eyelid closed; symmetrically smile; pucker.
8.	Poor hearing or symptoms of vertigo.

Cranial nerve testings (*Contd.*)

Nerve	Abnormal tests results
9.	Failure of uvula to elevate on the stroked side.
10.	Weakness in turning head against resistance.
11.	Deviation of tongue to one side on that side factors of extrinsic pathways = 1, 2, 5, 7, 10 = tested by PT.

- Factors of intrinsic pathways = tested by PTT.
- Vitamin K dependent factors = 2, 7, 9, 10 = tested by PT/PTT.
- Platelet inadequacy = tested by BT/platelet count.

SIGNS NOTED IN TRAUMA

Guerian's sign	Seen in Le Fort 1 fractures, near the greater palatine foramen.
Battle's sign	Seen in fracture of middle cranial fossa, near the mastoid area. (post-auricular region).
Sublingual hematoma	Seen in mandibular symphysial and parasymphysial fracture.
Subconjunctival haemorrage	Is red in colour due to the free oxygen influx and eflux (has no posterior limit).
Black eye	As compared to SUBCONJUNCTIVAL HAEMORRAGE has a posterior limit.
Periorbita breach	Leads to subconjunctival haemorrage.
Verill's sign	Partial ptosis, partial hooding of the eyes.
Mongoloid slant	Seen in naso-ethmoid fractures.
Anti-mongoloid slant	Seen in zygomatic complex fractures.
Tinnel's sign	Seen in nerve injuries.
Vertigo	Dizziness.
Nystagmus	Uncoordinated movement of the eyeball.

DIPLOPIA

LEFT SIDE PARALYSED RIGHT SIDE PARALYSED

LATERAL RECTUS

Diplopia on looking towards the paralysed side

MEDIAL RECTUS

Diplopia on looking towards the sound side

SUPERIOR RECTUS

Diplopia on looking up

INFERIOR RECTUS

Diplopia on looking down

SUPERIOR OBLIQUE

Diplopia on looking down

INFERIOR OBLIQUE

Diplopia on looking up

SUMMARY OF ANTIBACTERIAL PROPHYLAXIS

Prevention of endocarditis in patients with heart valve lesions, septal defects, patent ductus or prosthetic valve.

(A) Dental procedures under local or no anaesthesia

- ♦ Patients who have not received more than a single dose of a penicillin in the previous month, including those with a prosthetic valve (but not those who have had endocarditis).
  - **Oral Amoxicillin** 3 g 1 hr before procedure.
  - CHILD UNDER 5 YEAR—QUARTER ADULT DOSE.
  - 5–10 YEARS—HALF ADULT DOSE.
- ♦ Patients who are **penicillin-allergic** or have received more than a single dose of a penicillin in the previous month.
  - **Oral clindamycin** 600 mg 1 hr before procedure.
  - CHILD UNDER 5 YEARS—QUARTER ADULT DOSE.
  - 5–10 YEARS—HALF ADULT DOSE.
- ♦ Patients who have had endocarditis.
  - **Amoxicillin + Gentamycin**, as under general anaesthesia.

(B) Dental procedures under local general anaesthesia

No special risk (including patients who have not received more than a single dose of a penicillin in the previous month).

- Either i/v **Amoxicillin** 1 g at induction, and then oral amoxicillin 500 mg 6 hours later.
- CHILD UNDER 5 YEARS—QUARTER ADULT DOSE.
- 5–10 YEARS—HALF ADULT DOSE.

OR

1. **Oral Amoxicillin** 3 g 4 hours before induction and then **oral amoxicillin** 3 g as soon as possible after procedure.
2. CHILD UNDER 5 YEARS—QUARTER ADULT DOSE.
3. 5–10 YEARS—HALF ADULT DOSE.
4. or **oral amoxicillin** 3 g + **oral probenecid** 1 g 4 hours before procedure.

♦ **Special risk** (patients with a prosthetic valve or who have had endocarditis).

1. **i/v Amoxicillin** 1 g + **i/v gentamycin** 120 mg at induction, then **oral amoxicillin** 500 mg 6 hours later.
2. CHILD UNDER 5 YEARS—AMOXICILLIN QUARTER ADULT DOSE, GENTAMYCIN 2 mg/kg.
3. 10 YEARS—AMOXICILLIN HALF ADULT DOSE, GENTAMYCIN 2 mg/kg .

♦ **Patients who are penicillin allergic** or who have received more than a single dose of a penicillin in the previous month.

Either **i/v vancomycin** 1 g over at least 100 minutes then **i/v gentamycin** 120 mg at induction or 15 minutes before procedure.

CHILD under 10 year—**vancomycin** 20 mg /kg,

—**gentamycin** 2 mg /kg,

or **i/v teicoplanin** 400 mg + **gentamycin** 120 mg at induction or 15 minutes before procedure.

CHILD under 14 years—**teicoplanin** 6 mg/kg,

gentamycin 2 mg/kg

Or **i/v clindamycin** 300 mg over at least 10 minutes at induction or 15 minutes before procedure then oral or i/v clindamycin 150 mg 6 hours later.

CHILD under 5 years—QUARTER ADULT DOSE.

5–10 years—HALF ADULT DOSE.

VACCINATIONS

BIRTH	BCG OPV (1) HBV (1)
6 weeks	DPT–1 OPV–2 HBV–2
10 weeks	DPT–2 OPV–3
14 weeks	DPT–3 OPV–4
6–9 months	OPV–5 HBV–3
9 months	MEASLES
15–18 months	MMR DPT 1st booster OPV–6
5 years	DPP 2nd booster OPV–7
10 years	TT–3rd booster HBV–booster
15 –16 years	TT–4th booster
OPTIONAL	typhoid fever Hemoph influenza type–B Hepatitis A Varicella vaccine

TNM STAGING OF HEAD AND NECK CANCER

PRIMARY TUMOUR

Tx primary tumour cannot be assessed.

To no evidence of primary tumour.

Tis carcinoma in situ.

T1 tumour 2 cm or less in greatest dimension.

T2 tumour > 2 cm but < 4 cm in greatest dimension.

T3 tumour > 4 cm in greatest dimension.

T4 tumour invades adjacent structures (e.g. through cortical bone, skin, etc.).

LYMPH NODE

Nx regional lymph nodes cannot be assessed.

No no regional lymph node metastasis.

N1 metastasis in a single ipsilateral lymph node 3 cm or less in greatest dimension.

N2a metastasis in a single ipsilateral lymph node more than 3 cm but not more than 6 cm in greatest dimension.

N2b metastasis in multiple ipsilateral lymph nodes none more than 6 cm in greatest dimension.

N2c metastasis in bilateral or contralateral lymph nodes none more than 6 cm in greatest dimension.

N3 metastasis more than 6 cm in greatest dimension.

DISTANT METASTASIS

Mx presence of distant metastasis cannot be assessed.

Mo no distant metastasis.

M1 distant metastasis.

STAGE GROUPING

STAGE			
O	T is	No	Mo
I	T1	No	Mo
II	T2	No	Mo
III	T3	No	Mo
	T1	N1	Mo
	T2	N1	Mo
	T3	NI	Mo
IV	T4	No	Mo
	T4	N1	Mo
	ANY T	ANY N	M1

EMERGENCIES IN THE DENTAL OFFICE

1. **Syncope/fainting is the most common** emergency. It is due to cerebral hypoxia. Dilation of the SPLANCHNIC VESSELS causes a fall in BP with a decrease in cerebral blood flow.

   Treatment is = placing the patient SUPINE.
   - Head lower than rest of the body.
   - Spirit of ammonia as RESPIRATORY STIMULANT.
   - O_2 administration.
   - Airway maintenance.
   - **Trendelenburg's position.**
2. **Toxic reactions of LA** = initial excitation followed by marked depression.
   - Patient is talkative and anxious.
   - If given I/V–may lead to convulsions. It can be Rxed by I/V Diazepam; give adequate O_2 and **aspirate** before injecting.
   - If **Anaphylaxis** occurs due to LA—give **Adr,** which is vasopressor/bronchodilator and anti histaminic, it is the **drug of choice.** Dose in adults is 0.3–1.0 mg S/c or I/m. O_2, antihistaminics and corticosteroids are also given.
   - If BP is low–give vasopressor, e.g. phenylephrine 1–5 mg I/m.

- If tooth goes inside the larynx/tracheobronchial tree = the ABDOMINAL THRUST PROCEDURE/HEIMLEICH'S procedure to dislodge large objects from tracheobronchial tree is recommended.
- If tooth is not dislodged from the larynx—then CRICOTHYROIDOTOMY is done.

Tracheostomy/Cricothyroidotomy

Tracheostomy = is the surgical creation of an opening into trachea through neck, for insertion of a tube to facilitate respiration.

Tracheotomy = is the incision of trachea through skin and muscles of neck, for exploration, removal of foreign body or obtaining biopsy sample.

Emergency cricothyrotomy = is surgical creation of an opening into the larynx between the anterior inferior border of thyroid cartilage and anterior superior border of cricoid cartilage (in cricothyroid space). It is most accessible point inferior to the glottis.

Important points

- Molt's curet no. 5/Moon's probe is used to ascertain the depth of anaesthesia.
- Parade ground fracture.
- Knock out fracture.

S/s of Hypothyroidism

- Fatigue
- Constipation
- Dry brittle skin/hair/nails
- **Wt gain**
- Oedema

DISTRACTION OSTEOGENESIS (DO)

- It is a slow application of force to a bone cut thereby widening the gap and resulting in production of new bone as well as soft tissues.

- Used for Rx of growth deficiencies.
- Based on the principle of "LAW OF TENSION-STRESS".
- It is also called CALLOTASIS.
- Tensile forces are used for stimulation of callus and generation of new bone.
- There is simulteneous expansion of functional soft tissue matrix. It is called as distraction histogenesis.
- First decreased by codivilla and then propagated by Ilizarov.
- Synder et. al. (1972) used an mandible using extra-oral device.
- Michielli and Miotti (1977) used intra-oral device.

Advantages–are long term stability; simple; physiologic bone generation; 3D destruction; no grafts required; early result, etc.

6 types of DO

1. Unifocal distraction Re—to lengthen the mandible.
2. Monobloc advancement—to advance the midface.
3. Bifocal distraction—bone segment-transplantation.
4. Trifocal destraction—e.g. to reconstruct mandibular symphyseal defects.
5. Alveolar augmentation.
6. Distraction implantology.

Biological principles of DO

1. Atraumatre corticotomy/osteotomy.
2. Healing period or latency period or delay—is the time internal when corticotomy is done; untill the time the DO is started. It is 4–7 days.
3. **Rate of DO**—i.e. the no. of mm/day at which bone surfaces are stretened @ 1 mm/day is normal.
4. **Rhythm**—no. of distractions/day divided in equal increments, e.g. 0.35 mm four times a day.
5. Healing index/consolidation period = 6–10 weeks.

Stages of bone formation in DO gap

1. Stage of fibrous tissue.
2. Stage of extending bone formation.
3. Stage of bone remodelling.
4. Stage of mature bone.

Vectors of DO—Vertical; horizontal and oblique.

Types of distractors—Extra-oral; intra-oral; subcutaneous; hybrid; monodirectional; bidirectional and multidirectional.

BIORESORBABLE OSTEOSYNTHESIS

- Polyglycolic acid (PGA), polylactic acid (PLA) and PGA–PLA copolymer are bioresorbable materials used for fractures fixation.
- No 2nd surgery required, as is required with metallic implant.
- Maintain their strength till 4–6 weeks and then degrade.
- Eliminate STRESS-SHIELDING PHENOMENON, and hence maintain bone density.
- Metallic implants in children cause growth restrictions, so PGA/PLA should be used.
    - Indicated for Re of comminuted fractures of naso ethmoidal area, lacrimal and frontal sinus bone, infra-orbital margin, paediatric patient, etc.
    - Self reinforced (SR) technique has improved mechanical properties by 5 times.
    - Sterile abscess may develop in vicinity of bioresorbable plates placed subcutaneously.

4

Prosthodontics

Fixed Partial Dentures

Crown = is an artificial replacement, which restores the morphology, function and contour of coronal part of the tooth.

Full veneer crown

Partial veneer crown

Intracoronal cast restoration—fits within the crown largely.

Inlay = intracoronal restoration with mild/moderate extensions.

Onlay = intracoronal restoration with an occlusal veneer is known as onlay.

Bridge = FPD—Permanently attached to remaining teeth.

Abutment = tooth serving as an attachment for a bridge.

Pontic = artificial tooth suspended between abutments.

Retainer = i.e. restorations which are cemented to the prepared abutment teeth.

Connecter = i.e. between pontic and retainer.

HISTORY OF THE PATIENT

1. Reactions to drugs especially LA and antibiotics.
2. Uncontrolled HT = No Rx till controlled.
   - Patients with HT/coronary heart disease = No adranline should be given, because adrenaline leads to = BP/increased HR.

3. Rheumatic fever = then premedicate the patient.
4. Epilepsy = provide Protection.
5. Diabetes = leads to Periodontal breakdown/Abscess formation.
6. Hyperthyroidism = should be controlled to avoid stresses.
7. TMJ S/S.

Diagnostic casts

1. Should be mounted on semiadjustable articulator.
2. Mandibular cast should be set in most retruded position.

Abutment

It bears additional forces (which were normally absorbed by missing tooth).

Ideally = it should be VITAL tooth.

Ante's law = PDL surface area of supporting teeth should be more than the teeth being replaced.

C:R ratio = ideal is 1:2; but 1:1 is acceptable.

Dislodging forces on a bridge retainer act in MD direction.

Dislodging forces on a single restoration act in BL direction.

Secondary abutment

- To bolster the primary abutment.
- To solve C:R ratio problem.
- Must have at least as much RSA root surface area and as favourable C:R ratio as the primary abutment.
- The retainers on secondary abutments will be placed in tension when pontic flexes and primary abutment acts as fulcrum.
- To avoid torquing, the secondary retention should extend a distance from primary inter-abutment axis equal to the distance that the pontic lever Arm extends in opposite direction.

Pier abutments = i.e. tooth having edentulous area on both sides.

- **Rigid connectors** = i.e. solder joints is preferred method of FPD.
- Bucco-lingual movements range from = 56–108 microns.

- Intrusion movement ranges to = 28 microns.
- **Non-rigid connector** = is a broken stress mechanical union of retainer and pontic, most commonly used is T-shaped key (on pontic) with dovetail key–way on retainer.

The location of stress-breaker on pier abutment—5 unit FPD = should be placed on the middle-abutment = it prevents it to act as a fulcrum.

- Keyway of the connector should be placed within the NORMAL DISTAL CONTOURS OF MIDDLE abutment.
- And the key should be placed on the mesial side of first molar pontic = it helps to seat the key into key way in mesial movement of teeth under occlusal leads.
- Rx of choice for a mesially tilted tooth = orthodontic uprighting.
- Long axes of the prospective abutments should converge by no more than 25–30°.

Canine replacement bridge = V. difficult.

- Maxillary lateral incisor and first premolar are weakest teeth.
- Maxillary canine bridge is subjected to more stresses than mandibular canine bridge, because forces are transmitted labially (outward) in the maxillary arch against the inside of the curve (i.e. its weakest point).
- On mandibular canine, forces are directed inward/lingually against the outside of curve (i.e. strongest point).

Cantilever bridge—which has an abutment's at one end only.

- Used only when there is minimum/no occlusal contact on the pontic.
- e.g. maxillary lateral incisor FPD with maxillary canine as abutment.
- But it is destructive.

Simple bridge = is one which replaces a single tooth.

Absolute maximum number of posterior teeth, which can be safely replaced with a bridge = 3 (except upper and lower incisors).

A C:R (crown to root ratio) of 3:1.0 is desirable.

OCCLUSION

Mandibular movements = are 3 dimensional.

1. Horizontal = i.e. in sagittal plane, when retruded mandible produces PURE ROTATONAL opening/closing movement around the hinge axis, extending through both condyles.
2. Vertical = occurs in horizontal plane, when mandible moves in lateral excursion. C rot. is a vertical axis extending through the **working side condyle.**
3. Sagittal = on lateral excursion, the non-working side condyle travels downward and forward, a downward arc rotating about an AP/sagittal axis passing through the **non-working condyle**.
   - **Pure rotational movement** = occur in lower compartment of TMJ.
   - Also some **gliding/translation** = occurs in the upper compartment of TMJ.
   - **Lateral movement** = non-working condyle moves medially and forward and downward.

Working condyle moves laterally/slightly posteriorly = it is known as **Bennett movement.**

Determinants of mandibular movement

- Anteriorly = U/L teeth
- Posteriorly = TMJ
- Overall = neuromuscular system
- Posterior teeth = provide vertical stops for mandibular closure; guide mandible into position of maximum inter cuspation.
- Anterior teeth = guide the mandible in Right and Left lateral excursions and in straight protrusive movements.
- Dentist has no control over posterior determinants.
- Dentist has direct control over the teeth determinants by orthodontic tooth movements selective grinding; so ICP and (AG) anterior guidance can be altered.

- The closer to a determinant a tooth is located, the more it will be influenced by that determinant. A tooth placed near the anterior region will be influenced greatly by AG and less by TMJ.

OCCLUSAL INTERFERENCES = 4 types:

- Centric
- Working
- Non-working
- Protrusive

1. **Centric interferences** = is a Premature Contact which occurs when mandible closes with condyles in a retruded, superior position in the glenoid fossa.
2. **Working interferences** = i.e. when there is a contact between maxillary and mandibular posterior teeth on the same side of arches as the direction, in which mandible is moved.
3. **Non-working interferences** = occlusal contact between maxillary and mandibular teeth on the side of arches opposite the direction, in which mouth has moved in lateral excursion.
4. **Protrusive interference** = a Premature Contact between the mesial aspect of mandibular posterior teeth and distal aspect of maxillary posterior teeth.

Normal maximum ICP is approx 1.25 ± 1 mm forward of the RCP (Retmdeol cuspal position).

- **Optimal occlusion** = i.e. which requires a minimum of adaptation by the patient.
- In normal occlusion = reflex function of neuromuscular system guides the mandible in CO.
- **Articulator** = the principle employed is the mechanical replication of the path of movement of posterior determinants, i.e. the TMJ.
- **Border movement** = the outer limits of all excursive movements made by mandible. They are controlled by ligaments.
- **Nonadjustable articulator** = is capable of only a HINGE opening; it is of smaller size.

- **Semi-adjustable articulator** = larger size; it reproduces the direction and end point, but not the intermediate track of some condylar movements (Anatomical distance of axis of rotation with the teeth is closely natural as compared with the smaller in nonadjustable articulators). Intercondylar distance does not have total adjustability. Used for bridge work.

Fully adjustable articulator—reproduces:

- Entire border movements.
- Curvature and direction of condylar movements.
- Immediate side shift.
- Completely adjustable intercondylar distance.
- Used for extensive Rx only.

Arcon articulator

- Condylar element is on lower member of articulator.
- Mechanical fossa on the upper member.
- Good for FPD but not for CD.
- Centric position is less easily maintained on arcon.

Non-arcon

- Condyle element on Upper part.
- Condylar path on Lower part.
- Best for CD.

Transfer of hinge axis

- Done by face bow.
- Most accurate method = trial and error method.

Hinge axis = at a point 13 mm anterior to the middle of the superior edge of tragus on a line from tragus to outer canthus of eye.

Pantograph tracings = for recording the condyle movement and border movements of mandible.

- Best done with fully adjustable articulators.

Definitions

1. **Bilateral Balanced Occlusion**
   - Maximum number of teeth should contact in all exclusive positions of mandible.
   - Esp. used in CD where contact on non-working side is important to prevent tipping of denture.
   - But not in natural teeth, because it leads to excessive wear and stresses on teeth.
   - Based on work of Spee and Monsoon.
2. **Unilateral BO** = widely accepted and used.
   - Based on work of Schuyler.
   - Cross arch balance is not necessary in natural teeth.
   - Here, all teeth on working side should be in contact during lateral excursion, and no contact on non-working side.

- ♦ So the group functions of teeth distributes LOAD on working sides.
- ♦ It also saves CENTRIC HOLDING CUSPS (which are mandibular buccal/maxillary lingual cusps) from excessive wear.

3. **Mutually protected occlusion**—also known as canine—protected occlusion or organic occlusion.
   - Based on the work of Stuart, Stallard, Lucia, etc.
   - Here, the anterior teeth bear all the load and posterior teeth get discluded in many excursion movements of mandible and vice versa.
   - Position of maximum inter-cuspation coincides with retruded position of mandible.
   - MOST-WIDELY ACCEPTED occlusion because of greatest ease of fabrication and patient tolerance.
   - But if Periodontal bone loss of anterior teeth is there, the mouth should be protected to group functions (i.e. unilateral balance).

PRINCIPLES OF CROWN PREPARATION

(a) Preservation of tooth structure = minimal cutting; maintain marginal topography of tooth.

(b) Retention and resistance.
(c) Structural durability.
(d) Marginal integrity.

Retention

- Prevents removal of restoration along the path of insertion or long axis of tooth preparation.
- Axial walls of preparation must be parallel or slightly tapered to permit the restoration to seat.
- A taper of 6° is optimal between opposing walls (2.5–6.5°).
- There is an INVERSE relation between taper and retention.
- Greater the surface area of preparation greater is the retention.
- Larger teeth have better retention than smaller teeth.
- Increase Surface Area by making grooves/boxes, etc.
- Retention increases by geometrically limiting the no. of paths of insertion. Maximum retention is with one path only.
- Basic unit of retention = 2 opposing axial walls with a 6° taper.

Resistance

- Prevents dislodgement of restoration by the forces directed in apical/oblique direction and prevents any movement of restoration under occlusal forces.
- The walls of preparation should be at right angle to the direction of forces for better resistance.
- Buccal and Lingual walls of the proximal box must meet the wall at 90°.
- A flare/bevel is added at cavosurface margins if gold is used. It helps in burnishing and adaptation of the restoration.

Path of insertion—An imaginary line along which the restoration will be drawn off or inserted on preparation.

- In maxillary posterior area = it should be parallel to long axis of tooth.
- In anterior teeth = should be parallel to incisal half of labial surface.

- Mesiodistal path should = parallel to the contact areas of tooth.

Structural durability—For adequate bulk of metal in restoration:

- There should be 1.5 mm occlusal clearance on functional cusps (i.e. lingual upper and buccal lower cusps).
- On non functional cusps = 1.0 mm.
- **Functional cusp bevel** = a wide bevel on LINGUAL inclines of maxillary lingual cusps and buccal inclines of mandibular buccal cusps to provide space for an adequate bulk of metal in the area of heavy occlusal contact.
- If bevel is not used = an over cut axial surface will occur.
- Offset; occlusal shoulders; isthmus; proximal grooves, boxes provide rigidity and durability.

Isthmus—Connects the boxes.

Offset—Ties the grooves together.

MARGINAL INTEGRITY

- For cast gold restoration—The finish line should be acute-angle = good for burnishing and adaptation.
- BUTT joint/shoulder finish line is poorest for Au (gold).
- For veneer gold restorations = best is **CHAMFER;** it exhibit LEAST stresses.
- **SHOULDER** = for porcelain—jacket crowns; wide ledge provides resistance to occlusal forces and minimizes stresses. Not good for gold.
- **BEVEL** = (modified) SLOPING shoulder; does not meet the axial walls and cavosurace at 90°, but makes an obtuse angle with axial wall; Good for porcelain fused to metal crowns. Good for labial finish lines for PFM in aesthetic areas. Less stress conc. on PFM.
- As gingival finish line on proximal box of inlays/onlays and MD 3/4 crowns; labial finish line in PFM.
- But more cutting of axial wall is required for this type of finish line as compared to shoulder, to give bulk for both metal and porcelain.

KNIFE EDGE = or feather-edge.

- Permits acute margin of Gold and seems to be the IDEAL FINISH line, but can create problem—because WAX–UP is difficult for V. Thin margins;
- Can result in over-contoured restorations.
- Used on LINGUAL of mandibular posterior and on teeth with very convex axial surfaces.

FINISH LINE for Bucco-occlusal margin of maxillary partial veneer crown **and MOD onlays:**

- Narrow finishing bevel perpendicular to path of insertion.
- A contra-bevel = if heavy functions.

LOCATION OF FINISH LINE

- In areas approachable for cleaning and finishing.
- Mesial extensions = should be conservative for good cosmetic effect.
- Should be placed in enamel if possible.
- Subgingival lead to periodontitis.

Cutting should be done with HIGH SPEED AIR TURBINE; low speed cause injury to tissues and overextends the preparation.

PARTIAL VENEER CROWN (PVC)

Electric pulp testing can be done on PVC, but not on fully coverage.

Most commonly used additional retentive feature in PVC is PROXIMAL GROOVE.

The occlusal finish line in maxillary teeth terminates near the bucco-occlusal angle; in mandibular teeth the finish line is approx 1 mm gingival to the lowest occlusal contact.

FOR Maxillary PVC

- First step is occlusal reduction alone.
- Reduction at functional cusp = 1.5 mm.

- Reduction at nonfunctional cusp = 1.0 mm.
  - Functional cusp bevel is given.
  - Proximal grooves placed in the more inaccessible proximal surface of molar (Distal) or more aesthetically critical surface of PMs (mesial).
- 2 grooves are joined by occlusal **offset** on the lingual inclines of buccal cusps. It reinforces the margins.
  - Bucco-occlusal finish line bevel = 0.5 mm.

Features and their functions

Chamfer	For marginal integrity
Axial reduction	Retention and resistance structural durability
Axial cusp bevel	Structural durability
Occlusal reduction	Structural durability
Occlusal offset	Structural durability
Buccal bevel	Marginal integrity
Flare at buccal proximal line angle	Marginal integrity
Proximal groove	Retention, resistance, structural durability.

Mandibular posterior PVC–(1) Occlusal reduction.

Clearance = 1.5 mm on buccal cusp/1.0 mm on lingual cusp.

Functional cusp bevel = terminates at bucco-occlusal finish line.

Occlusal shoulder = on buccal incline of buccal cusp; 1.0 mm wide; 1.0 mm gingival to the lowest occlusal contact on buccal surface.

No offset placed on lingual inclines of buccal cusps. 0.5 mm bevel on occlusal shoulder = for BO finish line.

Functional cusp bevel	Structural durability
Occ. shoulder	Structural durability
Buccal bevel	Marginal integrity
FLARE in prox. grooves	Marginal integrity
DCP reduction	Structural durability
Axial	Structural resistance pretension
Prox. grooves	Structural resistance pretension
Chamfer	Marginal integrity

7/8th PVC—Where distal/DB cusp is to be covered; mostly used in maxillary molars.

Reverse 3/4th crown

- Mostly done on mandibular molars.
- On teeth with severe lingual inclination.
- Nonfunctional cusps left uncovered.

Proximal half crown

- A PVC which has been rotated 90° so that **the distal surface**, rather than buccal, left intact.

Anterior 3/4th crown

- Path of insertion = parallel to incisal 1/3–2/3rd of labial surface (rather than long axis of tooth).
- Proximal grooves = should be lingually inclined. If inclined labially, then over-cutting of labio-incisal occurs.
- Cingulum reduced for clearance of more than 0.7 mm.
- Proximal grooves = connected by incisal OFFSET placed near the opposing occlusal contact.

FULL VENEER CROWN

It is the most retentive preparation.

- It should not be used in mouths with uncontrolled caries.

First step = occlusal reduction

- 1.5 mm clearance on functional cusps.
- 1.0 mm clearance on nonfunctional cusps.
- A wide bevel is placed on functional cusps (Buccal inclines of mandibular buccal cusps and lingual inclines of maxillary lingual cusps).
- **Chamfer line =** ***best for bulk*** required for strength and for good adaptation also.
- **Final step** = placement of seating grooves, which prevent any MD rotation of casting also. It is placed in axial surface with greatest bulk (i.e. buccal surface of mandibular and lingual surface of maxillary teeth).

For Porcelain–Fused to metal preparations

- **Coping** = metal casting which fits over the tooth.
- Has more strength than porcelain alone.
- Deep/more reduction done on facial surface of tooth to provide space for both Porcelain and Metal (1.2 mm).
- Reduce labial surface in 2 planes to avoid pulp exposure or over contouring; parallel to gingival half and parallel to incisal half.
- Ist step = orientation grooves followed by incisal reduction.
- Labial reduction is done extending to 1 mm lingual to the proximal contacts
- **Wings** = formed on proximal surface, where labial reduction (1.2 mm) ends and lingual reduction (0.7 mm) begins, its sole aim is **to conserve tooth structure**.
- Lingual reduction = 0.7 mm; do not over reduce junction between cingulum and lingual wall.
- Shoulder with bevel (0.2–0.3 mm bevel) is finish line on labial.
- Chamfer finish line on proximal and lingual surfaces.

- Mesial and Distal incisal notches placed for edges of coping to be rounded over for structural durability.
- **Shoulder alone** = to minimize gold collar at labiogingival margin.

Functions of different features

Gingival bevel	Marginal integrity
Shoulder	Structural durability
Wing	Preservation of tooth structure
Chamfer	Marginal integrity
Axial reduction	Retain, resistance, structural durability
Incisal notch	Structural durability
Functional cusp bevel	Structural durability
Occlusal reduction	Structural durability

For porcelain jacket crowns:

- Give best cosmetic effects; done only on INCISORS.
- But susceptible to fracture as it is brittle.
- Preparation should be long for better retention.
- If short preparation—the **half moon fracture occurs** due to stress concentration in labiogingival areas.
- **Finish line**—shoulder of approx 1 mm; it provides bulk to the porcelain and thus helps to resist forces.
- Do not use if there is edge-to-edge bite. Porcelain being harder, tends to abrade the natural teeth in its contact.
- Do not use if opposing tooth occludes in cervical 5th of lingual surface.
- 1.5–2.0 mm reduction on incisal edge.
- Shoulder finish line = 0.8–1.0 mm; for marginal integrity (i.e. 90° angle with cavosurface margin).
- Lingual axial reduction = wall should form a **6° taper** with gingival portion of labial wall.

INTRA-CORONAL RESTORATIONS

- Intra-coronal inlay = is the **simplest cast restoration**.
- Intra-coronal restoration = uses WEDGE type of retention; which exert outward pressure on the tooth.
- Inlay = can only be used if there is a large bulk and tooth structure is intact.
- It rarely replaces the lost tooth structure without protecting the remaining tooth.
- Inlay should be modified (with occlusal coverage) to distribute the stresses to a wider area.

Class II inlays—MO/DO

Occlusal outline should avoid occlusal wear faces and occlusal contacts. Otherwise inappropriate masticatory stresses get accumulated on the restorations.

Walls of isthmus = should have 6° taper.

Isthmus = no reverse curve is required, where the buccal part of isthmus blends with proximal box.

Bevel on occlusal isthmus = begins at the junction of occlusal 1/3 and gingival 2/3rd of isthmus wall and extends outward at 15–20°.

Class V inlay

- Retention = augmented by pins in M and D sides.
- Occlusal wall = at the HOC/height of contour of crown.
- Proximal walls = till the bucco proximal line angle.
- Walls should diverge slightly to conform with the directions of enamel rods and for easy removal of wax pattern.
- Axial wall is gently curved to follow buccal surface—otherwise it may lead to over-cutting and pulp exposure.
- Pin holes = placed near the junction of occlusal 1/3rd and gingival 2/3rd of axial surface; made 2 mm deep; help in retention.
- 45° narrow bevel at walls of preparation all around; 0.5 mm wide, (for marginal integrity).

MOD ONLAYS

MOD onlay is an inlay + occlusal surface cover to prevent stress concentration.

- Should not be used as bridge retainers.
- Maxillary tooth: 1.5 mm clearance on lingual cusps and 1.0 mm clearance on buccal cusps.
- Wide bevel on lingual inclines of lingual cusps on the functional cusp.
- Occlusal shoulder = 1.0 mm wide; 1.0 mm gingival to lowest occlusal contact on lingual cusp at the level lingual-occlusal finish line.
- **In Md. teeth** = functional cusp bevel and occlusal shoulder are on buccal cusp.

MANAGEMENT OF ROOT CANAL TREATED TOOTH

Post/Dowel core preparation

- Initial step is axial reduction.
- Canal preparation = by Peeso reamer (for removing GP and enlarging the canal).
- Post/Dowel should be = 2/3–3/4th the length of the root or at least as long as the clinical crown.
- A min. of 3 mm of RC filling should remain at the apex.

Peeso reamer size	Used for
1.2 mm diameter	• Mandibular incisors • Maxillary premolars • Molars
1.4 mm diameter	• Maxillary lateral incisor • Mandibular canine
1.6 mm diameter	• Maxillary central incisor • Maxillary canine • Mandibular premolars

- Key way prepared in RC at occlusal margins. It helps in preventing the rotation of the restoration.
- **Keyway placed** at the greatest bulk; 1 mm deep; 4 mm long.
- **Contra bevel** = around occlusal external periphery of preparation; prevents fracture of tooth structures.

In maxillary premolar = there are 2 roots, Main dowel placed in BUCCAL RC and stabilizing keyway in LINGUAL RC.

In maxillary molar = Dowel is placed in PALATAL RC.

In mandibular molar = Dowel is place in DISTAL RC.

IMPRESSIONS

Gingival cord = acts by chemical + pressure.

Contains 8% Adrenaline = local vasoconstriction; gingival shrinkage. or-Alum (aluminium potassium sulfate).

Adrenaline is contraindicated in—CVS diseases; in patients on ganglionic blockers, etc.; Hyperthyroidism; Hypersensitivity to Adrenaline. In such cases, use Alum.

Force of packing instrument should be directed towards the cord previously packed.

Impression materials

Material	Features
Agar	• Agar is a ***polymer of galactose***; obtained from seaweed; **sodium tetraborate** increases strength of gel; and viscosity of sol. • It is approx 85% water. • Least expensive; but requires special expensive instruments. • Can loose water by **SYNERESIS** (water seeping from surface). • Can absorb water by **imbibition.** • Impression can be stored in 2% K2SO4, water bath, etc. but impression starts distorting when it is removed from mouth.

Impression materials (*Contd.*)

Material	Features
	• **SO Pour immediately.** • Setting of **gypsum is RETARDED** in contact with gel; and BORAX can enhance it, a SOFT CAST formed. • So K_2SO_4 added = accelerates and hardens the stone.
Polysulfide	• also known as mercaptan/Thiokol. • Accelerator = **lead peroxide** with sulfur and oil. • Polymerization is **exothermic.** • Polymerization affected by moisture and temperature. • Has much greater dimensional stability. • Polymer contracts as curing occurs, so impression should be **poured with in 1 hr**. • **Hydrophobic** = so no moisture should be there on the prepared tooth when impression is taken.
Silicone rubber base	• Most commonly used rubber base impression material. • **Reactor** = ethyl silicate and tin octoate. • **Bye-products** = Methyl and ethyl alcohol, whose evaporation causes shrinkage. • It has **less dimensional stability** than polysulfide. • Impression should be **poured as soon as possible**. • Limited shelf life due to instability of alkyl silicates in presence of organo-tin compounds.
Polyether rubber base	• A copolymer of 12-epoxy ethane and tetra-hydro-furan. • Esterification reaction = by unsaturated acid. **Sulfinate** = as **cross-linkage agent**.

Impression materials (*Contd.*)

Material	Features
	• Much larger volume of base is used than the accelerator (slightly less than 8:1). Has ***excellent D-stability*** = can be poured after a long time also. • Material has affinity for water; impression should not be stored in humidor/moist atmosphere.

Type	Advantages	Disadvantages
Reversible hydrocolloid	• No custom tray required • Some **moisture tolerated** in sulcus • Clean and pleasant • Easy to pour • **Inexpensive**	• **Must be poured immediately** • Finish lines difficult to read
Polysulfide rubber base	• No special equipment required • Finish lines easily read • **Cast pour can be delayed to 1 hr** • Can be **silver plated** • **Can be poured more than once**	• Custom tray required • **Hydrophobic** • **Objectionable odour** • Messy–clothes can be ruined by contact • Requires special care in pouring
Silicone rubber base	• No special equipment required • **Superior strength** in deep sulcus • Finish lines easy read • Pleasant odour and appearance	• **Must be poured immediately** • **Hydrophobic** • Easily distorted • **Expensive**

(*Contd.*)

Type	Advantages	Disadvantages
Polyether	• No special equipment required • Fast setting • Finish lines easy read • **Pouring cast can be delayed** • **Can be poured more than once**	• Custom tray required • **Expensive** • Severe undercuts must be blocked • Requires special care in pouring

Working cast = is the cast, which is mounted on the articulator.

Die = is a model of the individual prepared tooth, on which the margin of wax pattern are finished.

Articulation of casts

- U/L arches relationship should be developed with the condyle in most posterosuperior position in glenoid fossa (CR).
- Mounting for diagnosis is done with the mandible in retruded position.
- Mounting for limited Rx is done in inter–cuspal position (to avoid interferences).
- **INDEXING** = soft wax placed against upper arch and patient is asked to bite lightly to get the impression of cusp tips.

CONDYLAR GUIDANCE/CG

- TMJ influences the movements of mandible.
- CG = not under the control of operator.
- Occlusal morphology of restoration should be in harmony with movements of mandible to prevent trauma form occlusion and premature contacts (TFO and PC).

Wax patterns (Also refer to the section of dental materials in Vol. II.)

- Indirect technique is better than direct = as chair side time is avoided; margins are directly visible for finishing.
- Type I wax = for making intraoral wax patterns.

- Type II wax = for extra-oral wax patterns.
- The wax patterns should be SLIGHTLY OVERSIZED mesiodistally = s.t. the finished casting will have adequate proximal contacts.
- Proximal contacts are located slightly to the facial of middle of the posterior teeth, except between max 6, 7, which is centred facio-lingually.
- So the lingual embrasures are slightly larger than the facial.
- HOC on facial surfaces of all posterior teeth = in cervical 3rd.
- HOC on lingual surface of max PMs and Ms = cervical 3rd.
- HOC on mandibular teeth = in middle 3rd.
- Over contouring of surfaces promotes gingival inflamers (by collection of plaque); the under contouring does not.

Occlusal morphology

- Waxing of occlusal surface is done in the last after axial surface waxing is complete.
- Lingual cusp of upper and buccal cusps of lower posterior teeth occlude in occlusal fossa or the marginal ridges of opposing teeth. These are also known as **FUNCTIONAL cusps.**
- Buccal cusps of upper and lingual cusps of lower are also known as **nonfunctional cusps**; protect soft tissues; prevent food from overflowing.
- **2 types of occlusal schemes** = cusp-fossa and cusp-marginal ridge.

Cusp-fossa	**Cusp-MR**
Tooth contact is occlusal fossa only	In occlusal fossa and MR.
Tooth-to-tooth contact.	Tooth-to-2 teeth contact
Occlusal forces parallel to long axis of tooth; near the centre of tooth.	
Used for full mouth/several teeth.	Most cast restorations done in restoration daily practice.
Rarely present in natural teeth.	MOST NATURAL TYPE occlusion, in 95% of adults.

MANDIBULAR CUSP PLACEMENT

Mandibular buccal cusp	Maxillary occlusal surface	
	Cusp MR	**Cusp fossa**
First premolar	MMR of first premolar	Mesial fossa of first premolar
Second premolar	DMR of first premolar, MMR second premolar	Mesial fossa of second premolar
MB cusp of first molar	DMR second premolar, MMR first molar	Mesial fossa of first molar
DB cusp of first molar	Central fossa of first molar	Central fossa of first molar
Distal cusp of first molar	Non functional	Distal fossa of first molar
MB cusp of second molar	DMR of first molar, MMR second molar	Mesial fossa of second molar
DB cusp of second molar	Central fossa of second molar	Central fossa of second molar
D cusp of second molar	Not present	Non functional

MAXILLARY CUSP PLACEMENT

Maxillary lingual cusps	Mandibular occlusal surface	
	Cusp MR	**Cusp Fossa**
First premolar	Distal fossa of first premolar	Distal fossa of first premolar
Second premolar	Distal fossa of second premolar	Distal fossa of second premolar

MAXILLARY CUSP PLACEMENT (*Contd.*)

Maxillary lingual cusps	Mandibular occlusal surface	
	Cusp-MR	**Cusp-Fossa**
ML cusp of first molar	Central fossa of first molar	Central fossa of first molar
DL cusp of first molar	DMR of first molar + MMR of second molar	Distal fossa of first molar
ML cusp of second molar	Central fossa of second molar	Central fossa of second molar
DL cusp of second molar	DMR of second molar	Distal fossa of second molar

- ♦ Lingual cusp of maxillary premolars fall in Distal fossa of mandibular PM.
- ♦ ML cusps of maxillary molars fall in central fossa of mandibular teeth.
- ♦ DL cusps of maxillary molars fall at DMR of mandibular molars and distal fossa of mandibular molars.

Triangular ridges

- ♦ Extend from central groove to cusp tip. Are known as triangular, because they are much wider at their base than at the cusp tips.
- ♦ Buccolingual dimension of each occlusal table formed by the ridges should be approx 55% of the overall BL dim. of the respective tooth.
- ♦ In working movement = the buccal cusp of each maxillary PM passes distal to the buccal cusp of its counterpart in the mandibular arch. So a concavity is placed in the distal inclines of buccal cusps of mandibular premolars. This depression is the **THOMAS NOTCH**.
- ♦ During working, the MB cusp of maxillary molar passes through the buccal groove, distal to the MB cusp of mandibular molars

and DB cusp of maxillary molar pass the DB groove mandibular molars.

- Also, the lingual cusps of mandibular molars should be short enough such that they do not collide with cusps of maxillary molars.
- **Fish's mouth** = is so named because of the appearance of cusp and MR at this point.
- TRIPOD contact should be formed about the cusp tips and in the fossa. The contacts should be the point contacts.
- In non-working movement, the ML cusp of maxillary molar passes distal to DB cusp of mandibular molar (i.e. through DB groove). So a notch is formed on distal incline of DB cusp.
- Also, **DB cusp** of mandibular molar moves in a ML direction across of the buccal incline of ML cusp of maxillary molar. So a groove is placed in ML cusp of maxillary molar, directed mesiolingually from central fossa. It is the **STUART'S GROOVE.**

Rules

1. Cusp height depends on inclination of protrusive path (condyle).
   If inclination is steep-longer cusps required.
   If inclination is less steep-shorter cusps required.
2. Deep bite (I G)-longer cusps required (CH).
   If less bite (I G)-shorter cusps required (CH).
3. Overjet if more-shorter cusps required.
   If overjet less-longer cusps required.
4. If protrusive condylar path is shallow and cusps must be made short, the longer cusps can be used if anterior guidance is increased.
5. A pronounced immediate side shift-shorter cusps required.
   A gradual side shift-longer cusps required.
6. A pronounced immediate side shift requires shorter cusps if little IG is there. But CH can be increased if IG is increased.
7. Angle between working and non-working path is greater on the teeth located farther from condyle.

INVESTING and CASTING (Also refer to the section of dental materials in vol. II.)

- Gold alloy shrink = 1.5% during solidification = known as solidification shrinkage.
- Gypsum bonded investment.

  Type I = uses thermal expansion.

  Type II = hygroscopic.
- Matrix = gypsum (a-$CaSO_4$ 1/2 H_2O = 30–35) acts as binder.
- Refractory filler = Silica (quartz/cristoballite) 60–65%.
- Chemical modifiers.

Dimensional compensations = uses setting expansion SE + thermal expansion TE.

SE = is due to normal crystal growth; it can be augmented by allowing the setting to occur in presence of H_2O producing HSE; this replaces the water used during HYDRATION process and so the space between crystals is maintained and they can continue to expand outwards; maximum HSE is by immersing the ring in 100°F water bath.

TE = is achieved through normal expansion which occurs upon heating the silica and phase changes, which occur in the material.

3 purposes of investment:

1. Precisely detailed reproduction of anatomical form.
2. Strong enough to withstand the heat of burnout.
3. Compensation expansion equal to the solidification shrinkage of molten alloy.

SPRUE: 10–12 gauge.

- It provides inlet for the molten metal into the casting.
- Attached at a point of greatest bulk.
- At an angle to allow free flow of incoming molten metal.
- If used at thin areas or very small size = may lead to SHRINK SPOT POROSITY.

- For uniform expansion = the pattern should be placed in the centre of the ring and should be surrounded by a uniform thickness of the investment.
- Sprue should be long enough— s.t. highest point of wax pattern is 6 mm from the end of the ring.
- For adequate solidification = the sprue itself should not be longer than 6 mm.

Investing

- 1 mm thick ASBESTOS—to act as buffer zone. It allows expansion outwards to enlarge the mold. If it is not there the expansion forces will occur towards the mold leading to contraction/distortions.
- Liner should be 3 mm shorter on both ends of the ring so as to restrict expansion near the open end of the ring.
- Wet asbestos gives extra expansion of HSE type.
- Double layer provides more expansion.
- Invest under vacuum to avoid BUBBLES.
- W/P ratio should be controlled; more water means less expansion.
- Over spatulation increases the TE.

Burn out

- To remove the wax.
- Prepares the mold for molten metal.
- Allows TE to occur.
- Higher heat technique = at 1200°F for TE.
- For HSE = 1000° F used
- First burn out at 600° F × 30 min.
- Put in inverted position, s.t. wax comes out.
- Then place at 900° or 1200° F for 1 hour.
- Allow oxygen to contact the ring for 10 min before casting is made = to ensure complete wax elimination.
- The casting should be done within 30 sec; any delay may lead to heat loss and mold contraction.
- Give 3 winds to the right hand of casting machine.

USE blue/reducing/hottest zone of flame to heat the alloy.

On proper heating—the alloy is straw yellow colour; wiggles easily; appears shiny and mirror—like; and moves with the flame.

Put some flux in molten metal—to increase fluidity and to prevent oxide formation.

Quench the ring—helps to anneal the metal for better working qualities and also disintegrates the investment for easy removal.

Pickling—done to cleanse the casting.

Phosphate bonded investment

- Used for non precious alloys and for gold-platinum alloy for PFM restorations.
- Temperature = 2100° F used (If gypsum bonded is used at higher temperature, the $CaSO_4$ is disintegrated and sulfur is released which contaminates the mold).
- Mg PO_4 + Ammonium PO_4 form Mg–Ammonium PO_4 = provide STRENGTH at room temperature.
- At high temperature = silico-phosphates produced give more strength.
- Liquid = of ***colloidal silica suspension*** is used.
- Graphite and silica are present in powder.
- More silica sol + less water = more expansion.
- Less silica sol + more water = less expansion.
- Usual ratio = 3:1 = silica sol to water ratio.
- Overall liquid powder ratio = 9.5 C.C/60 gm powder.
- It possesses poor surface—wetting characteristics.
- Setting allowed for 1 hour on bench.
- HSE (0.7%) if required = place in 100° F H_2O.
- Then at 600°F × 30 mm.
- Then at 1300°F × 1 hr.
- A silica crucible should be used, without asbestos, instead of clay crucible.
- Heat the alloy till white/shiny and then cast it.

FINISHING AND CEMENTATION

Beilby layer—During polishing, minute amounts of abraded surface materials are filled in the surface irregularities, forming a microcrystalline surface layer.

Abrasives—Should be much harder than the material on which it is used.

Substance	KHN
Dentin	68
Amalgam	110
Type III gold	145
Enamel	343
Cr-Co-alloy	350
Porcelain	460
Sand (flint)	800
Al_2O_3	2000
Emery	2000
Si-carbide	2500
Diamond	8200

Material	Features
Diamond	Hardest; Should be used on hard, brittle substances, e.g. Enamel/porcelain. The soft/ductile substance, e.g. Au tend to choke the abrasive particles.
Silicon carbide	Very commonly used e.g. carborundum discs; separating discs/joe-dandy discs; wheels/points/green stones.
Emery	Is a mixture of Al_2O_3 and Fe_2O_3. Bound to paper disc. Used on gold/porcelain.

Material	Features
Aluminum oxide	Al_2O_3 is produced from bauxite 400 grit. Used in white polishing stones known as **POLY-**STONES.
Garnet	Red in colour. Silicates of Al and Fe with Mg. Co. Mn, etc. Used for metal/porcelain.
Sand	Quartz known as flint is used. Sharp cutting edges. Various grits of sand paper available.
Tripoli	Fine siliceous powder with wax. Used for initial polishing steps.
Rouge	Iron oxide Fe_2O_3. Is finest of polishing agents used on gold casting. Used on crocus discs also.

Occlusal adjustment

- U/L anterior teeth should not touch in CR; the gap should be = 0.0005″.
- Non-working side adjustments are done by removing contacts on buccal incline of maxillary lingual cusp and lingual inclines of mandibular buccal cusps.
- Working side adjustments are done by removing contacts on lingual inclines of maxillary lingual cusps and buccal inclines of mandibular lingual cusps.
- Contacts between lingual inclines of maxillary buccal cusps and buccal inclines of mandibular buccal cusps should be removed if mutually protected occlusion is required and should not be removed if group function occlusion is required.

- Protrusive interferences are removed by adjusting mesial inclines of mandibular teeth and distal inclines of max teeth.
- Surface roughness on the margin is found approx 40 micron, which can be decreased to 8 micron by petrolatum and cuttle disc polishing on a white stone. Green stone should not be used.

PONTICS

- Area of contact between ridge and pontic should be small.
- Part of pontic which is near the ridge should be CONVEX and smooth.
- Pontic should exert no pressure on ridge.
- Mesial, distal, and lingual embrasures should be WIDE open for easy cleaning.
- Pontic is narrower (esp. from lingual surfaces) than the natural tooth so as to align it on the inter-abutment axis. It helps in preventing the torquing of abutments/retainers and also plaque accumulation.

Designs of pontics

Design	Features
Saddle	• Replaces all contours of missing tooth. • Fills embrasures and overlaps the ridge with a large concave contact. • Impossible to clean. • Should never be used.
Ridge lap	• Has all CONVEX surfaces for easy cleaning. • Used in appearance zone, i.e. U/L anteriors for esthetics.
Hygienic	• No contact with the tissues; 2–3 mm gap. • Also known as SANITARY pontic. • Esp used in nonappearance zone (mandibular posteriors). • Restores occlusal function; stability of teeth;

Designs of pontics (*Contd.*)

Design	Features
	• Occlusogingival thickness should not be less than 3 mm.
Conical/bullet/ spheroidal modified ridge lap	• Cleanable, but triangular space around the tissues may collect debris.

PIN FACINGS

Reverse pin facing = has good retention where a deep bite would force the use of very short pins in the conventional facing.

PFM facing = used when maximum esthetics is required esp in anterior teeth.

Harmony facing = is most frequently used for fabricating the maxillary posterior pontics. Is not useful if occlusogingival dim. is short.

Pin facing = is used where occlusogingival space is limited.

Modified pin facing = made by adding porcelain to the lingual gingival area of a pin facing.

Junction between gold and porcelain should not cross the facet of wear, otherwise heavy forces may cause dislodgement of facing.

At least 1 mm clearance should be there between porcelain and the opposing facial cusp.

SOLDERING

- **Soldering** = is joining of metal parts by a filler metal/solder.
- Bonding occurs due to wetting of joined surfaces by the solder and not by the melting of metal components.
- **Welding** = the metal parts are joined by melting and fusing together, without solder.
- **Flux** = displaces gases, removes corrosion products by either combining with them or reducing them.

- **Flux** = 55% Sodium pyroborate + 35% Boric acid + 10% Silica.
- Paste of flux should be made with petrolatum, as it burns off without leaving any residue.
- Paste made with water tend to effloresce when they are heated; it produces pits in the joints and weaken them.
- **Antiflux** = used to outline the area to be soldered to limit the flow of solder, e.g. graphite pencil; rouge suspended in chloroform.
- **Karat** = i.e. parts per 24 of a metal which is gold.
- **Fineness** = i.e. parts per 100 of solder which is gold.
- However, with solder, 18 karat means that it's to be used with 18 K gold casting alloy.
- Actual precious metal content of a solder is given by = its fineness rather than karat.
- **580 fine is the minimum fineness,** which should be used for corrosion resistance.
- Solder should have fusion range about 100–150°C below that of the metal being soldered.
- If base metal % age is increased in solder, it leads to PITTING of the joint.
- Solder should be free flowing. Ag makes it free-flow and Cu makes it sluggish.
- Soldering investment = is made of quartz with low setting expansion, should be one inch thick.
- Used to solder pontic with retainers in a bridge.
- Gap between retainer pontic should be approx 0.005″, and their surface should be parallel to each other; the solder flows in the gap by capillary action. If no gap, it leads to distortion. If wide gap, then no proper flow of solder occurs.
- Solder is fed from lingual side; buccal side is used for heating the casting during soldering.
- Preheat the invested casting to 1500°F.
- Blue zone of flame is used.
- **Do not quench** or thermal stresses/distortion may occur.

- If kept for bench cooling to room temperature—crystallization and grain growth is excessive and so weaker joint occurs.
- **Best procedure is to** bench cool for 5 min. and then quench. Minimum distortion occurs; ordering heat Rx occurs, strength and hardness increase.
- Polishing rouge, i.e. (Fe_2O_3) is also an anti-flux for soldering—so do not use it before soldering.
- In non-rigid connectors, the path of the insertion of key way is aligned with the distal abutment.

PORCELAIN

- Most aesthetic material.
- Non-crystalline glasses having Si and O_2.
- It should be low fusing. The fusing temperature is decreased by reducing cross linking between Si and O_2 with the help of glass-modifiers (e.g. Potassium oxide, Na_2O and Ca-oxide but they decrease viscosity).
- So Al_2O_3 is used to maintain viscosity.

Types	Temperature in F	Temperature in C
High fusing	2350–2500 F	1290–1370
Medium fusing	2000–2300 F	1000–1260
Low fusing	1600–1950 F	860–1070

High fusing

- Used for making porcelain teeth.
- It has feldspar (70–90%) + quartz (11–18%) + Kaolin (1–10%).
- **Feldspar**—glassy, translucency, matrix.
- Quartz—refractory.
- Kaolin—Binder.

Low and medium fusing porcelains—are produced by:

- **FRITTING**
- Addition of metallic oxides (Zr, Tr, Sn) make the porcelain OPAQUE—used to mask metal coping in PFM restorations.
- Yellow colour to porcelain is given = By In
- Pink colour to porcelain = Cr/Sn
- Black colour to porcelain = Fe
- Blue colour to porcelain = Co

Porcelain jacket Crown

- 0.001″ Pt foil is adapted on the die.
- Porcelain **firing** = started at 1500° F and reach at 1900°F in six minutes—under vacuum.

PFM restorations = stronger than porcelain.

- Combine strength and accuracy of metal + esthetics of porcelain.
- Coping = is the metal casting which fits over the prepared tooth. Porcelain is fused to the coping.
- Coping is covered with 3 layers of porcelain.

1. **Opaque**—Covers metal underneath.
2. **Body** —Makes the bulk of restoration.
   —Provides most of the colour/shade.
3. **Incisal area**—Translucent layer in incisal part.

- Bonding of porcelain to metal is through OXIDE LAYER, and is adhesive.
- Bond strength increases when firing is done in oxidizing atmosphere.
- Failure occurs in porcelain rather than at Porcelain—metal interface.
- Coeff of thermal expansion of Au alloy = 14×10^{-6}/°C.
- Coeff of thermal porcelain = 2–4 × 10^{-6}/°C.
- The ideal difference should be 1×10^{-6}/°C, as a difference of 1.7×10^{-6}/°C can produce shear stresses.
- So coeff of porcelain is increased by ALKALI (e.g. lithium carbonate) to 7–8 × 10^{-6}/°C.

- Coeff of metal is decreased by adding Pd or Pt to 7–8 × 10^{-6}/°C.
- Min. different between MP of metal and porcelain should be 300–500°F to avoid flow/creep of metal. So MP of porcelain should be lower than metal.
- Most satisfactory metals with porcelain have high gold (83–87%) + Pt (6–16%).
- Also ***Sn is there to form OXIDE layer,*** which gives bonding strength.
- Absolute min. thickness of porcelain is 0.7 mm and optimum thickness is 1.0 mm.
- Outer junction of metal with porcelain should be a butt joint to provide bulk to the porcelain and hence strength.
- For proper strength and rigidity—the coping should be 0.3–0.5 mm thick.
- **Occlusal contacts** = should be placed on the metal on all posterior restorations and should be **away from P-M junction,** otherwise porcelain may get fractured.
- On maxillary anteriors on lingual side, the junction should not be placed in the vicinity of those contacts with mandibular teeth. But approx 2.0 mm from the contact.
- P–M junction should not be too far incisally or porcelain may fracture and also **translucency decreases.**
- Porcelain is stronger in compression.
- Proximal contact for anterior teeth should be on porcelain for better esthetics.
- On maxillary posterior teeth, the buccal porcelain covers cusp tips and 1/3rd the lingual inclines of buccal cusp.
- On mandibular teeth = the entire occlusal surface should be in **METAL.**
- On first premolar, the mesial half of occlusal surface can be covered with porcelain, because contact is only in DISTAL FOSSA.
- Proximal contact on posterior teeth should be in **metal** except mesial surface of maxillary first premolar.

- In PFM bridges—porcelain is extended on the tissue surface of pontics to avoid plaque accumulation. The thickness should be 0.5 mm.
- Surface contaminants are removed by pickling the casting in 52% HF acid for 20 min. in a sealed polyethylene container in an ultrasonic cleaner.
- **Degassing**—removes H_2 gas from coping surface so as to avoid bubbles in porcelain. Place the coping in furnace at 1200°F in vacuum till 15 min.
- Opaque porcelain is applied first to mask the metal and to give proper shade. A 0.5 mm thickness is fired from 1200°–1750°F.

Body porcelain

- Incisal 1/3rd of restoration is built up with incisal porcelain, which has less colour and more translucency.
- The restoration should be over-contoured by 1/5th to compensate for 20% shrinkage during firing.
- Glazing = from 1200° to 1800° F firing.

SHADE MATCHING

- Should be done under more than one type of light.
- **Metamerism** = is a phenomenon of an object appearing to be of different colour when viewed in different light sources.
- **Hue** = quality which distinguishes one colour from another.
- **Chroma** = is saturation or strength of a hue.
- **Value/brightness** = is relative amount of lightness or darkness in a hue. It is the single most important factor in shade matching. Higher value means lighter shade and vice-versa.
- Observation of shade should be quick (10–15 sec.) to avoid **fatiguing** the cones in retina.
- Observer should glance at **BLUE** object while resting his eyes.
- Shade should be matched by value, saturation and hue (VSH) in that order.
- Shade should be matched before the tooth preparation is started. The tooth gets dehydrated during preparation.

Complete Dentures

General features and important points

- **Bennett movement** = condyle of working side moves laterally.
- **Bennett angle** = condyle on non-working side moves forwards and mesially.
- **Working side** = the side towards which the mandible deviates in lateral excursive movements.
- **Non-working side** = the side away from which the mandible deviates in lateral excursive movements.
- Restorations are usually built in RCP as this is the most reproducible position.
- In 80–90% of the population, RCP = is < 2 mm posterior to ICP.
- **Terminal hinge axis** = an axis passing through the lower part of the condyles, about which the condyles rotate when they are in their uppermost centred position in the glenoid fossa.
- **Retention** = is the resistance to displacement of a denture **away from the ridge**.
- **Support** = is the resistance of **vertical movement** of a denture towards the ridge.
- **Stability** = is the ability of a denture to resist displacement by functional stresses. It gives physiological comfort.
- **Saddle** = that part of the alveolus from which teeth are missing.

Overdenture—is a prosthesis that gains support form one or more abutment teeth by enclosing them beneath its fitting surfaces.

Immediate denture = is a prosthesis used to replace one or more teeth and inserted on the day of extraction of the tooth or teeth.

Complete denture

- The principal functions of periodontium are support and positional adjustment of the tooth, together with the secondary and dependent function of sensory perception.
- The most prominent feature of physiological occlusal forces is their intermittent, rhythmic and dynamic nature.
- The greatest forces acting on the teeth are normally produced during mastication and deglutition.
- Deglutition occurs about 500 times a day and tooth contacts during swallowing are of longer duration than those occurring during chewing.

Total time calculated during 24 hrs during chewing

1. Actual chewing time per meal = 450 sec.
2. Total chewing time for 4 meals = 1800 sec.
3. Each second 1 chewing stroke = 1800 strokes.
4. Duration of each chewing stroke = 0.3 sec.
5. So total chewing time = 1800 × 0.3 = 540 sec. = 9 min.

Total duration of swallowing in 24 hrs

1. Duration of 1 deglutitional movement during meals = 1 sec.
2. During chewing 3 × per minute 1/3 of movements with occlusal forces only = 30 sec.
3. Between meals, in day time is 25 per hr for 16 hrs = 400 sec.
4. During sleep, 10 per hr for 8 hrs = 80 sec.
5. So total = 540 + 30 + 400 + 80 = 1050 sec = 17.5 min.

- So the total time during which the teeth are subjected to functional forces of mastication and deglutition during an entire day amounts to ***approx 17.5 min***.
- **Masticatory forces**—44 lbs; it is very much less than can be produced by conscious efforts.

- Maximum masticatory **forces by complete dentures** = 13–16 lbs.
- The mean **denture bearing area in maxillary** edentulous arch = 22.96 cm^2.
- The mean **denture bearing area in mandibular** edentulous arch = 12.25 cm^2.
- The **areas of PDL of natural teeth** = 45 cm^2 in each arch, which is more than 3.5 times the average area of the basal seat of a mandibular complete denture.
- Alveolar bone supporting natural teeth receives tensile loads through a larger area of PDL; but the edentulous residual ridge receives vertical, diagonal, and horizontal loads applied by a denture having less surface area.
- Denture wearing is almost invariably accompanied by an undesirable bone loss.
- Oro-facial and tongue ms play an important role in retaining and stabilizing the CD. It occurs by setting the teeth in the **neutral zone** in the area of the ms functional balance.
- **Centric relation**—is the most posterior relation of the mandible to the maxilla at the established vertical relation. It coincides with a reproducible **posterior hinge position** of the mandible. It depends on both structural and functional harmony of osseous structures, the intra-articular tissues, and capsular ligament of TMJ.
- Unconscious swallowing is carried out with the mandible at or near the CR position. Unconscious or reflex swallow is important during the developing dentition.
- The contact of the inclined planes of the teeth aid in the alignment of the erupting teeth.
- **Centric occlusion**—the most functional natural tooth contacts occur in a mandibular position anterior to that of CR, which is known as CO.

Morphological changes associated with edentulous state

1. Deepening of the nasolabial groove.
2. Loss of labiodental angle.

3. Decrease in horizontal labial angle.
4. Narrowing of the lips.
5. Increase in columella-philtral angle.
6. Prognathic appearance.
7. Lip pursing.

TISSUE RESPONSE TO CD

- Soft tissue hyperplasia occurring around the borders of the CD = is fibrous; known as **epulis fissuratum**; it occurs in free mucosa ***lining the sulcus or the junction of attached and free mucosa***, due to chronic irritation from ill-fitting or overextended denture;
- **Denture stomatitis** = is chronic inflammation on basal seat; it occurs due to trauma from ill-fitting denture or a parafunctional habit. Candidal infection or irritation from residual monomer is

Changes in the size of the basal seat

Maxillary arch	Mandibular arch
Bone reduction is **upward and inwards.** Resorption from outer cortex is greater and more rapid as it is more thinner.	**Anterior area** = bone resorption occurs on labial and alveolar area; so the ridge migrates lingually and inferiorly. **Posterior area** = bone resorbed on lingual side so the ridge moves buccally.
Denture bearing surface/ basal seat becomes smaller in all dimensions.	**The mandibular arch becomes wider posteriorly**; so the failure to place the artificial teeth in the natural teeth site may hamper denture support and stability.
Maxillary arch becomes narrower with time both anteriorly and posteriorly.	Outer cortex is thicker than the lingual cortex except in the molar area.

also a cause; it is ***more common in maxillary arch***; it may be granular known as ***papillary hyperplasia*** or papillomatosis.

- To take an impression of hyperplastic tissues, ***the mucostatic impression materials*** should be used.
- ***Denture sore mouth*** = is mainly due to the result of an underlying abnormal metabolic or hormonal function or nutritional deficiency.

HOUSE'S CLASSIFICATION OF PATIENTS

Types	Features
Philosophical	• *Accept the judgement of their dentist without questions.* • *Have* **ideal situation for successful Rx.** • *They know that dentist will do best.*
Indifferent	• Have ***little concern for their oral health.*** • Seek Rx on the insistence of family members. • Give up the Rx easily if problems arise.
Critical	• ***Find fault in everything*** done for them. • ***Never happy*** with previous dentist as he did not follow their instructions. • Must not be allowed to direct the Rx according to them.
Skeptical	• Had bad results with previous dentist. • Doubtful that any other can help them. • Are often in poor health, e.g. severely resorbed ridges. • Dentist should take more time than usual for examining such patients.

Hard and soft tissue areas in maxillary basal seat

Ideal layer should be **firm and resilient**.

1. **Torus palatinus**—should be relieved or removed.
2. **Incisive papillae**—relieve denture here to avoid pressure on blood vessels and nerves.
3. Flabby maxillary tuberosity—should be surgically removed.
4. Zygomatic process of maxillary bone as it crosses the buccal vestibule on both sides.
5. Pterygomaxillary notch—is very important for the maximum breadth to the PPS area of the CD.

Hard and soft tissue areas in mandibular basal seat

1. **Torus mandibularis**—mostly in premolar areas on lingual side = relieve or remove.
2. Hard areas of the attachment of **mentalis ms,** which come to lie close to the alveolar crest in badly resorbed ridges—**no surgery** is indicated to remove them; relieve them by modifying the denture bases.
3. **Buccal shelf**—is made of ***cortical bone***; lies on the body of mandible b/w the buccal frenum and retromolar pad and b/w the residual ridge crest and external oblique line. It has a covering of the suctorial pad and attachment of **buccinator ms.**
4. **Retromolar pad area**—***cannot supply support***; but covered to provide border seal; should not be displaced from relaxed position as some movable structures, e.g. **buccinator, superior constrictor m, and pterygomandibular raphe** pass through it. Also fibbers from temporalis ms and some mucous glands are present.
5. **Fibrous cord like ridges**—should not be displaced; do not provide any support to the CD; its surgical removal can be problematic as it detaches mucosa from the mandible, and so the mucous membrane over the ridge can get pulled forward by lip and backward by tongue.

- Teeth replacement in case of Class II and Class III m.o. requires that ***the artificial teeth should be in the position of natural teeth***.

RIDGE FORM

- Ideal ridge has a broad top and parallel sides.
- When the mandibular ridge is sharp and has sharp bone spicules then = **selective pressure impression technique** is used so that more force is placed on buccal shelf area.
- When the sharp ridge has disappeared = use **minimum pressure technique** so that occlusal forces are distributed more evenly.

RIDGE RELATIONS

- Bones of maxilla resorb primarily from the occlusal surface and the buccal and labial surfaces, so that upper residual ridge **becomes shorter Antero-Posteriorly and narrower from side-to-side**.
- Mandibular ridge resorbs primarily from occlusal surface, so mandibular **ridge in posterior part becomes wider**, because the inferior border of mandible is broader than the occlusal part. The cross section shrinkage in mandible is downward and outward;
- The cross shrinkage in anterior part is D and B first; later on the basal seat moves forward.

SHAPE OF PALATAL VAULT

- ***Most ideal form*** = which has a medium depth with a well-defined incline of the rugae area in the anterior part of the palate.
- A **flat palatal vault** = gives insufficient resistance to a forward movement of upper denture.
- A **high narrow V-shaped vault** = unfavourable for the retention of the CD.

TONGUE

- Tongue becomes larger if a loose denture is there in the mouth as the patient uses it to hold the denture in place.
- A small tongue causes a problem for mandibular CD = the small tongue drops back away from the lower anteriors and thus break the border seal.

SALIVA

- ***Ideal saliva*** = moderate flow of serous saliva.
- Excessive saliva = complicates the impression making.
- Absence of saliva/***Xerostomia*** = ***affects retention***; so reduced retention. Also the lips and cheeks stick to the denture.
- Thick and ropy saliva = gets build up below the denture bases and can force the CD out of its correct position. Also complicates impression by making voids in the cast; may cause gagging.

Pre-prosthetic considerations

- **Upper labial frenum** may have a strong band of ***fibrous connective tissues*** that attaches on lingual side of the crest of residual ridge = should be removed surgically.
- **Hyperplastic maxillary tuberosity** should be removed for better base; to reduce undercuts; avoid opening in maxillary sinus.
- **Mandibular tori** should be surgically removed to prevent undercuts; and to improve border seal.
- High mandible and low maxillary attachments reduce the denture bearing area and affect the border seal; so the **vestibuloplasty** is advised. It is restricted to interpremolar area as in the posterior area, buccinator m does not give any problem. **Most frequent site is the anterior part of the body of mandible and the mentalis m** attachment migrates to the crest of the residual ridge obliterating the labial sulcus.
- Obliterated pterygomaxillary fossa/**hamular notch** = undermines the retention and PPS; so it should be deepened surgically.
- **Mental foramen** = due to extreme resorption, it comes to lie on the crest having sharp edges 2–3 mm higher than adjacent bone; **best way** is to provide relief in the denture so that no pressure fall on the nerves.

Basal seat—foundation of the denture is known as basal seat.

Fibrous connective tissues are present in those areas, where the external forces are applied; but glandular tissues are not found in those areas.

Support for the maxillary denture

- Use that impression technique which equalizes the pressure distribution.
- Midline palatal suture and raphe = should be relieved.

Stress bearing areas

- **Primary SBA** = residual ridge; is covered with fibrous connective tissues.
- **Secondary SBA** = rugae; it can resist the forward movement of the denture; it shouldn't be distorted during impression.
- Glandular area in posterior part of palate on either side of the midline = aids in retention; should not be subjected to significant occlusal forces.

Stress bearing areas	**Maxillary**	**Mandibular**
Primary SBA	Crest of the residual alveolar ridge	Buccal shelves
Secondary SBA	Rugae	Slopes of the alveolar ridges
Non SBA	Incisive papillae mid-palatal raphe	*Crest of alveolar ridge*

Incisive papillae (Refer selection of teeth also.)

- Lies behind and b/w the central incisors.
- Foramen carries the nasopalatine nerves and vessels; it ***should be relieved in denture*** to avoid disruption in blood and nerve supply.
- With resorption, it comes near to the crest of the alveolar ridge.
- Its location indicates the amount of the resorption.
  - **Zygomatic/malar process** = located **opposite the first molar region**. ***Relief*** is required to aid in retention and prevent the soreness.

- **Maxillary tuberosity**—if excess fibrous tissue is there, it prevents the proper location of occlusal plane.
- **Torus palatinus**—hampers in retention; ***should be relieved*** in denture; if large then it is removed surgically.
- **Maxillary labial frenum**—is a **fold of mucous membrane** in the median line; ***has no muscles***; no action of its own; should be ***relieved*** in denture.
- **Orbicularis oris m**—its tone depends on the support provided by the labial flange; its fibres pass horizontally through the lip and anastomose with fibres of buccinator m.
- **Buccal frenum**—caninus m (***levator anguli oris***) is attached below it; requires more clearance for its function. It is affected by 3 ms, i.e. orbicularis oris, buccinator, caninus.

Buccal vestibule

- Extends from buccal frenum to hamular notch; used for the buccal flange of denture.
- Its size varies with the contraction of **buccinator**.
- Thickness of distal end of buccal flange is adjusted to accommodate the ramus and coronoid process and masseter m during functions.
- ***Masseter m on contraction under heavy pressure*** reduces the size of the space available for distal end of buccal flange.
- This space is usually higher than any other part of the border.
- It is altered by lateral movement of the mandible.
- Zygomatic process is unyielding and **requires relief**.

Pterygomaxillary/hamular notch

- Is b/w tuberosity of maxilla and hamulus of medial pterygoid plate.
- Is used as boundary of posterior border of maxillary denture back to the tuberosity.
- *No ms or ligament is present.*
- PPS is placed through the centre of this notch.

Palatine fovea

- Are formed by the collection of several ***mucous gland*** ducts.
- Are close to the vibrating line; are always in soft tissues.
- Acts as ***ideal guide for location of posterior border*** of denture.

Vibrating line of the palate

- Marks the beginning of the motion in the soft palate when patient says AH.
- PPS passes 2 mm in front of fovea palatine.
- It is not the junction of hard and soft palate; ***is always in the soft palate***.
- Vibrating line on soft palate contains glandular tissues.
- Higher the vault, the more abrupt and forward the vibrating line.
- In Flat vault—it is placed posteriorly.
- Denture should extend 1–2 mm posterior of this line.
- Denture must cover the tuberosities and extend in the hamular notch.
- Overextension of denture in hamular notch = interferes with pterygomandibular raphe, which extends from hamulus to the top inside back corner of the retromolar pad, RMP.
- On wide opening of mouth = pterygomandibular raphe is pulled forward, which dislodges the denture.
    - **Submucosa**—is devoid of fat or glandular cells; in edentulous mouth is thicker than in the attached gingiva of the dentulous mouth.
    - **Compact bone**—is best able to provide primary support for the upper denture.
    - **Mucous membrane**—on the slope of the upper residual ridge; less stress is placed on the moveable tissue of the slope of the ridge.
    - **Soft tissue of hard palate**—anterolaterally is the fatty/adipose zone; postero-laterally is glandular zone; these tissues are recorded in **resting condition**.

- **Submucosa of median palatal suture**—non resilient; little or no stress can be placed; highly sensitive; **proper relief** is provided.
- **Incisive papillae**—nasopalatine nerve and vessels; **relief** to avoid pressure on them.
- **Vestibular space**—lining mucosa is non-keratinized; elastic fibres in submucosa.
- Natural ms activity in the lips and cheeks is important for the development of the borders.
- Hamular notch contains loose areolar tissues; additional pressure can be placed on this tissue to complete PPS.
- Increased amounts of keratinized material are present in edentulous ridges, when clinical quality of the denture is good.
- Removing the dentures from the mouth for 6–8 hrs a day esp during sleep allows keratinization to increase and the signs of inflammation are reduced.

RELATED ANATOMIC STRUCTURES

Muscles of soft palate

- Levator veli palatini; tensor veli palatini; musculus uvulae; glossopalatinus; pharyngopalatinus;
- Wall of soft palate is formed principally by the pharyngopalatinus ms.
- Posterior border of maxillary denture, which forms the PPS, rests on the soft palate upto the place where the soft palate becomes moveable.

Muscles of pharynx

- Main ms are superior, middle, inferior constrictors; stylopharyngeus; salpingopharyngeus; palatopharyngeus.
- **Superior constrictor** is the muscle of kinetic chain during **swallowing**.
- **Superior constrictor** is separated from buccinator by pterygomandibular raphe just above the buccinator m.

Nerve and blood supply

- Maxillary denture foundation gets blood from—descending palatine and posterior superior alveolar A.
- Mandibular denture—from inferior alveolar A and its branches.
- Tongue—lingual A.
- Nerves of maxillary area—nasopalatine; anterior palatine; middle palatine; inferior nasal nerve on palatal side; by anterior-middle-posterior superior alveolar nerves on buccal side.
- Mandibular area—inferior alveolar and its branches, i.e. mylohyoid; dental, incisive and mental.
- Buccinator/long buccal n supplies—buccinator, vestibule, cheeks.
- Anterior 2/3 rd of tongue by lingual n; posterior 1/3rd by 9th n.

MAXILLARY IMPRESSION

- Definition—**impression** is a record of negative form of tissues of the oral cavity.
- **5 objectives of the impression**—retention; stability; support; esthetics; preservation/health of the tissues. (PRESS)
- **Retention**—is its resistance to removal in a direction opposite of its insertion; it resists the forces of gravity and is ***in vertical direction***.
- **Stability**—is the resistance ***against the horizontal movement*** and forces.
- **Denture support**—is the resistance to vertical components of mastication and to occlusal or other forces applied in a direction towards the basal seat.
- **Factors of retention**—adhesion; cohesion; interfacial surface tension; capillarity; atmospheric pressure; oral and facial ms. (CATCAM)
- **Adhesion**—is the physical attraction ***of unlike molecules*** to each other.
- A watery saliva is quite effective; thick ropy saliva gets built up and literally pushes the denture out of position (as hydraulic pressure of saliva is more than force of adhesion).

- Amount of retention supplied by adhesion is directly proportional to the area covered by the denture.
- **Cohesion**—is the physical attraction ***of like molecules*** to each other. It occurs in the layer of saliva b/w mucosa and denture. It is directly proportional to the area covered by the denture.
- **Interfacial ST**—is the resistance to separation possessed by the film of liquid b/w 2 well-adapted surfaces; directly proportional to the size of basal surface of the denture. For best results, the impression should be minimal distortion and displacement.
- **Capillarity**—is force developed because of surface tension, it causes retention of denture, because a thin film of saliva acts as a capillary tube. It is directly proportional to the area of basal seat of the denture.
- **Atmospheric pressure**—is **14.7 psi**; the retentive force by atmospheric pressure is directly proportional to the area covered by the denture.
- **Musculature**—teeth are placed ***in neutral zone***; shape of buccal and lingual flanges should be in harmony with the movement of the ms; buccal corridor.
- **Contraction of the buccinator ms** will tend to **seat both dentures** on their basal seats.
- **Occlusal plane/OP** must be at the correct level.
- Insufficient space may be present b/w the ridges esp in the tuberosity regions. It is due to excessive fibrous tissue covering the tuberosity; it should be **removed surgically**.

Impression

- Softer materials displace the soft tissues less and require less force in their molding.
- During making the special tray, ***1 mm thick spacer*** is placed, which provides space for the final impression material. The PPS area is not covered with the spacer.
- **Border molding**—is the process by which the shape of the borders of the tray is made to conform accurately to the contours of the buccal and labial vestibules.

- ***Holes*** are placed in median palatal raphe and anterolateral and posterolateral regions of palate to provide relief.
- Distobuccal angle of the buccal flange = is molded by asking the patient to move mandible side by side.

Posterior palatal seal (PPS)

- When properly formed it will be about **1 mm thick** and about **4 mm wide.**

Making space in the tray

- Is provided for final impression material.
- Entire surface is scraped for—1 mm except PPS.
- 1.5–2.0 mm relief is given at—median palatal raphe.
- Buccal and labial borders—shortened by 1.5 mm.

MANDIBULAR IMPRESSION

- Total basal area of mandible is less than maxilla.
- With teeth loss, bony base of mandible becomes shorter vertically and narrower bucco-lingually.
- Total width of bony foundation and mandibular basal seat—becomes **greater in molar area,** because the width of the inferior border of mandible from side to side is greater than the width of mandible at the alveolar process.

Buccal flange area or buccal shelf

- Is the area b/w mandibular buccal frenum and the anterior edge of the masseter muscle.
- Is ***bounded by*** external oblique ridge laterally and by RMP distally.
- Formed by smooth ***compact bone***.
- It is the principal bearing surface of the mandibular denture (***primary stress bearing area***).
- BFA is at right angle to the direction of vertical occlusal forces.

- Some buccinator ms fibres are located under it. The fibres run antero-posteriorly parallel to bone and the denture does not resist the contracting forces of this muscle. Its contraction does not lift the denture.
- Requirements of mandibular impression—best by a **selective pressure technique**.
- Short flanges in labial anterior area—because of the attachment of various ms to the rest of ridge. These ms act nearly at right angles to the flange.
- In posterior region—crest of greatly resorbed ridges is at the level of the mental foramen, which should be relieved.

Mylohyoid ridge

- Mylohyoid ms—attaches close to the inferior border of mandible ANTERIORLY and near the superior surface of the residual ridge POSTERIORLY.
- Angle of the **posterior part of lingual flange of denture** in molar region is affected by angle of mylohyoid m. while **anteriorly, only the length of the flange** is affected by it.
- MH m moves **outward and upwards** during contraction, so the denture should not be extended into the undercut below MH ridge.
- In mandible with flat residual ridge, mylohyoid ridge is very sharp; so ***relief is provided*** in denture to avoid soreness.
- **Mental foramen**—should be ***relieved*** to avoid impingement on mental N and vessels in case of severe resorption.
- Insufficient space b/w mandible and tuberosity—angle of mandible is frequently made more obtuse with early loss of the posterior teeth and retention of anterior teeth.
- Removal of posterior support destroys the necessary counter-balance against the muscle pull at the angle of mandible. This reduces the space b/w upper and lower posterior areas.
- **Direction of ridge resorption**—maxilla resorbs upward and inward to become smaller/**narrower progressively** due to the direction and inclination of roots of upper teeth.
- In mandible, becomes **wider progressively** with age; it inclines outward.

Buccal and labial border anatomy

- Mandibular denture should be wide posterior to buccal frenum; and narrow in anterior labial region.
- Mandibular labial frenum contains a ***band of fibrous CT,*** which helps to attach the orbicularis oris m, so the frenum is active and sensitive.
- **Mandibular labial flange**—is the part b/w labial frenum/notch and the buccal frenum/notch; it is limited, because the fibers of orbicularis oris and incivus labii inferioris ms run closely to the crest of the ridge.
- **Buccal frenum**—the denture should be trimmed functionally and less extended in this area because, buccal frenum connects as a continuous band through the modiolus to the buccal frenum in maxilla.
- Tone of the skin of the lip and orbicularis oris m depends on the thickness of the flange and position of the teeth.
- **Labial flange**—no muscle extends from the residual ridge to the lip b/w the 2 triangularis ms; so the labial flange can be extended in length and thickness to supply the necessary support for the lip.

Buccal vestibule

- **Ante's law** = the PD surface area of the abutment teeth should be at least equal to the teeth replaced. Ideal ratio is 2:1.
- **Ideal C:R ratio** = should be 1 : 2. but recommended is 2:3 ideal; the ratio should be at least 1:1.
- Maxillary first molar has the maximum root surface area/RSA, i.e. 433 sq. mm; the RSA of mandibular first molar is 431 sq. mm.
- Maxillary canines have maximum RSA among the anterior teeth, i.e. 273 sq. mm.
- Mandibular first premolar has the least RSA among the posterior teeth , i.e. 180 sq. mm.
- Mandibular central incisors have least RSA among all the teeth, i.e. 154 sq. mm.

- **Canine replacement** = occlusal scheme should be designed to provide group function in lateral excursions to avoid stresses and never the canine guidance scheme.
- **Resin bonded bridges** = panavia-21 cement is used; it has dual affinity, i.e. it chemically bonds to both enamel and non- precious alloys.

ARTICULATORS

- An articulator is a mechanical device which represent TMJ and Jaw members, to which maxillary and mandibular casts may be attached.
- Movements of articulator should simulate mandibular positions or movements of the patient within the range of normal functional contacts.
- Condylar path is governed partly in its shape and function by the MENISCUS and it moves forward during mandibular movements under lateral pterygoid muscle.
- Path is also controlled by the shape of glenoid fossa.
- Edentulous patients give only one controlling factor (CG) to the movement of mandible.
- IG provided by anteriors is an important part of control.
- IG is always UNDER CONTROL of the DENTIST.
- IG is controlled by overjet and overbite.
- IG is more influential to control mandible movements than the CG because the condylar paths are further away from the cusp incline.

ECCENTRIC RELATION RECORDS

- Ideal amount of protrusion required for making this record is to bring anterior teeth in END-TO-END relation.
- The shape of mandible fossa is an OGEE curve, rather than a straight line.
- Mechanical limitations of most of the articulators required a protrusive movement of at least **6 mm** for adjusting CG.

- For complete registration, the lateral records are necessary to indicate the limit of range of movement as shown by GOTHIC ARCH (needle point) tracing.
- Required lateral movement is to place upper buccal cusps over the lower buccal cusps.
- When needle point of the tracing device is 6 mm from the apex-the mandible in first molar region will be approx 3 mm lateral to its CR.
- During lateral movement—the gap between occlusal surfaces of posterior teeth is more on balancing side than on working side.
- A protrusive record of 6 mm is made, because with a shorter distance, the condyle does not move down its path sufficiently to be recorded properly.

POSTERIOR PALATAL SEAL _____/ details

- Extends between pterygomaxillary/hamular notches.
- Vibrating line of soft palate is a guide for ideal posterior border of denture and is located slightly anterior to the fovea palatinae.
- CD can extend posterior to vibrating line because of the gradual slope of palate.
- A narrow PPS is attained if soft palate is more sloppy and forward in the mouth.
- A wide PPS is attained if soft palate is backwards and gradually sloping.
- Width of PPS seen as a BEAD on CD = 1.0–1.5 mm high; 1.5 mm wide; and 2 mm anterior to the posterior border of CD.
- A wide PPS can displace soft tissues more and so CD is unstable during function.

POSTERIOR TEETH ARRANGEMENT

- BO is the bilateral contact of teeth during function, regardless of mandibular position; used for stability of CD. It is essential during mandibular movements when no food is in the mouth.
- Unbalanced occlusion of CD can lead to breakdown of supporting structures.

- Dr can establish all the factors of occlusion, except the CG, which is the presentation of condylar anatomy.
- Concept of flat OP allows maximum horizontal mandibular movements with the use of NEUTRAL or ZERO DEGREE IG.
- When proper appearance of patient requires an overbite, then cusped posterior teeth should be used, e.g. C_2D_2 type of occlusion.

Factors of centric occlusion details

- CO = position of U/L arches when teeth are in maximum contact.
- CO is the normal termination of masticatory closure.
- CO and CR are same in a child; but with age, the mandible takes a different position for CR there is a difference of approx 1 mm.
- During LIGHT chewing—mandible is in habitual eccentric occlusion, which may be protrusive or lateral or combination.
- But during resistant food chewing—the mandible is completely RETRUDED.
- CR = most posterior relation of mandible to maxilla at the established VR and from which lateral movement can be made at a given degree of jaw separation.
- Eccentric occlusion–is the protrusive and lateral contacts of inclined planes of teeth when jaw is not moving.
- Articulation–is relation of teeth during movements into and away from eccentric position while the teeth are in contact. It is occlusion **IN MOTION.**

Arrangement of posterior teeth

- Vertical overlap and IG are already established in natural teeth but in CD—it is partly in the **HANDS OF DENTIST.**
- Inclination of condylar path on balancing side is in harmony with the inclines of posterior teeth on working side.
- 2 controlling factors considered in CD occlusion are—CG and IG.
- Other controlling factors are in dentist's control within the limit of esthetics.

- The more closely the IG angle approaches zero degree, the more stable the CD due to reduction of lateral inclines.

Laws of protrusive occlusion—also known as Hanau's quints

1. Inclination of CG (CG).
2. Inclination of IG (IG).
3. Orientation of OP (PO).
4. Inclination of cusps (CI).
5. Prominence of compensating curves. (CC).
    - CG and IG control the movements of the articulator and are determined before other 3 factors, i.e. OP/CC/IC.
    - OP, cusps inclination, CC can be changed by the DENTIST to attain harmony.
    - CG is the ONLY FACTOR FIXED BY PATIENT. It is obtained by protrusive registration.
    - IG is set BY DENTIST and is influenced by amount of horizontal and vertical overlap.
    - The greater the horizontal overlap—the more it reduces the angle of inclination.
    - Less the vertical overlap—the less will be the angle of inclination.
    - Posterior teeth are closer to the action of incisal inclination than they are to the condylar inclination, so greater influence is exercised on the teeth by IG than by CG.
    - With shallow vertical, the cuspal inclinations are lowered and the rotational centre of mandible is above the level of OP. The denture is more stable.
    - With steep vertical overlap and so steep cusp inclination, the rotational centre of mandible is below OP and posterior to mandible and this tends to push denture forward.
    - Rotational centre is determined by drawing the lines at right angle to the IG and CG surfaces.
    - OP orientation is also the **third fixed factors** of occlusion; because lowering/raising its level can lead to aesthetic and mechanical troubles.

- Cuspal inclination of tooth is the angle between the total occlusal surface of the tooth and the inclination of the cusp in respect to that surface.

$$BO = \frac{CG \times IG}{CI \times CC \times PO}$$

- If CG increases, the CC increases.
- Basic inclination of cusp is steeper when distal end of lower tooth is set higher than mesial end.
- CI can be decreased when the distal end of lower tooth is set lower than mesial end.
- The factor of CC is variable as it allows the dentist to alter CH without changing form of the teeth.

LAWS OF LATERAL OCCLUSION

- 2 end factors are:
  - (a) CG incline on balancing side.
  - (b) Lingual inclines of maxillary buccal cusps and buccal inclines of lower lingual cusp on the working side.
- These inclines must be harmonious with the path of lower canine to meet upper canine end to end.
- Rational centre in latero-trusion is established by the lines drawn perpendicular to working side inclines, balancing side inclines and balancing side condyle.
- Lateral shift of mandible may occur due to movement of condyles along the lateral inclines of mandibular fossa. This translatory movement is known as **Bennett movement**.
- 15° is the average Bennett movement.
- Angle of inclination on working side is less in posterior area and greater towards the incisal area.
- Also inclination on working side is less compared to balancing side.
- CG is not so great a factor as the amount of IG (as it is selected by Dentist).

- Reduction of cusp inclination is a great stabilizer for CD.
- Since condyles do not move horizontally, there should be some inclination of occluding surface to harmonize with the downward movement of mandible. This cuspal clination should be as flat as possible for stability of CD.
- Cusped teeth give vertical closing forces for mastication. Zero degree cusps cannot shear food. Patients do most of the chewing in CO. A cuspless occlusal scheme eliminates the possibility of deflective occlusal contacts.
- To avoid excess forces falling on the ridge, the lateral and protrusive inclines of CD teeth should be smaller than the natural teeth.
- Teeth with steeper CI should be used with steeper IG.
- An area of freedom should be provided anterior and lateral to CR for any occlusal scheme.
- Primary consideration is to set the first PM to follow the form of residual ridge and should be set slightly buccal to canine.
- Each mandibular tooth is set s.t. the perpendicular at buccal side of crest of residual ridge would bisect the buccal cusp.

When upper teeth setting is done first

- Then the lingual cusps should fall on line indicating the crest of mandibular ridge.
- Mandibular Ist PM is last tooth to be placed, as it may require grinding.
- Also, it has only buccal cusp in occlusion and does not affect the esthetics on grinding.
- The mild spaces are left between maxillary posterior teeth s.t. mandibular teeth may be fitted properly.

Cuspless teeth setting

- Should contact maximally on a CC.
- IG should be zero.
- Protrusive lateral balance is achieved by using second molar ramp.

- No vertical overlap of anteriors.
- 3 point balance effect is achieved.
- If overbite is necessary for esthetics then overjet should also be incorporated.
- CG—zero for cuspless teeth.
- IG–should be zero.
- Posterior limit of mandibular teeth is the point at which the mandibular ridge begins to curve upward. If teeth are to be placed on this slope, they should not contact their antagonist.

Appearance and functional harmony of denture bases

3 factors concerned with functional harmony are:

1. Basal surface
2. Leverage position and occlusal surfaces of teeth.
3. Shape/form of polished surface of dentures.

Most important factor is—the occlusal surface.

Inclination of polished surfaces is determined by 2 end factors, viz.

(a) Width of the border.

(b) Buccolingual position of teeth.

- Buccal surface of mandibular dentures in the first PM region should be shaped carefully so as not to interfere with the action of modiolus.
- Fullness of buccal/labial surfaces of U/L dentures is desirable and the palatal surface should be thin to allow all the space for tongue.
- Lingual flange of mandibular CD should be least bulky except at borders. It should be concave s.t. tongue has a seating action. The buccolingual width should be smaller than the natural teeth for providing space for tongue and also for less occlusal forces to be transmitted to the basal bone.
- Roots of maxillary canine > centrals > laterals.
- But roots of mandibular canine > laterals > centrals.
- Palatal surface of upper CD should be waxed approximately 2.5 mm thick.

- Lingual contours of U/L teeth should be carved in wax to provide a natural feel to the tongue.

Complete rehabilitation of the patient: i.e. occlusal settling

- The occlusion should be checked on the very first touch, when teeth are closed together.
- Old dentures should be kept outside for 24 hours s.t. new CDs are seated on healthy, undistorted tissues.
- Errors in occlusion appear in CDs due to polymerization shrinkage and warpage of acrylic resins.
- Maxilla mandibular relations are bone-to-bone relations.
- Bone is more plastic than mucosa and so any occlusal errors.
- Also inclined plane relation of cusped teeth may change if resins absorb the water.
- The errors should always be located on remounted CDs in articulator. Soft tissues being resilient, the CDs may shift/move during closure in the mouth and may increase the occlusal errors.
- In CR = the jaw should close slowly till the first contact of a back tooth. No pressure should be applied on mandible to retrude it.
- Position of left hand should be: Thumb and fingers are partly between occlusal surfaces of U/L CDs and provide slight resistance to the closure; keep CDs seated; provide tactile sensation to know any shifting of CDs.
- Palm covers the eyes of patient s.t. he is not able to see and react to the expression of dentists.

Inter-occlusal records for remounting CDs

- Errors of occlusion should be removed in articulator after remounting and not in the mouth.
- Protrusive inter occlusal records—mandible brought forward and to bite easily on front teeth. Closure is stopped before any anterior teeth make contact.
- CR record is made by pulling of the mandible backwards and the closure must be stopped before any teeth touch.

Articulator adjustment

- The lateral CG is set after setting horizontal CG (H) by the formula:

$$L = \frac{H}{8} + 12$$

To eliminate occlusal errors

- Articulating paper should be of minimum thickness.
- During centric grinding process—the incisal guide pin should be slightly away from the table to allow for slight reduction of VD.
- Lateral errors are checked, if the IG pin rises during lateral movement—then
  ⇒ Buccal cups of upper teeth (working).
  ⇒ Lingual cusp of lower teeth (working side) **(Bull rule)** are reduced.
  ⇒ On balancing side—lingual side of buccal cusps of lower teeth.
  ⇒ Grinding to treat occlusal errors in lateral occlusions are limited to—lingual inclines of upper buccal cusps and buccal inclines of lower lingual cusps on working side and lingual inclines of lower buccal cusps on balancing side.
  ⇒ Lingual upper and buccal lower cusps should not be ground to maintain VDO. These are the **centric cusps**. Other names of the cusps.
  ⇒ Also, grinding is to be done only in fossae and not on the cusps.
  ⇒ After completion—there should be uniform contacts on U/L teeth shown by articulating papers.
  ⇒ Carborundum (abrasive) paste should not be used for it, as VDO will be reduced; area of contact of tooth surfaces is increased; decreased number and size of sluice ways occurs.

Types of errors in occlusion

- Occlusal errors in CO = 3 types.
- Working side occlusal errors = 6 types.
- Balancing side errors = 2 types.

Occlusal errors in non-anatomic teeth

- Grinding is done on occlusal surfaces of teeth which appear tipped/displaced during processing.
- In eccentric occlusion—DB portion of mandibular 2nd molar is not ground.
- All balancing side grinding is done on lingual portion of occlusal surface of upper 2nd molar.
- Abrasive past can be used here.
- BO helps in maintaining even pressure in all parts of the arch, which maintain the CD stability in functional and para-functional activities.
- Mastication with new CDs is learnt properly in 6–8 weeks.
- Tongue helps in stability of lower denture.
- **Food is pushed inward and upward** to break it with CDs (as cp. to ***Downwards and outward in natural teeth***).

Rest to oral tissues

- Is very necessary for health.
- CDs should be left out of mouth at night to relieve stresses.
- Soft tissues should be cleaned with brushes and finger massage for stimulation and circulation.
- Adhesives and home reliners should not be used—as they change the position of CDs and lead to inadvertent stresses on residual ridges.

Follow up of CD Patients

- First appointment—24 hours after insertion.
- Check shift of CDs—if the teeth touch and slide, there is an error in CO.
- Pressure on **mental Foramen**—numbness in the lower lip at the corner of mouth.
- Pressure on **incisive papilla**—numbness in anterior part of upper jaw.

- **Gagging**—mainly due to making/breaking on PPS during function. Posterior border of upper denture should not be extended more than 2 mm past the vibrating line.
- Retromylohyoid fossa lesion = may be due to pressure due to extended borders.
- **Falling upper CD** on wide opening of mouth—it is **due to DB flange** is very thick and interferes with coronoid process of mandible during opening and lateral movement function.
- If **upper CD loosens** during smiling, it is due to excess thickness or height of flange in the region of buccal notch or posterior to it.
- Acrylic resin base material of CD absorbs water and can change size and occlusion.
- **Soreness** due to occlusal shift—is mostly on the lingual side of mandibular ridge in respect to, canine and first premolar. Its cause is mostly the deflective occlusal contact on the balancing inclines of lower 2nd molar.

TOOTH SUPPORTED CD

(a) Overdenture

- PO healthy PDL helps maintain alveolar ridge form and bone.
- Roots are maintained in bone by RCT, etc.
- Apply fluoride solution (1% NaF neutral pH on prepared abutment teeth).
- For abutment teeth, the anterior teeth are preferred over posteriors, because the anterior alveolar ridge is more vulnerable to bone resorption/reduction.
- Also **mandibular overdenture is preferred** over maxillary teeth.

(b) Immediate denture are the dentures made before removing all the remaining teeth and is inserted immediately after the removal of the teeth.

- It acts as splint after surgery; prevents humiliating period of healing and aesthetic concern, remaining teeth can act as guide for tooth selection.

- Major changes in denture supporting tissues takes 8–12 months. Bony reduction is related to denture-wearing habits and the loading of denture bearing tissues.
- It acts as a splint over the surgical area and prevents breakdown of blood clot.

(c) **Delayed dentures**—prepared dentures are inserted 1–2 weeks or more after extractions. Its objective is to prevent bacteremia during early postoperative period.

(d) **Transitional dentures**—are the interim intermediate dentures, which are given until the stability of denture supporting tissues is achieved and then a new denture is made.

- All posterior teeth are removed except bilateral opposing premolars, which serve as centric stops and prevent decrease of inter-arch distance.
- ***Dual impression technique*** is used for the impression making.
- PO posterior teeth helps determine the level of OP.
- After making a cast, the alternate teeth are cut away and replaced, starting from the central incisors.
- ***Distance between the labial surfaces of the canines*** on the cast is measured to replicate on the teeth setting for proper lip support.
- A deep overbite requires steep IG and hence sharp inclines in all anterior and posterior teeth.
- After delivery, the final occlusal corrections are not made till the healing of tissues, esp 48 hrs to 2 weeks.
- Early pressure should not be placed in the area of immediate extractions especially in anterior area which is more vulnerable to resorption.
- Patient FU is done every 3 months to determine the amount of change.
- Socket calcification takes 8–12 months after extraction, approx 20–30% of bone volume of ridge decreased during 8–12 months. Only then final refitting of denture is done.
- Extensive alveolectomy is done in Angle's $C_2 D_1$ type of teeth set.

Single CD opposing natural teeth

- In such cases, the objective of BO cannot always be met without altering natural teeth inclines or OP.
- Maxillary CD opposing mandibular natural teeth is more common and safer; but mandibular CD is harmful to upper natural teeth.
- Most common cause of difficulty with occlusion of maxillary denture and mandibular natural teeth is due to inclination of some parts of OP (which occur due to supra-eruption of remaining teeth) of natural teeth, which may cause the maxillary CD to rotate.
- Cross–arch balancing contacts should be developed by teeth preparation for stability.
- If IG is more horizontal, the cuspal inclines are to be decreased more and so more stable will be the CD.
- If RPD/FPD is present in lower arch and maxillary CD—then all the prosthesis should be placed at the same appointment for optimal control and OP development.
- One of the major problems with CD opposing natural teeth is ABRASION. e.g. porcelain in CD can abrade gold/Ag/acrylic and natural teeth.
- Single mandibular CD opposing a natural maxillary arch poses more problems, as leverage leads to undue resorption of mandibular bone.
- Area available in maxillary denture = 45 cm^2.
- Area available in mandibular denture = 12 cm^2.
- **Relining** = denture base material, i.e. acrylic resin is added to the existing denture base, thereby refitting the denture. Done if there is mild to moderate changes in based seat.
- **Rebasing** = the CDs require refitting and reorientation; also to compensate for vertical and horizontal changes in both dentures orientations.
- Shrinkage of bone of maxilla permits upper CD to **move U and B** in respect to the original position. But the occlusion may force maxillary CD forward.
- Lower denture moves **D and B** in respect to the mandible with shrinkage. Mandible moves forward and upward, causing abnormal stresses due to occlusal prematurities.

IMPLANTS

Types of the casts

1. Working cast.
2. Study/Diagnostic cast = poured by dental stone.
3. Refractory cast.
4. Master cast = by die stone.

Advantages of casts

1. Occlusion from LINGUAL SIDE can be seen.
2. Reference of work progress comparison.
3. Discussion with patient about the Rx plan.
4. Topographic survey of dental arch.
5. Diagnostic wax up.
6. Less chair time—Lab work without patient.
7. Records.
8. For patient awareness/presentation/lectures.
9. Discussion with other Doctors.
10. Permanent patient record.

Tissues	Important properties/features
Mandibular labial frenum	• Has a band of **fibrous CT** which helps to attach orbicularis oris muscle, it must be trimmed. • Mandibular denture should be wide posterior to buccal frenum and narrow in anterior labial region.
Mandibular labial flange	• Part of denture between labial frenum/notch and buccal frenum/notch is known as **mandibular.** **LABIAL FLANGE** • It is ***limited by fibres of orbicularis oris*** and incisivus labii inferiors run close to crest of ridge.

Tissues	Important properties/features
Buccal frenum	• Mandibular Buccal frenum passes through the modulus to maxillary BF; these pull actively across the denture borders and surfaces and teeth. So denture ***should be extended less*** in this region and functionally trimming done. • **Thickness of labial flange and position of lower teeth.** • Affect the lower lip; tone of skin of lip and orbicularis oris m.
Labial flange	• Can be extended in length and thickness for supporting the lip. • Because **no muscle extends** from residual ridge to lip between 2 TRIANGULARIS Ms.
Buccal vestibule	• From buccal frenum to outside back corner of RMP area and from crest of ridge to cheek. • Buccinators from modiolus to pterygopalatine raphe; lower side attached in molar region in buccal shelf area, i.e. between ridge and external oblique line. • ***Action of buccinator is in horizontal direction*** and so cannot lift the denture.
Buccal flange	• Extends from buccal frenum to ant. part of masseter; is wide in cheeks; approx ***at right angles to biting forces***. • Provides GREATEST RESISTANCE to vertical occlusal forces. • ***External oblique ridge does not govern*** the extension of buccal flange.
Masseter muscle area	• Distobuccal corner of lower buccal vestibule of mandibular denture is trimmed by action of masseter m., otherwise denture gets displaced.

Tissues	Important properties/features
	• Anterior fibers of masseter m. pass outside the buccinator here. • Pushes inward against buccinator and suctorial pad of cheek.
Distal extension of mandibular impression	• Is defined by ramus, buccinator and retromandibular fossa/RMF. • Buccinator passes from buccal to lingual. • Buccinator attaches to pterygomandibular raphe with superior constrictor. • RMF is formed by continuation of internal and external oblique ridge.
Retromolar region and pad	• RMP must be covered by mandibular denture for perfect seal. • RMP contains glandular tissues + temporal tendon fibres + buccinator + superior constrictor + RM raphe.
Lingual border	• Should be extended below mylohyoid ridge. • Should be made parallel to mylohyoid m. during contraction.
Floor of mouth	• MH m arises from whole length of MH line. • Extends from 1 cm back of distal end of MH ridge to lingual anterior part of mandible at symphysis. • Posteriorly, its fibres continue to the hyoid bone. • MH m lies deep to sublingual gland and other structures in premolar region. • Posterior part of MH m in molar region affects lingual impression during swallowing and tongue movements. • MH m is attached more superiorly on mandible in posterior region and so it **affects the slope of lingual flange** in molar area and so flange slopes towards the tongue.

Tissues	Important properties/features
	• Lingual flange is ***extended below the palpable part*** of MH ridge to avoid direct pressure on this sharp edge of bone to reduce soreness. • Also, lingual flange completes seal in retromylohyoid fossa and guides the tongue on the top of flange. • MH is also known as ORAL DIAPHRAGM. • Sublingual glands lies above the MH m.
Lingual frenum	• Should be registered in function by functional trimming, as it comes close to the crest of the ridge.
Lingual flange	• Its lower border runs parallel to the lower edge of mandible from lingual frenum to posterior end of denture. • It is shorter in anterior part and longer in posterior part. • Posteriorly, extension is bounded partially by glossopalatine m, which lies at distal extension of RMP. • Occupies alveolo-lingual sulus (ALS). • Distal ends of ALS ends at RM curtain. • RMC is pulled forward when tongue is thrust out. • Distal end of lingual flange is partly limited by glossopalatine arch. • GP arch is formed by GP m and lingual extension of sup. constrictor m. • Lingual flange is influenced by MH m in molar region. • Ant. part of lingual flange over the sublingual gland is shallow because mobility of tissues are controlled by MH m.

Tissues	Important properties/features
	• Lingual flange is of **S shape curve** as: 1. From midline, it curves outwards following curve of residual ridge. 2. At pre-mylohyoid eminence, the flange curves away from mandible to accommodate MH m. on contraction. 3. At distal end of MH ridge, the flange turns laterally towards ramus to fill retro-mylohyoid fossa. • Distal end of lingual flange is known as retromylohyoid eminence.
Alveolo-Lingual sulcus and its 3 areas	• Is space between residual ridge and tongue; occupied by lingual flange. • Extends from lingual frenum to retro-mylohyoid curtain. • **Anterior region** = from lingual frenum to pre-mylohyoid fossa/eminence. • **Middle region** = from mylohyoid fossa to the distal end of mylohyoid ridge. 1. Sulcus curves mesially from the body of mandible. 2. Curvature is caused by prominence of MH ridge. 3. The part slopes towards the tongue which rests on the flange and helps stabilizing the lower denture. • **Posterior region** = is retro-mylohyoid space/fossa. 1. Extends from end of MH ridge to retro-MH curtain. 2. Bound by anterior tonsillar pillar on lingual side; by RMH curtain and sup. constrictor muscle on distal end; and by MH m, ramus and RMP on buccal side.

Tissues	Important properties/features
	• Denture border should contact RMH curtain. • In the border of lingual flange is a **S-shape curve**.
Buccal shelf	• Located posterior to buccal frenum and extends from crest of ridge to external oblique ridge. • Fibres of buccinator run horizontally in submucosa immediately overlying the bone. • ***Bone of buccal shelf is COMPACT bone.*** • It is ***most suitable PRIMARY STRESS BEARING AREA.*** • Impression tray is in direct contact with mucosa here and so soft tissue is slightly displaced and so additional load can be placed on the supporting tissues.
RMP area	• Non-keratinized epithelium. • Submucosa contains = glandular tissue + buccinator fibres + sup. constrictor m. fibres + pteryomandibular raphe + terminal part of tendon of temporalis m. • It should be **registered in a resting position**.

Classification of mandibular impressions

1. **Pressure impression**
   - No space for the final impression material.
   - Denture may cause ***rapid resorption of residual ridge***.
2. **Selective pressure impression**
   - Space for final impression material in some places than other.
   - Spaces with less relief will transmit more pressure in favourable part of bone, i.e. buccal shelf and vice-versa.
3. **Pressureless impression**
   - i.e. with ***least possible displacement*** of soft tissues.
   - Taken with ***very fluid type of impression materials***.

Impression making

- Metal tray selected—which provides approx 6 mm (1/4 inch) bulk of impression material over the entire basal seat area.
- A wax spacer approx 1 mm thick is placed over crest and slope of ridge.
- Buccal shelf on each side and retro—MH spaces are left uncovered –s.t. More pressure can be placed in primary stress bearing area.
- Special tray of 2–3 mm thick is made of acrylic.
- 2 additional handles, one each in molar region are placed, to be used as finger rests.
- Lingual flange is shorter anteriorly than posteriorly.
- Flange becomes longer and extend below the level of mh line in canine-premolar region at pre-mh fossa.
- Lingual flange must slope towards the tongue parallel to the fibres of MH ms in molar region.
- Distal end of lingual flange is 1 cm distal to the end of MH ridge. It turns laterally towards ramus below the level of rmp and MH ridge.
- The distal end of lingual flange is activated by mouth opening and tongue protrusion to activate superior constrictor m. in retromolar/RM curtain.
- On closing the mouth against resistance, the medial pterygoid m. Gets activated against rm curtain and limits the space for border in RM fossa.
- Holes about 1/2 inch about are placed in the tray in the centre of alveolar groove.
    - In retromolar fossa.
    - Help to relieve pressure on crest of residual ridge and RMP.
- Border of tray should be 0.5–1.0 mm short for final impression material.
- Minimum tissue displacement and pressure.
- Existing dentures are left out of mouth for 24 hrs to allow the tissues of buccal seat to return to health and undistorted form.

- **Boxing**—wax should extend about 9–15 mm to provide appropriate thickness to the base of cast.
- Tongue is protruded out = to determine distal extent of lingual flange.
- Wide opening of mouth = pulls pterygomandibular raphe forward against the lingual side of part of retromolar pad—i.e. distal extension of occlusal part is defined.
- Closing month against resistance—activates medial pterygoid.

ANATOMICAL CONSIDERATIONS

- Mandibular fossa is 1″ long antero-posteriors and 3/4 inch in width mediolaterally.
- Condyles project out beyond the distal part of the fossa and can be felt in the soft tissues.
- Fossa is divided into 2 parts by the petrotympanic fissure, in which anterior tympanic branch of internal maxillary A passes.
- Chorda tympani nerve passes through the canal of Huguier (iter chordae anterius).
- Anterior part of mandibular fossa is the principal bearing surface on which the condyle presses through the disk.

Condyles (Also refer to the section of anatomy in Vol. I).

- 3/4″ wide × 1/2″ AP diameter.
- Does not fill the fossa to its AP limits.
- Condyles extend 1/2″ beyond the bony limits of the meatus laterally.
- Capsular ligament completely envelops the TMJ; attached to the rim of mandibular fossa and articular eminence to the neck of condyle; the fibers run Downward and Backward.
- **TM ligament**—fibres run Downward and Backward (D/B); extends from articular eminence and inferior border of zygomatic arch to the outer/posterior border of upper part of ramus. It limits the posterior movement of condyle.
- **Sphenomandibular ligament**—runs from the angle of sphenoid to lingula of inferior mandibular foramen; runs down on inner surface of ramus.

- **Stylomandibular ligament**—from styloid process to the medial side of angle of mandible and at its posterior border.

Articular disk (Also refer to the section of anatomy in Vol. I).

- Made of collagen fibres.
- Concavo-convex shape.
- Extends forward over the articular eminence.
- Position and movement are controlled by capsular ligament and lateral pterygoid m.
- It has extensive movements when mandible makes wider opening lateral protrusive movements.
- Disk can't move from side to side.
- TMJ is applied by auriculotemporal N (mostly, 90%) + deep temporal + masseteric N.

Muscles of mastication–4 (Also refer to the section of anatomy in Vol. I.)

- Masseter, medial pterygoid, Temporalis ms are closing ms.
- Lateral pterygoid is a guiding m/opening m.

Temporalis m

- ***Anterior fibres*** = run along coronoid process, anterior border of ramus and some fibres in RMP area.
- ***Posterior part*** = helps to retrude the mandible and braces the condyle during lateral movement.
- **Middle parts** = elevate the mandible in centric position.
- Temporalis m does not participate in biting force.

Masseter m

- 2 parts = superficial and deep.
- Elevates the mandible mainly.
- Deep fibres aid in retrusion also.
- Trim DB/disto-buccal corner of buccal flange of CD and border converges rapidly toward RMP.

Medial pterygoid m

- First part arises from medial surface of lateral pterygoid plate and the palatine bone.
- 2nd part arises from pyramidal process of palatine bone and posterior end of maxilla.
- Inserts on lower and posterior surfaces of ramus and into medial side of angle of mandible.
- Action = mostly ELEVATION; assists in lateral and protrusive movements of mandible.

Lateral pterygoid m—2 heads

- Superior belly = from greater wing of sphenoid bone.
- Inferior belly = from lateral pterygoid plate.
- Fibres run horizontally backwards and laterally.
- Superior belly = attaches mostly to disk and neck of condyle.
- Inferior belly = inserts at the neck of condyle.
- Principal action = protrusion of condyles.
- When one lateral pterygoid m. contracts, the mandible moves to opposite side.
- Helps in food to be engaged by the teeth.
- **Superior belly** = stabilizes/floxes the condyle/disk in specific position during elevation of mandible. But it does not elevate the mandible.

Ms of depression—3 groups of ms

1. Suprahyoid ms = digastrics, geniohyoid, mylohyoid, stylohyoid and platysma.

   –are the primary movers in opening of the mandible.
2. Infrahyoid group = stabilizes the hyoid bone s.t. suprahyoid group can be effective.
3. Lateral pterygoid ms = pull the condyles forward or medially.

Mylohyoid m—is the ***only muscle of these groups which affects the denture borders***.

- Originates from MH ridge.
- Extends from symphysis to distal aspect of 3rd molars.
- Closer to the crest of alveolar process in 3rd molar/posterior region on lingual side of mandible and travels forward.
- Runs medially and D and F.
- Inserts in midline and to the anterior cornu of hyoid bone.
- MH with geniohyoid muscles forms the floor of mouth.
- **Principal action** = assists in swallowing by raising the tongue.
- Also helps in opening of mandible.

JAW RELATIONS

- All jaw relations are BONE-TO-BONE relations.
- **Orientation relations**—establish the references in the cranium.
- **Vertical relations**—establish the amount of jaw separation.
- **Horizontal relations**—establish the front-to-back and side-to-side relation of one jaw to the other.
- **Orientation relations**—orient the mandible to cranium s.t. when mandible is in most posterior position, the mandible can rotate in sagittal plane around an axis passing through or near the condyles.
- **Face bow**—is used to record the relation of jaws to TMJ or opening axis of the jaws; the record is not a maxillo-mandibular record.

Arbitrary face bow—used in CD patients; locates approximate location of condyles axis.

- The rods are placed **13 mm in front** of external auditory meatus on a line from outer canthus of eye to top of tragus.
- It locates the axis within 5 mm of true centre of opening axis of the jaws.
- Fork of this face bow is attached to the maxillary occlusal rim.

Kinematic face bow

- The fork is attached to mandibular occlusal rim.
- Locates condylar axis MORE ACCURATELY.
- Mandible is then in CR position.
- Posterior terminal hinge axis (THA) can be located only when mandible is in its most posterior position.
- Since in edentulous mandible, the occlusal rim is not as stable when face bow is attached, so its more extensive use in edentulous patients is not possible.
- If the vertical separation/VD of casts or CD is to be reduced on the articulator, the face bow record is essential.
- Face bow transfer allows a more accurate arc of closure on articulation
- Kinematic face bow helps in finding the kinematic centre of jaw opening.
- **Hanau model face bow** and other arbitrary bows are located at a point 13 mm forward from external auditory meatus.
- **Whip mix face bow**—its ends are placed in auditory meatus instead of on condyles. THA is 15 mm anterior to the position of ends of the face bow.

VERTICAL RELATIONS

Are of 2 types – VR in occlusion VDO
– VR in rest position. VDR

VDR is **physiological rest position.**

- Established by ms and gravity.
- Is the postural relation of the 2 jaws.
- Teeth do not determine its vertical level.
- All the closing and opening ms are in minimum tonic contraction only to maintain the posture.
- *Position of Head* is important—must be upright and not supported by head rest.
- Helps as a guide to the lost VDO.

- ***Free way space***/inter-occlusal gap IOG is = VDR–VDO difference; is 2–4 mm in first premolar region.
- IOG is essential for health of PDL.
- If IOG is not there clicking of CDs occurs; rapid destruction of residual alveolar bone due to heavy forces; tissue soreness occurs, etc.

HORIZONTAL RELATIONS

- Basic horizontal relation is CR (centric relation).
- **Centric relation**/CR is the most posterior relation of mandible to maxilla at established vertical relation.
- **Eccentric relations**—i.e. deviations from CR, e.g. lateral; protrusive, etc. in horizontal plane; but changes also occur in vertical relations. It is also occur in vertical relations. It is known as ***CHRISTIANSEN phenomenon***. It develops spaces between U/L occlusal surfaces at posterior end of occlusion rim/CD.

Factors regulating jaw motion

- Rim system.
- Guiding influence of teeth.
- Mandibular ms.
- Occlusal surfaces of the teeth in c.d. should meet evenly on both sides during centric and eccentric jaw positions (***balanced occlusion***).
- It provides stability to dentures and mandible is not deflected.
- Inclined places of teeth should pass smoothly over each other and should be harmonious with other factors regulating jaw position.
- CG and IG should not be disrupted.

TMJ

- Upper compartment = primarily TRANSLATION movements occur.

- Lower compartment = primarily ROTATION movements occur.
- TRANSLATION means all points within the body move at the same velocity and in the same direction.
- Condyles can translate anteroposteriorly by approx 3/4″ (18 mm).
- During opening/closing movements—the mandible moves in SAGITTAL PLANE around a TRANSVERSE AXIS passing through both condyles.
- In lateral excursion—mandible rotates around a vertical axis which, passing through **working condyle** and the balancing/non-working condyle moves downwards, forwards and medially. It is a form of translation occurring in superior compartment of TMJ.
- Downward movement of balancing condyle causes working condyle to rotate around a sagittal axis.

Direct lateral side shift of mandible

- Occurs simultaneously with lateral movement of mandible (Bennett 1908), known as **Bennett movement**. It is due to mesial/inward movement of balancing condyle and lateral/outward movement of working condyle.
- Is an important component of lateral jaw movement.

MUSCLE ACTIVITY

Temporalis m

- Middle/Posterior part = activity increased during hinge openings and retrusion of mandible.
- Activity decreased during uncontrolled mandibular opening.
- Posterior part braces mandible during lateral excursions to the same side.
- **Temporal m** = posterior part is more horizontal than anterior and middle.
- **ISOTONIC** contraction of posterior fibres moves the mandible in CR or to hold it in most posterior position during terminal hinge movement.

Lateral pterygoid m

- Plays MAJOR ROLE in uncontrolled mandibular opening.
- It has very little role in hinge openings movements 3.
- It moves mandible forward or side ways.
- It remains inactive during mandibular terminal hinge opening movements.
- Responsible for forward movements of condyle and mandible during uncontrolled opening movements.
- Sup. belly of lat. pterygoid = fixes and stabilizes the condyle and disk during elevation of the mandible.
- It also helps in adjusting the horizontal CG and lateral CG/Bennett movement of the articulator.

Digastric ms are = very active in uncontrolled opening, retrusion and hinge opening movements of mandible.

Suprahyoid ms = produce rotary jaw movements around a transverse mandibular hinge axis.

Important points

- For CD patients, the occlusion of artificial teeth can be perfected better on articulator than in mouth, because CDs move on basal tissues, but not on articulator.
- There is only one true CR and it coincides with the most retruded position in skull.
- **Isotonic contraction** (ms fibres shorten in length during contraction and cause movement of a part) of posterior temporalis and in combination with suprahyoid ms—position the mandible in CR.
- **Isometric contraction** (ms maintain same length during contraction and fix a part in a particular location) = maintain mandible in CR during making an inter-occlusal CR records.

Neuromuscular regulation of mandibular movements

- Impulses from subconscious level including RAS also regulate muscle tone = plays a primary role in physiologic ***rest position*** of the mandible.

- Proprioceptors are located in PDL, mandibular ms and ligaments = provide information about ***location of mandible*** in space.
- Impulses from oral receptors travel to sensory nucleus of 5th N.
- Impulses from proprioceptors go to ***mesencephalic nucleus***.
- Impulses then can go to sensorimotor cortex (conscious level) to produce VOLUNTARY changes in mandibular position or to motor nucleus of 5th N and then to mandibular ms (in a reflex arc) causing INVOLUNTARY movements of mandible.
- Due to loss of receptors in PDL in edentulous mouth causes loss of control of mandibular position.
- **Mastication**—is a programmed event residing in a CHEWING CENTRE located in brain-stem (in reticular formation of PONS).

CEREBELLUM

- Acts as feed back control.
- Does not initial mandibular movements.
- Compares information from outer cortex, etc. to the sensory information received form periphery.
- Sends signals back to motor cortex to excite antagonist ms and inhibit agonist ms—to generate a coordinated response from muscles.

Parallelogram of forces

- Direction of pull of posterior temporalis = Upward and Backward.
- Direction of pull of anterior temporalis = more Upward and Forward.
- Direction of pull of superficial masseter and direction of pull of medial pterygoid = more Upward and Forward.
- Direction of pull of deep masseter m = more Upward and Backward.
- Direction of pull of resultant forces = exerted in line with long axes of teeth.

ENVELOPE OF MOTION IN SAGITTAL PLANE—i.e. maximum border movements. It is roughly **teardrop shaped**.

- Tracing starts at most protruded position of mandible with teeth in contact.
- Dip in top line of tracing occurs as incisal edges of U and L anterior teeth pass across each other, when mandible is moved posteriorly.
- As CO is reached = U/L posterior teeth get maximally intercuspated.
- At CR = mandible is further retruded.
- Single restorations are generally made in harmony with CO; while multiple restorations and CD are made with their occlusion in harmony with CR.
- On opening mandible from CR, i.e. when mandible is most retruded position, opening can be done in this retruded position ***without any condylar translation*** till MHO (Maximum Hinge Opening) position.
- Any opening beyond MHO = condyle moves Downwards and Forwards; translation occurs.
- The track CR–MHO is known as ***posterior terminal hinge movements***. It is used to locate transverse hinge axis.
- At maximum opening—the jaws are separated maximally and condyles are in most anterior position in the mandibular fossa.
- Pathways of masticating cycle occur anterior to the line representing the terminal hinge movement.
- For edentulous patients, the teeth should contact evenly throughout the normal range of function.
- Mandibular rest position occurs somewhere downward and slightly forward from CR.
- At habitual rest position—the only ms activity is minimal tonic contraction required to support the mandible against the force of gravity.

Envelop of motion in FRONTAL PLANE

- Is **shield shaped.**
- Dip in upper line is seen = as U/L canines pass edge to edge.

- Masticatory cycle contacts the superior border of envelop at CO—it shows that opposing teeth penetrated the bolus and contacted each other.

BIOLOGICAL CONSIDERATIONS OF VERTICAL RELATIONS

VDR is assumed when ms of jaws are ***in a state of minimal contraction*** to maintain posture of mandible.

Physiological rest position—controlled by ms and force of gravity; posture of head should be upright and unsupported.

Physiological rest position = allows supporting tissues to take rest and so health is maintained, otherwise destruction/resorption of alveolar bone occurs due to continuous pressure.

Masseter, medial pterygoid and temporalis ms are closing ms to establish vertical jaw relations.

Opening ms are inframandibular and suprahyoid ms + Digastric + Platysma + GRAVITY = all help to control the TONIC BALANCE and rest position.

IOG is essential for closing ms, opening ms and gravity to be in balance when ms are in minimum tonic contraction.

Establishing VR

A. Excessive interarch distance (VD) should not be there, it causes:

- Premature contact of teeth.
- Clicking of CDs.
- Bone resorption/destruction.

B. Reduced VD

- Decreases biting forces.
- But facial expression are not good.
- Over closure of mouth; purse-string appearance may occur.
- Lips loose their fullness; decreased ms tone.
- Creases appear at corners of mouth and may lead to PRELECHE due to candidal infections.

- Leads to loss of CUBICLE space of oral cavity.
- Push tongue in the throat and may block EUSTACHIAN TUBE, so hearing and ear problems may appear.
- TMJ Trauma—may cause decreased VDO and its S/S are = clicking, headache, neuralgia, obscure pain and discomfort.
- **Rx denture**—VDO should be built/increased gradually, in successive sets of CDs.

METHODS TO DETERMINE VERTICAL RELATIONS

Mechanical methods

(a) Ridge relations

- Incisive papilla is a stable landmark.
- Incisive papillae is **4 mm** from incisal edge of lower anteriors, in normal natural dentition.
- Incisal edge of maxillary CI is **6 mm below** the incisive papilla.
- Average vertical overlap of U/L Central incisors = 2 mm.
- Correct amount of jaw separation = according to Sears, is paralleling of U/L ridges plus a 5° opening in posterior region.
- The residual ridges in the posterior region are parallel to each other.
- Crest of U/L residual ridges are parallel to each other at VDO, which provides ideal situation for denture stability.

(b) Physiological rest position tests

- Help to determine vertical relation of mandible to maxilla.
- Patient is asked to swallow and let the jaw relax.
- IOG should be 2–4 mm at rest position when seen in premolar region.

(c) Phonetics/Esthetics as Guides

- **Ch, s, j, sounds** brings the U/L anterior teeth very close together, almost (but without) touching them.
- If teeth click = VDO is probably too great.

- Contour of lips depends on contour of labial surfaces of occlusion rims/AP position of teeth and contour of base of CD.

(d) **Esthetic guide** = selection of teeth the same size as natural teeth and estimation of amount of tissue loss from alveolar ridge.

(e) **Swallowing Method**

- On swallowing, the teeth come together with a very light contact at beginning of the swallowing cycle.

BIOLOGICAL CONSIDERATIONS OF HORIZONTAL JAW RELATIONS

- ♦ For best stability of CD, the opposing teeth should meet evenly on both sides within normal final range of mandibular movements. It is known as balanced occlusion.

Centric relation is a:

- ♦ ***Bone to bone relation***.
- ♦ Is a type of horizontal relation.
- ♦ **CR** is the most retruded unstrained position of condyles in glenoid fossa at a given degree of opening.
- ♦ Is the most posterior relation of the mandible to maxilla at established VR along the pathway of THM.
- ♦ Is a reference relation, which is **constant for each individual patient**.
- ♦ Is a mandibular position determined by the nm/neuromuscular reflex learned when primary teeth are in occlusion.
- ♦ Centres of vertical and lateral motion are in their posterior THP.
- ♦ Posterior and middle parts of temporalis and suprahyoid m (geniohyoid and digastric ms) move and fix the mandible in its most retruded relation to the maxilla.
- ♦ Masseter, medial pterygoid and temporalis ms/(MMT) ms elevate the mandible to a particular vertical relation with maxilla.
- ♦ Lateral pterygoid/LT m shows little activity when mandible is in its CR.

Centric occlusion/CO is a **tooth-to-tooth relation** of U and L teeth.

- ♦ Edentulous patients cannot control mandibular movements or avoid deflective occlusal contacts in CR due to loss of receptors in PDL.
- ♦ CR must be recorded for edentulous patients to establish CO in harmony.
- ♦ Upper cast is accurately oriented to the opening axis of articulator by location of a physiologic terminal hinge axis/THA and a face bow transfer.
- ♦ At THA—there is NO TRANSLATION movement occurs.
  - is within THM/terminal hinge movements.
  - mandible is most retruded in respect to maxillary.
  - THM are those posterior border movements, which occur without translation.
- ♦ A VDO should be established between 2 jaws to provide adequate inter occlusal gap/IOG and allow the mandibular ms to function at their optimal physiologic length.
- ♦ With face bow-casts should be mounted to a physiologic THA to correspond with THA of articulator.
- ♦ CR serves as a references relation for establishing an occlusion. CR is a HORIZONTAL relation used to orient the lower cast to the upper cast for CD patients.
- ♦ Edentulous patients use CR closures in mastication and in other functions, e.g. Swallowing.
- ♦ CR permits ***proper adjustments of CG***/condylar guidance for control of eccentric movements.
- ♦ CR orients the lower cast to the opening axis of articulator and orients CR to hinge axis of articulator and mandible.
- ♦ CR records can be made either by minimal closing pressures or under heavy closing pressures.
- ♦ If minimal closing pressures is used, the occlusion should be tested under heavy pressure.

- Minimal pressure teeth produces the BEST results for most patients.

REALEFF—is the tissue resiliency.

- Known as **phase resiliency and like effect.**
- Undue pressure in securing the relation must be avoided to eliminate the possibility of excessive displacement of soft tissues.
- Materials used for minimal pressure technique are—soft POP, ZOE or soft wax.
- Minimal pressure should be applied to avoid distortion of soft tissues and especially if the tissue depth is uneven and opposing ridge relation or size is not normal.
- Temporal m. shows reduced functions when the mandible is in a protruded position.

Recording CR

- **Static methods** = advantage is that it causes minimal displacement of recording bases on the basal seat.
- **Functional methods**—involve functional activity/movement of mandible at the time of recording. The disadvantage is that it causes lateral and AP displacement of recording bases.
- Swallowing procedure establishes both proper vertical and horizontal relation of mandible to maxilla.

Extra-oral tracings

Gothic arch tracing/arrow point tracings

- Are made ***in horizontal plane*** to record the relation of U/L jaws.
- To find out ***true retruded position of mandible, indicated by sharp apex*** of tracing.
- This centre point varies at different levels of VDO.
- Extra-oral tracings are preferred over intra-oral tracings, as I/O tracings are very small and not clear.
- Central bearing point should not be used when ridge relation is not normal or when there is excess soft tissue on the ridges.

- **Neutral zone** = given by Fish; is a portion of equilibrium of tongue, lips and cheek forces. It is occupied by the teeth and polished surface of CD.

Level of occlusal plane/OP

- Incisal plane is parallel to **interpupillary line**.
- Height should be adjusted to allow for the length of natural tooth and the amount of tissue resorption.
- **2 mm below** the border of upper lip.
- OP posteriorly should be parallel to the **ala-tragus line**.

- **Occlusal table** = i.e. mandibular occlusal surfaces; is an area bounded by cheek, tongue, pterygomandibular raphe and its overlying tissues posteriorly, and the contraction of corner of mouth anteriorly.
- **Modiolus = 8 muscles meet** at the corner of mouth; becomes fixed when buccinator contracts; presses corner of mouth at premolars to close the occlusal table in front/mesially; food can not escape at corner of mouth unless 7th damaged (e.g. Bell's Palsy).
- RMP are relatively **STABLE posterior landmarks** even in patients with advanced ridge resorption.
- Mandibular first molar = is at a level corresponding to ***two-thirds of the way up*** the RMP.
- To test the correct VDO—the ***average speaking space*** or interocclusal/inter-rim space is observed on making **'S' sound** (e.g. sixty-six).
- This speaking space between posterior teeth is not related to inter-occlusal space of rest position.
- This space is 1.5–3 mm for most of the patients.
- Patients with Class II m.o. have large space (3–6 mm).
- Patients with Class III m.o. have small space = 1 mm.

Arch form

- Natural teeth are in a zone of equilibrium/neutral zone, which is the resultant of all the forces acting on it [**Buccinator mechanism**].

- **Best guide** = consider pattern of bone resorption and use stable anatomic landmarks.

Mandibular Arch form

1. Pattern of Bone loss

- From labial side of anterior residual ridge.
- Equally on buccal and lingual sides of the ridge in PM region.
- Mainly on lingual side of ridge in MOLAR REGION, because mandible is wider at its inferior border than at ridge crest.
- Residual ridge becomes more lingually in anterior region and more bucally in posterior region.
- Lingual surfaces of posterior teeth should be placed on a line joining lingual side of RMP to a point just lingual to crest of ridge in PM region.
- Corners of mouth determine approx location for C and First PM.
- In cases of advanced anterior ridge reduction, when mentalis m migrates to the crest of ridge = surgical labial sulcus deepening is done.

Maxillary Arch form

Bone loss occurs at

- Labial and buccal areas of maxillary residual ridge.
- So ridge is usually PALATAL to the original location of the natural teeth.
- **Incisive papilla** is a very stable landmark on the palate.
- Incisal edges of max. CI are = **8–10 mm anterior** to the centre of incisive papilla.
- Tips of canines are ± 1 mm in front of the CENTRE of papilla.
- Canines should be located in a coronal **plane passing through posterior border of the papillae**.

Degenerative changes in skin appear if not proper lip support is there as:

- Deep vertical lines in body and margin of lips (**Purse-string appearance**).

- Shortening and thinning of lips.
- Tendency for lip margins to roll inwards.
- Nasolabial fold changes direction; becomes continuous with the groove at the corner of mouth.
- Cheek support is not affected as much as lip, because buccinator m is stretched between modiolus and pterygomandibular raphe.
- Anterior part of maxillary occlusal rim is gently caressed by the lower lip during pronunciation of the letter **'f'**.

4 jaw relations are transferred from the patient to the articulator— It helps to simulate jaw movements.

1. Relation of jaws to opening axis.
2. Vertical separation of jaws.
3. Horizontal relation of U/L jaws in CR.
4. Relation of lower jaw to upper jaw when incisors are edge to edge.

ARTICULATOR—is a mechanical device to which U/L casts may be attached, to represent TMJ and Jaw members.

Theories of occlusion—3:

1. **BONWILL THEORY**
   - Teeth move irt each other as guided by condylar controls and incisal point.
   - Also known as ***theory of equilateral triangle.***
   - **4″ (10 cm)** inter-condylar distance and between each condyle and the mid-incisal point.
   - Its articulator allows lateral movement also.
   - But CG is not adjustable, so movement permitted were in horizontal plane.
2. **CONICAL THEORY**
   - Lower teeth move over surfaces of upper teeth as over the surface of a cone, at a **generating angle of 45°**.
   - Central axis of cone is tipped at a 45° angle.
   - Teeth with 45° cusps are necessary for making CD on Hall–articulator.

3. **SPIERICAL THEORY**—By Monson (1918).
   - Lower teeth move on the surface of upper teeth, as over the surface of a sphere with a **diameter of 8″** (20 cm).
   - Centre of sphere is located in the region of glabella.
   - Surface of sphere passes through the glenoid fossa along the ARTICULAR EMINENCES.
   - Based on relation of teeth with skull observed by von Spee.

TYPES OF RECORDS ON ARTICULATOR—3 classes of records for transferring maxillo-mandibular relations are taken:

1. **Inter occlusal record adjustment**
2. **Graphic record adjustment**
   - Graphic records consists of records of extreme border positions of mandibular movements, which are in CURVES.
   - Articulator must be capable of producing equivalent of these curved movements.
3. **Hinge axis location for adjusting articulators.**
   - H.A. of patients should be correctly located for correct adjustment of the articulators, e.g. transograph.

Selection of articulators

1. If occlusal contacts are to be perfected in CO only = A HINGE TYPE of articulator or one-dimensional instrument, without lateral/protrusive movement is enough.
2. If denture teeth are to have cross-arch and cross-tooth balanced occlusion/BO = A SEMI-ADJUSTABLE articulator is required, e.g. Hanau; whip-mix, etc.
3. If complete control of occlusion is required = A FULLY ADJUSTABLE articulator is required.
   - But these articulators are problematic because of RESILIENCY OF BASAL SOFT TISSUES.

HANAU—is semi-adjustable, arcon type articulator.

- ♦ Is a modified 2–D instrument.
- ♦ Hanau face bow = U shaped; 2–3″ away from face in front and wide enough not to touch side of the face.

- Condyle rods are placed 13 mm in front of external auditory meatus, on a lateral canthus tragus line.
- The condylar rods will be located with in 2 mm of true centre of opening axis of the jaws.
- Horizontal CG is adjusted by = inter-occlusal protrusive record.
- Lateral CG = adjusted by right and left lateral inter-occlusal records.
- IG table = to adjust lateral incisal guidance.
- Incisal pin on Hanau is adjustable and allows for vertical changes.
- Inter condylar distance is adjustable, though this adjustment is rarely done in CD construction, but is required in FPD construction.

RELATING patient to whip mix articulator.

- Is semi adjustable, arcon type articulator.
- Upper and lower members are not mechanically connected.
- Inter condylar distance is semi-adjustable to small (88 mm), medium (100 mm) and large (112 mm) (i.e. a difference of 12 mm b/w each type).
- Vertical axis of rotation of mandible can be approximated.
- Lateral plates of adjustable incisal guide table can be adjusted for later IG.
- Balancing condyle moves D/F/M and working condyle moves laterally (i.e. Bennett shift).
- Face bow is anteriorly located in the region of infra orbital notch.
- Nasion relator determines vertical position of face bow anteriorly and establishes axis-orbital plane on the patient.
- Metal rods of face bow are located = 6 mm posteriorly from actual transverse axis of articulator to compensate for the location of ear posts in auditory meatus, which are roughly the same distance posterior from mandibular THA of the patient.

OCCLUSAL RIM

- Size and form of rim represents the dental arch of natural teeth plus part of ridge resorbed.

- Occlusal rim may be slightly above the Vermillion border of the upper lip if the lip is long.
- In normal lip–U rim is 2 mm visible below the relaxed upper lip.
- OP is made parallel to ALA TRAGUS line.
- Lower occlusal rim anteriorly at the level of corner of mouth and posteriorly at the level of post. 1/3rd of RMP. This height approximates level of OP.

TEETH SELECTION

- Best way to find colour/form/size of teeth is = By trial in patients mouth.
- Diagnostic cast of the natural teeth are most RELIABLE guide in selection and arranging the anteriors.
- Photos = width of teeth and outline form can be seen.
- R/G images = slightly enlarged and distorted due to divergence of x-rays.
- Women's teeth are smaller than men's teeth, especially LI.
- Approximately canines are placed at the corners of the mouth.
- Apex of maxillary natural canine is found by extension of parallel lines from the lateral surfaces of the alae of nose on to middle of the labial surface of upper occlusal rim.
- Greatest bizygomatic width divided by 3.3 = overall width of upper 6 anteriors.
- Ratio of cranial circumference to the width of upper anteriors = 10:1.
- Av. width of upper anteriors = 48–52 mm

  < 48 mm = Small teeth.

  > 52 mm = Large teeth.

FORM OF ANTERIOR TEETH

- Should harmonize with the shape of patients face, e.g. square/tapering/ovoid.
- Shape of LABIAL surface is more important than the outline form.

- Grinding should be done on anteriors according to age of the patient.
- Labial face of tooth viewed from proximal aspect = should show PROFILE/CONTOUR OF FACE, i.e. convex/straight/ concave.
- Labial surface of tooth as viewed from incisal edge = should be similar to contour of face as seen from under the chin.
- **LEON–WILLIAM'S RULE.**
- Broad contact areas look more natural, because long contact surfaces give a truer appearance of age.
- **SPA concept**—i.e. **dentogenic concept** is based on sex/ personality/age of the patient.

♦ Squareness of tooth form = MUSCULANITY.

♦ Rounded incisal and proximal contours = femininity.

♦ LI smaller than CI feminine.

♦ LI almost equal to CI musculine.

COLOUR OF TEETH—colour of face and teeth came from the effects of reflected light on the rods and cones of retina.

♦ Colour of **most concern to dentists** is = **yellow band** in spectrum, because colours of face and teeth are primarily yellow.

4 qualities of colour are:

(a) Hue

(b) Saturation (chroma)

(c) Brilliance (value)

(d) Translucency

HUE—is the specific colour produced by a specific wavelength of light acting on retina.

♦ It is the COLOUR itself.

♦ Must be in harmony with face.

CHROMA

♦ Amount of colour per unit of area of an object, i.e. same colour but different shade/concentration.

VALUE—i.e. brilliance (Light or Dark).

- Is the lightness or darkness of an object.
- Variance is produced by **dilution of the colour** (i.e. hue) by black or white.
- It must correspond to the lightness/darkness of the patient's face.
- In fair people = teeth are of less colour; Colours are less saturated; teeth are lighter in colour.
- In dark people = darker teeth.

TRANSLUCENCY

- Property of an object which permits passage of light through it, but cannot give any distinguishing image. It is a characteristic of enamel.
- Translucency of teeth has the effect of mixing of various colours (hues) of porcelain in the teeth with changing colours within the oral cavity.
- Teeth appear darker when mouth is nearly closed than when it is open wide.
- ***Blue is the complementary colour of yellow.***
- So stare at blue cloth for 30 sec. before colour matching for better observation.
- Colour of face is the BASIC GUIDE to the colour of the teeth.

AGE—colour of natural teeth becomes progressively DARKER with age (especially incisal edges of lower anteriors).

- So darker teeth are better for older patients and lighter teeth in young patients.
- Extracted teeth are valuable for selection of size and form of teeth but not the colour, because of the loss of colour and H_2O from the extracted tooth.

COLOUR SELECTION OF ARTIFICIAL TEETH—is done in 3 positions:

1. Outside the mouth alongside of the nose = to establish basic hue, brilliance and saturation.

2. Under the lips with only incisal edges exposed = to reveal effect of tooth colour when patient's mouth is relaxed.
3. Under the lips with only cervical end covered and mouth open = to simulate tooth exposure during smiling, when light is reflected through the teeth from inside of mouth.
   - Colour of teeth should be selected on a bright day; patient sits close to natural light; should be observed in artificial light also (i.e. **2 sources of light** used).
   - **SQUINT TEST** = to correlate tooth colour with face colour. The colour which fades away from the view first is least conspicuous in comparison with colour of the face.

Most common error in selection of anterior teeth = is to select teeth which are too small in size and too light in colour. They create DENTURE–LOOK.

POSTERIOR TEETH SELECTION

- ♦ Occlusal surfaces of artificial teeth should be modified.
- ♦ 2 types of teeth—anatomic, non-anatomic.
- ♦ **Anatomic teeth**—used for those posterior teeth that more nearly resemble the teeth of a dentition.
- ♦ BL width of artificial teeth should be greatly reduced from the width of natural teeth they replace.
- ♦ Narrow posterior teeth enhance the development of correct form of polished surfaces of CD by allowing buccal and lingual flanges to slope away from occlusal surfaces.
- ♦ Helps denture stability on ridges.
- ♦ Also decreases stresses falling on basal seat.

MD lengths of posterior teeth

- Area available for artificial posterior teeth is = from distal surface of canine to the beginning of RMP.
- **Mold No.** = total MD width of four posterior teeth in mm.

- ♦ Posterior teeth should not be placed too close to the posterior border of maxillary denture = to avoid cheek biting.

- If mandibular ridge slopes up sharply at its distal end = DO NOT PLACE POSTERIOR TEETH on this slope, otherwise lower denture will SLIDE FORWARD during working.
- Posterior teeth SHOULD NOT BE placed on RMP; because soft tissue of RMP is easily displaced and hence, CD tips during function.

VERTICAL LENGTH OF POSTERIOR TEETH

- Should correlate with inter-arch space and to the length of anterior teeth.
- Length of maxillary first PM should be comparable to canine = for proper esthetic effect.
- Dental arch form should be as nearly same as possible to the NATURAL ARCH FORM; should be in neutral zone.

Types of posterior teeth

- **Resin teeth**, wear faster and stain easily than porcelain teeth, because they are softer.
- Resin teeth are used against natural teeth/resin teeth/gold covered teeth—to minimize abrasion of enamel/gold.
- Porcelain teeth should be used against porcelain only; so that no abrasion of natural teeth occurs.
- Porcelain teeth used against natural teeth/gold restoration leads to enamel/metal abrasion, because porcelain is harder than enamel.
- Resin teeth also required if inter arch space is less, as it can be decreased in height during set-up but porcelain cannot.
- Resin posterior teeth should not be used with porcelain anterior teeth on CD, because posterior teeth will wear more and will create excessive and destructive forces at anterior part of basal seat, which is least able to bear increased forces.
- Cuspal inclines of posterior teeth depend on plane of occlusion.
- IG = is in control of dentist.
- CG = is in control of anatomy.

- With deep overbite + low posterior teeth inclines = anterior teeth are set with increased overjet.
- With a flat/nearly horizontal IG the posterior tooth inclines should be SHALLOW.
- In CD, IG is determined by the Dr, so posterior tooth inclines are decided after settling the overjet.

Types of posterior teeth are:

1. Anatomic = 33° teeth.
2. Semi anatomic = 20° teeth.
3. Non anatomic = 0° teeth.
   - Cuspal inclination is the angle formed by incline of MB cusp of lower first molar with the horizontal plane.
   - 33° teeth = give maximum opportunity for fully BO (Best for BO).
   - But final effective height of the cusps is related to many factors, e.g. inclination of teeth, IG, height of OP and COS/COM/COW curves, i.e. curves of spee, Monsoon and Wilson.

Curves	**Features**
Curve of Spee	• Is the AP curve which begins at the tip of lower canines and follows cusp tips of premolars and molars follows an arc through condyle. • It may form a circle of 4 inches diameter if extended.
Curve of Monsoon	• It is formed by extending the curve of spee and curve of Wilson to all cusps and incisal edges.
Curve of Wilson	• It contacts the buccal and lingual cusp tips of the mandibular posterior teeth. • It is mediolateral on each side of arch. • It occurs due to inward inclination of the crowns of lower posterior teeth. • It helps to align the teeth parallel to the **direction of medial pterygoid ms.**

- **Shallow IG** and esthetics allow as **little cusp height** as possible of posterior teeth for BO and so lateral forces are reduced on residual ridge.
- Anatomic teeth are healthy to support tissues than other teeth.
- **20° teeth** = wider BL dimension than 33° teeth; they have less cusp height.
- **0° teeth** = used ONLY if CR record is set on articulator and no BO is to be established.

Or when it is impossible to record CR/ or in abnormal jaw relations.

TEETH SETTING: Use setting instructions; **Andrews keys**; Fenn-also.

According to Andrews, there are 6 keys to normal occlusion as given below:

Key	Features
I. molar relation	MB cusp of upper first molar falls in the MB groove of the lower first molar; the ML cusp of upper first molar falls in the central fossa of lower first molar; the distal surface of distal marginal ridge of upper first molar contacts and occludes with the mesial surface of MMR of lower second molar.
II. crown	The gingival portion of long axis of each crown angulation; MD tip is distal to the occlusal part of the axis.
III. crown inclination; torque	The angle b/w a line 90° to the OP and a line tangent to the middle of the labial or buccal surface of the clinical crown.
IV. rotations	Should not be there.
V.	Tight contacts.
VI.	Curve of spee; normal depth is 1.5 mm.

Guidelines

1. Amount of bone resorption is proportional to the time of teeth loss.
2. Amount of resorption and the time of edentulousness indicates the distance the teeth should be set from the residual ridge, (should replace natural positions).
3. If natural teeth oppose/occlude a CD then more bone loss occurs in the residual ridges; due to heavy forces.
4. OP of the CD should be in same position as occupied by natural teeth.

Incisive papilla

- Has a constant relation with natural CI.
- Acts as a guide for teeth setting.
- Present in lingual embrasure between CI in midline.
- Labial surfaces of CI = 8–10 mm in front of it.
- Papilla moves distally with severe vertical resorption of ridge.
- Distance of labial surfaces of teeth from papilla may become increased with much vertical bone loss.

Reflection of soft tissues

- Labial surfaces and incisal edges of teeth should be anterior to the tissues at the reflection, where the denture borders would be placed.
- There is an OBTUSE angle between labial surface of root of CI and the clinical crown of the tooth.
- A thin layer of bone exists over the labial surface of root of CI.
- Labial surface of ridge acts as a guide to determine the proper inclination of anterior teeth; but becomes LESS-ACCURATE with extreme resorption.

AP position of dental arch

- Governed by orbicularis oris, its supporting ms; and tone of skin of lips.

- Orbicularis ORIS is affected by 7 other ms at MODIOLUS which are

- ♦ Quadratus labii superioris.
- ♦ Caninus (levator anguli oris).
- ♦ Qudratus labii inferioris.
- ♦ Zygomaticus.
- ♦ Resorius.
- ♦ Triangularis (deeper anguli oris).
- ♦ Buccinator.
- ♦ Zone and action of these ms depends on AP support provided by teeth and denture base materials.
- ♦ MAXILLARY anterior alveolar process is at an angle to the labial face of maxillary incisors and its direction is Upward and Backward. So ridge CREST is more posterior than in recently extracted case.
- ♦ Imaginary roots of the teeth should extend into the residual ridge (before resorption).
- ♦ Position of teeth should resemble NATURAL TOOTH POSITION for best support and esthetics and health of tissues.
- ♦ If horizontal overlap of natural teeth is decreased to develop contacts in CO, unfavorable forces are applied on the anterior residual ridge.
- ♦ Relation of U/L anterior ridges has an influence on AP position of U/L anterior teeth.
- ♦ AP position of teeth should vary with AP relation of ridges, e.g. Class II, Class III.
- ♦ In Class III, i.e. prognathic mandible, the incisors can be placed end-to-end, but never labial to lower anteriors. Incisal edges of U/L teeth should cut at an angle, which have a seating action on maxillary denture.
- ♦ Insufficient space between ridges indicates that either artificial teeth are LONGER than natural teeth or the VD of face is too short.

- Fibrous tissues of maxillary tuberosity should be SURGICALLY removed for better stability.

MANDIBULAR ANTERIOR TEETH

- Roots of mandibular incisors should be seen to be coming out of mandibular alveolar process.
- Mandibular natural teeth are mostly LABIAL to the apices of their roots. It is because the pattern of bone resorption in mandibular anterior region is on labial side.
- The long axis of all natural mandibular teeth if extended apically seem to DIVERGE, while that of maxillary teeth seem to converge.
- Overbite of U/L incisors = 1.5 mm.
- Overjet of U/L incisors varies with sizes of U/L Jaws.
- Upper teeth should be related to the upper jaw and lower teeth to lower jaw, for BEST positioning and stability.

OCCLUSAL PLANE

- Posterior end of OP should be at the level of junction of middle and distal 3rd of RMP.
- This level is BEST familiar to the TONGUE, which then helps in the stability of denture and mastication.
- OP level is anterior region is influenced by—length of lips, ridge fullness, ridge height, maxillo-mandibular space, incisal guide angle.
- If OP is too low anteriorly and/or too high posteriorly, then the mandibular denture slides forward under biting pressure.
- Level of OP should be placed as nearly as possible to position of natural O.P.
- Most reliable guides for OP height are corners of mouth and RMPs.

Bucco-lingual position of posteriors

- Determined anteriorly by position/arch form of anterior teeth and posteriorly by the shape of the basal seat of MANDIBLE.

- Should be properly related to supporting bone and to the soft tissues which contact their buccal-lingual surfaces.
- Determined by NEUTRAL ZONE between cheeks and tongue, where these forces are in perfect balance.
- Forces provided by the tongue/cheeks and lips influence the alignment of teeth in dental arches. See forces from profit.
- Buccinator mechanism (Refer to orthodontics–section).
- Posterior teeth have most FAVORABLE LEVERAGE if set close to the residual ridge and LINGUAL to it.
- Amount of leverage exerted on OP depends on the distance the OP is above the ridge (i.e. Moment = Force × Distance).

Posterior Arch form

- Should conform the shape of residual ridge.
- Teeth should be placed so as to have erupted from the ridge.
- RULE = a perpendicular erected from buccal side of crest of ridge should bisect the buccal cusp of lower first molar.
- Form of each dental arch must be in harmony within itself and with its foundation.
- Posterior teeth are set between 2 lines extending posteriorly from the distal surface of canines to the buccal and lingual margins of RMP.
- 30° teeth are more effective for checking accuracy of jaw relations than 20° or 0° teeth.
- Most residual ridges are curved laterally between the position of canine and RMP.

Guidelines for CO

- Long axis of each upper tooth is DISTAL to long axis of corresponding lower tooth.
- Each tooth is opposed by 2 teeth except lower CI and upper LAST molar.
- Mandibular first molar is set such that it contacts both 2nd PMs and its buccal cusp would be bisected by a perpendicular on buccal side of crest of ridge.

- Alignment of lower buccal cusps should correspond with the curvature of arch form of the residual ridge.
- Distance between distal surface of lower canines and mesial end of RMP determines the total AP space, which may be covered by the teeth.
- Distal limit of posterior teeth is governed by incline of the lower ridge. If tooth is placed on this incline—the denture will slide forward if pressure is applied on that tooth.
- The BL width of posterior teeth should be narrower than natural teeth to decrease biting pressure and to increase tongue space.
- Anterior teeth play important role in 3 basic oral functions, i.e. ESTHETICS, INCISION, PHONETICS.
- So they should be of same size, shape, colour and position.
- They also help to regain TONE OF SKIN and lips and proper ms functions.
- Phonetics can serve as a guide to esthetics and to establish VR of the Jaws.

VERIFICATION OF JAW RELATIONS

- Patients should leave existing dentures out of the mouth for a minimum of 24 hrs before the jaw relation records are verified and try-in.
- It allows soft tissues of basal seat to take rest and come in the same form as they were at final impression.
- An error in CR will cause error in CO and produce contact of inclined planes of teeth. Amount of error is magnified by the effect of inclined plane contacts.
- Further closure causes teeth to slide in CO.
- Path of closure is an arc about posterior THA.
- There should be uniform and simultaneous contacts on both sides of mouth and in front and back, without any detectable touch and slide of teeth.
- SQUASH BITE is taken ST there are imprints of all posterior teeth, without perforation and penetration of wax.

- If perforation is there—it shows defective occlusal contacts and shifting of bases.
- Uniform contacts without pressure are less damaging to the tissues of basal seat, because the dentures do not get displaced.

FACIAL EXPRESSION AND HARMONY

- Appearance of lower half of face depends on

1. S/S of reduced VRO = thin, drooping, long upper lip; reduced vermilion border; so tense wrinkled lips show patient's efforts to hold in CD.
2. Premature aging appearance of lips is due to—lack of support for lips and cheeks; improper replacement.
3. Apparent extra fullness of lower lip = too broad mandibular arch. or elimination/reduction of mento-labial sulcus. It may also be due to lingual placement of lower anteriors or overextended/ thick labial flanges.

- **Nasolabial sulcus**/groove = from ALA of nose to just outside the level of rima-oris (corner of lip line).
- **Zygomaticus** m = origin from zygomatic bone, goes D and F; inserts in corner of mouth; produces nasolabial sulcus during smiling/laughing.
- Upper lip rests on labial surfaces of upper anteriors.
- Lower lip rests on labial surface of lower anteriors and incisal 3rd of the upper teeth.
- So edge of lower lip should extend upward and outward from mento labial sulcus.
- Clinical crowns of lower teeth are labial to the bone, which supports them.
- Many ms are inserted in modiolus and orbicularis oris m. at the corner of the mouth, and their functioning length depends on the function of orbicularis oris m.
- **8 ms** inserted in modiolus/orbicularis oris m are:
    - Mentalis
    - Zygomaticus

- Quadratus labii superioris
- Quadratus labii inferioris
- Levator anguli oris (caninus)
- Depressor anguli oris (triangularis)
- Buccinator
- Risorius

- If teeth are placed over the crest of ridge, it leads to the lack of lip support.
- Bone resorption in mandibular anterior region = moves the ridge first LINGUALLY and then LABIALLY, as resorption continues.
- **ORBICULARIS ORIS m** = is the m. of lips, attached by maxillary labial frenum to maxilla along the midline, and by mandibular labial frenum to the mandible.
- **Buccinator** = forms entire side-wall of cheek from the corner of mouth; reaches the lingual surface of ramus to join the superior constrictor of the pharynx at PTERYGOMANDIBULAR RAPHE.
- Buccinator ms and orbicularis oris form a FUNCTIONAL UNIT.
- If VDO is v. less and the teeth are placed far posteriorly, the ms sag at rest and are less effective on contraction. It is due to movement of INSERTION of THESE Ms closer to their ORIGIN. It gives senile appearances.
- If ridges are very much resorbed due to long-standing–the denture borders are made THICK to restore position of these ms.
- Position and expression of lips and face are BEST GUIDE = to determines proper AP position of teeth.
- Insufficient support of lips is characterized by drooping of corners of mouth, reduction of visible part of Vermillion border, drooping/deepening of nasolabial grooves, reduction of prominence of philtrum, vertical lines above the vermilion border.
- AP position of teeth must correspond to the positions of ridges, e.g. in prognathic patients—the anterior teeth can be set end-to-end, with incisal edges producing a SEATING ACTION as upper CD.

- Imaginary roots of teeth should appear farther in front of the crest of the ridge, if there is greater amount of resorption.
- Imaginary transverse line between upper canines should cross the middle of incisive fossa for proper AP width and position of 6 anteriors.
- During normal smile, the incisal and middle 3rd of max anteriors are seen.
- Incisal 3rd of mandibular anteriors are visible.
- Mandibular anterior teeth are seen more than maxillary anteriors during SPEAKING and are seen more in men than in women.
- Lower lip is a better GUIDE for vertical position of anteriors than the upper lip.
- Incisal edges of natural lower canines and cusp tip of mand first PM are at the level of lower lip at corner of the mouth when mouth is slightly open.
- U/L natural teeth occupy approx the same amount of inter-arch space, and should be replicated in CD.

PHONETICS ("from fenn also)

Sound	Examples	Features
Labial	**B, p, m**	AP position of anterior teeth and thickness of labial flange of denture affect them.
Labio-dental, e.g. fifty five	**F, v**	• Made between upper incisors and labio-lingual centre to the posterior 1/3rd of lower lip. • Relation of incisal edges to lower lip should be observed. • If upper teeth touch labial side of lower lip. • During f, v speaking, it shows too far forward placed upper teeth. • If lower anterior are placed too far forward, then lower lip tends to raise the lower CD.

PHONETICS ("from fenn also) (*Contd.*)

Sound	Examples	Features
Dental	**Th**	• Tip of tongue comes slightly between U/L anteriors. • If about 3 mm of tip of tongue is not seen, implies anterior teeth are probably too far forward (except $C_2 D_1$ malocclusion) for increased overbite. • If > 6 mm tip seen, it implies teeth are placed too far lingually.
Alveolar	**T, d, n, s, z**	• Tongue–tip contacts with anterior most past of palate. • If teeth are set lingually, the t will come like d. • If teeth are placed anteriorly, the d will sound as t. • Thick acrylic in RUGAE AREA has same effect.
Sibilants	**S, z, sh, ch, zh, j**	Are alveolar sounds. U/L incisors come end-to-end, without touching. Produced between rest and occluding position. If incisors do not come exactly end-to-end, it implies overjet error, e.g. Class II, Class III.
S-sounds		• S-sound can be considered as dental and alveolar sound. • S-sound is made with tip of tongue against the alveolus in rugae area, with small space for escape of air between tongue and alveolus.

PHONETICS (from fenn also) (*Contd.*)

Sound	Examples	Features
		• **Lisping** occurs if space is too broad and thin. • Frequent cause of undesired whistles with CD is. • A NARROW POSTERIOR DENTAL ARCH FORM, because tongue comes forward leaving a very small space for escape of air. • In 30% patients, S-sound occurs with tongue tip contacting lingual side of anterior part of lower CD, and arching against the palate to form desired size/slope of airway.
Palatal	**e.g. in year, vision; she; onion**	These do not present any problem in CD making.
Velar	**K, g, ng**	

Important points

- Sound of speech sounds is NOT A SAFE GUIDE for teeth setting.
- OBSERVING the position of lips and tongue to the teeth and CD bases when sounds are made is A SAFE GUIDE.
- Functional contouring of palatal surface of CD helps to attain a physiologic space for sounds.

INCLINATION OF ANTERIOR TEETH

- Roots of anterior teeth are parallel to and very close to the labial surface of the bone.
- An obtuse angle exists between bone and labial surfaces of the teeth.

- Profile of face also represents the inclination of anteriors, which is parallel to the profile line of face, e.g. in Class I, II, III malocclusion cases.

A. Harmony of arch form with residual ridge

- Anterior arch may be square/tapering/ovoid.
- CI in square arch form is more nearly on a line with canines; no rotations in incisors; harmonize with a BROAD-SQUARE FACE.
- In tapering arch form—CI are a greater distance forward from the canines; incisors are rotated/crowded due to less space in the arch; harmonize with a narrow-tapering face.
- In ovoid arch, CI are forward of the canines, in a position between square and tapering arch from; seldom rotated incisors; broader effect harmonious with ovoid face.

PALATAL VAULT

- If Broad and shallow = arch form SQUARE.
- If High and V-shaped = arch form TAPERING.
- If Rounded vault of average height = arch form OVOID.

BUCCAL CORRIDOR SIZE

- Is the space between buccal surfaces of upper teeth and corner of mouth, which is seen when patient smiles.
- It helps eliminate an appearance of too many teeth in the front of the mouth.

B. Harmony of long axes of CI and the face

- Incisal plane should be parallel to inter-pupillary line.
- Midline of arch should be at the centre of the face.
- Long axes of CI should be parallel to the long axis of the face.
- Midline position of CI is guided by position of incisive papilla.
- Lower CI, the imaginary line should pass between middle of lower denture and between lower CI.

C. Harmony of teeth with smiling line of lower lip

- Lower lip forms a pleasant curvature known as SMILING LINE, which is used to set upper anterior.
- Incisal edges of upper anteriors follow this smiling line during smiling.
- Vertical position of upper canines is mainly responsible for the shape of smiling line.
- When incisal edges of canines a slightly shorter than LI, the smiling line will tend to be parallel with the lower lip on smiling.

D. Harmony of opposing lines of labial and buccal surfaces

- There should be ASYMMETRICAL SYMMETRY in arrangement of the teeth to give NATURAL APPEARANCE.
- Long axes are the balanced opposing lines on either side of midline.
- Labial and buccal lines must have opposing equivalent angles.
- Labial and buccal lines of teeth and lines of the face should be harmonious.
- Square and ovoid faces should have teeth that have lines, which are more nearly perpendicular, and in tapering faces should have lines which are more divergent from the perpendicular.

E. Harmony of teeth and profile lines of the face

- Labial surfaces of maxillary CI are parallel to the profile line of the face.
- When maxillary CI are parallel to profile line, the LI should be set at an opposite angel to prevent parallelism from being dominant.
- Most predominant facial form can be helpful as a guide for teeth positioning.

F. Harmony of tooth wear and age

- Incisal edges and proximal surfaces wear with age, which should be incorporated in the artificial teeth.

- More lingually placed upper teeth or parts of teeth wear more than more labially placed upper teeth.
- Greatest amount of wear on lower anteriors occur on more labially placed lower teeth.
- Wear should be placed on teeth, where it would have occurred during function and also where it assists in mechanics of BO.

REFINEMENT OF INDIVIDUAL TOOTH POSITION

- Should be set with typical inclination and rotations for natural appearance.
- Labial surface of maxillary CI is parallel to profile line, which is approx perpendicular.
- Labial surface of LI is in at the cervical end more than adjacent teeth.
- Labial surface of canine is out at cervical end more than the other maxillary teeth.
- Degree to which cervical end of canine is out is in harmony with the lateral lines of the face.
- Labial surface of mandibular CI is in at cervical end more than LI or canine.
- Mandibular LI is out at cervical end more than CI such that it is almost perpendicular.
- MD inclination
  - CI is almost perpendicular.
  - LI is inclined distally at CEJ.
  - C is inclined distally at CEJ less than LI; more than CI.
- Mandibular canine is out at CEJ same as maxillary.

Location

- CI is slightly rotated from parallelism to a tangent of the line of arch contour.
- LI rotated to have its distal surface turned lingually at a larger angle to the tangent.

- Canine rotated to half its DISTAL half in the direction of posterior arch form.
- Mandibular incisor are generally parallel to tangent of arch contour.

VERTICAL POSITION

- ♦ Max LI and C are slightly above the level of the inclined plane.
- ♦ Mandibular 1, 2, 3 are at the same level.

HARMONY with SPA features of patients

- ♦ **Femininity** = curved surfaces/softness in form of dentition/ prominent smiling line.
- ♦ **Masculinity** = boldness/vigor and squareness of dentition/ straightness of incisal line of teeth.

Esthetics and IG = best plan for CD STABILITY is:

- With SHALLOW IG.
- If overbite is decreased, then increase overjet.
- Protrusive balance is less important than lateral balance.
- Angle of IG for lateral occlusion must be adjusted so that the posterior teeth contact at the same time the U/L canines are end-to-end.
- Also, U/L anterior teeth should not be in contact when posterior teeth are in CO to avoid excess pressure and bone resorption of anterior ridge.

Removable Partial Dentures

Kennedy classification

Classification	Features
I	Bilateral edentulous areas located posterior to remaining teeth.
II	A unilateral edentulous area located posterior to remaining teeth.
III	A unilateral edentulous area, with natural teeth remaining anterior and posterior to it.
IV	A single, bilateral, i.e. crossing the midline edentulous area, located anterior to remaining teeth.

Kennedy's classification of edentulous spaces

- Class I bilateral free end saddle.
- Class II unilateral free end saddle.
- Class III unilateral bounded saddle.
- Class IV anterior/across the midline.

Rules

- The most posterior edentulous area's determine the classification.
- There can be no modification areas in Class IV arch.
- Class I RPD—tooth and tissue supported. 3 features required for it are—adequate support for distal extension, flexible direct retainers; and some provision for indirect retention; mostly support is TISSUE–borne; FUNCTIONAL impression is required, relining required.

- Class III PD—entirely tooth borne RPD; no Indirect Retainer required; no functional impression required; total metallic; no relining required.
- Class II PD (with modification areas) is in between Class I and III and has design features of both Class I and III; combination of tooth bone and tissue borne PD; distal extension is made of acrylic.
- Modification spaces—are edentulous areas in the arch, other than the main area describing the classification.
- Maximum % age is of Kennedy Class I; Class II; Class I mod 2; Class II mod 1 = 72% and Kennedy Class III; Class III mod 1 (14%).

COMPONENTS OF RPD

1. Major connector.
2. Minor connector .
3. Rests.
4. Direct retainers.
5. Reciprocal/stabilising components.
6. Indirect retainers.
7. Bases.

Major Connectors

- Connects the part of prosthesis located on one side of arch with those of opposite side.
- All parts are directly/indirectly attached to it.
- Must be RIGID—for proper distribution of forces.
- **RIGIDITY**—important requirement; resists flexing and torque.
- Superior border of a lingual bar connector should be located at least 4 mm below gingival margins and its width should be at least 4 mm.
- It should be free from movable tissues.
- There should be minimal gap between MC and tissue in mandible to avoid overgrowth of tissues.

- There should be no gap in maxillary arch for wider force distribution.
- In upper arch-border of palatal connector should be 6 mm away from gingival margin and parallel to their mean curve.
- All MINOR connectors should connect the major connectors at RIGHT angle.
- Anterior border should avoid interference with tongue and should follow the valleys between rugae.
- Posterior border should be just anterior to the vibrating line.
- Most important property of an RPD esp of major connector is RIGIDITY.

Lingual Bar

- Half pear shaped with more bulk at lower border, above the moving tissues.
- **Continuous bar retainer** = located on or slightly above the cinguli of anterior teeth.
- **Linguoplate** = should be thin; should not extend above the middle 3rd of lingual surface.
- **Labial bar** = is used when there is extreme lingual inclination of lower incisors and PMs.

Maxillary major connectors–4:

1. **Single palatal strap**
   - Most widely used but least logical.
   - Must be rigid.
   - Bilateral tooth borne RPD of short spans especially posterior edentulous areas may be connected with broad palatal strap.
   - Used mostly in Class III type.

2. **U-shaped palatal connector**
   - Least desirable.
   - Used only if large torus or for replacing several anterior teeth.

- Lacks rigidity.
- Does not provide good support.

3. Combination of Anterior and Posterior palatal strap–type connectors

- Most RIGID.
- Posterior palatal bar should be half oval in shape and placed posteriorly to avoid interference with tongue and movable tissues.
- Anterior strap should avoid Rugae coverage and tongue interferences.
- Should cross midline at right angle.
- Used mostly in Class II and IV types.

4. Palatal plate type

- Used in Class I situations.
- Located anterior to PPS; not on soft palate.

Release of inherent strains in resin base of CD requires some provision to maintain intimate contact of posterior part of denture and tissues. It is achieved by scoring the master cast to a depth of 1 × 1 mm as PPS.

♦ So beading (not more than 0.5 mm) is done to maintain the tissue contacts.

MINOR CONNECTORS

♦ Join the major connector with other parts of RPD.

♦ Also help to transfer functional stresses to the abutment teeth. It is ***prosthesis-to-abutment function***.

♦ It transfers effects of retainers; rests and stabilizing components to rest of the RPD. It is its ***abutment-to-prosthesis function***.

♦ Should be RIGID.

♦ Should be located in embrasure and so least irritating to the tongue.

♦ Should be thickest towards the lingual surface and tapering towards the contact area (V-shaped) (BUTT JOINT).

- Should be at right angle to major connectors.
- Contacts the guiding plane surfaces of abutment teeth and is 2/3rd the width b/w tips of buccal and lingual cusps.
- Extends from marginal ridge to 2/3rd the length of enamel crown, and is TRIANGULAR SHAPED when seen from above.
- Should not be located on convex axial surface of abutment.
- Minor connectors for mandibular distal extension base should extend posteriorly about 2/3rd the length of edentulous ridge and have elements on both lingual and buccal surfaces.
- Minor connector for maxillary distal extension should extend the ENTIRE length of the ridge and should be of a ladder like and loop design and extended to pterygomaxillary notch.

TISSUE STOPS

- Help in retention of acrylic resin bases.
- Prevent distortion of framework during resin processing.
- Should engage buccal and lingual slopes of the ridge for stability.
- Finishing index tissue stop = is located distal to the terminal abutment and is a continuation of minor connector contacting the guiding plane.
- Finishing lines should make an angle of less than 90° and should restore the natural palatal shape. It should minimize the bulk of acrylic resin attaching the artificial teeth.
- Junction of major and minor connectors at palatal finishing lines should be located 2 mm medial from an imaginary line, which would contact the lingual surfaces of missing posterior teeth.
- If OPD is not removed for a long period the mm may get changed in CT so the RPD should be removed at right s.t. tissues may rest.
- Most important property of RPD especially major connector is—RIGIDITY.

RESTS AND REST SEATS

- To provide VERTICAL SUPPORT.
- Prevents settling of denture and impingement of soft tissues.

- Direct forces along the long axis of abutment teeth.
- Must be RIGID.
- Rest seat should be rounded, triangular shape, with the apex towards the centre of the occlusal surface, inclined apically from marginal ridge.
- Base of the seat at MR should be at least 2.5 mm for bulk.
- MR is vertically decreased to 1.5 mm for bulk and to assist occlusal interference.
- Floor of seat should be **concave/spoon shaped**.
- Angle formed by occlusal rest and vertical minor connector from which it arises **should be less than 90°**—for avoiding slippage of RPD.
- Lingual extension of rest seat helps to provide strength.
- It is like a 'BALL and SOCKET JOINT'.

POSSIBLE MOVEMENT OF RPD—3 types:

1. Rotation about an axis through most posterior abutments. (i.e. **Fulcrum line**).
2. Rotation about a longitudinal axis as the distal extension base moves in a rotary direction about the residual ridge. It is resisted by RIGIDITY OF MAJOR CONNECTOR.
3. Rotation about an imaginary vertical axis located near the centre of dental arch. It is resisted by stabilizing components.
   - Occlusal rest should provide only OCCLUSAL SUPPORT; all movements of RPD other than in gingival direction should be resisted by other components.
   - In a tooth borne RPD, only HORIZONTAL rotation is of any significance, which is resisted by STABILISING components.
   - Canine is preferred over incisors for rest placement, because it is a strong tooth.
   - Lingual rest is preferred over incisal rests because of = ESTHETICS.
   - Lingual rest is also better, because it is placed near the horizontal axis of rotation (tipping) of abutment and so will have less tendency to tip the tooth.

- Rests seats in crowns and inlays are made deeper and larger than those in enamel.
- Incisal rests are placed at incisal angles of anterior teeth; it is least desirable. Used mainly as INDIRECT RETAINERS or auxiliary rests. It is more applicable to MANDIBULAR canine.
- It is better than 3/4 crown aesthetically.
- Rest seat inclined s.t the deepest part should be apical to incisal edge = it helps to direct the forces along the long axis of teeth.
- Slight labial bevel is also given.

Functions of different components of the RPD

Components	Functions
Occlusal rest Residual ridge Denture base	Support Stability against horizontal movements
Rigid connectors IR Other stabilizing components	
Retaining elements Intimate relationship of denture bases and maxillary major connector with tissues	Retention against dislodging forces

Retention—depends on:

- Accuracy of impression.
- Accuracy of fit of denture bases.
- Total area of contact.

Retentive forces are:

1. **Adhesion** = saliva to denture and tissues.
2. Cohesion = saliva to saliva attraction.
3. Atmospheric pressure.
4. Tissues around the polished surfaces of denture.
5. Gravity.

- Adhesion and cohesion are effective if there is PERFECT APPOSITION of impression surface of denture to mucosal surfaces.
- Atmospheric pressure acts as rescue force when extreme dislodging forces are applied to the denture. It depends on perfect BORDER SEAL.
- These 3 factors are directly proportional to the AREA COVERED by denture.
- Plastic molding of tissues around the polished surfaces helps to perfect the BORDER SEAL and also provide MECHANICAL lock.

DIRECT RETAINER—is a unit of RPD, which engages an abutment to RESIST DISPLACEMENT of RPD away from the basal seat.

- ♦ **Intracoronal retainers** = depend on frictional resistance for RETENTION of RPD.
- ♦ **Extracoronal retainers** = the clasp type retainer engages external surface of abutment cervical to HOC. Here, no frictional resistance is used. A flexible arm or a spring device produces resistance to removal.
- ♦ **Internal attachments** are better from aesthetic point of view.
- ♦ An internal attachment should not be used with tissue supported distal extension denture bases, unless a stress-breaker is used between them.

EXTRACORONAL DR

Component	**Function**	**Location**
Rest	Support	Occlusion, lingual, incisal
Minor Connectors	Stabilisation	Proximal surfaces, from MR to 2/3rd height of crown
Clasp Arms	Stabilisation	Apical part of middle 3rd of crown.
	Reciprocation	Apical part of middle 3rd of crown.
	Retention	Gingival 3rd of crown in measured undercut.

- **Angle of cervical convergence** = is the angle formed by tooth surface (at HOC) to the vertical blade of surveyor.
- Greater angle requires placement of clasp terminus nearer the HOC. Uniform clasp retention depends on the degree of tooth undercut, rather than on the distance below HOC, at which clasp terminal is placed.
- Area below HOC/infrabulge—for retentive arm; flexible component.
- Area above HOC/suprabulge = for reciprocating /stabilizing arms.
- Clasp retention is based on the **resistance of metal to deformation** (i.e. Proportional Limit), which is proportional to FLEXIBILITY of the clasp arm.
- **Guiding planes** = rigid parts of RPD contact these parallel tooth surfaces during path of insertion and removal; act as additional retention.
- Clasp should be PASSIVE with teeth except when a dislodging force is applied.
- Retention is provided mainly by FLEXIBLE PART of clasp assembly
- It depends on retentive clasp arm as:
  - (a) **Length** = longer arm is more flexible; should be tapered uniformly; tip is 1/2 thick than base.
  - (b) **Diameter** = more diameter means less flexible.
  - (c) **Cross section form** = one–direction flexible is half round form. UNIVERSALLY FLEXIBLE form is the ROUND FORM.
  - (d) **Contour.**
- **Type of alloy.**
- **Location and depth of undercut** = is the most important single factor to select a clasp for use with DISTAL EXTENSION RPD.
- Should be tapered in 2-dimensions, i.e. (length and width wise).
- Cast gold alloy has greater resiliency than cast chromium alloys.
- Wrought wire clasp arm, i.e. drawn in wire, has more toughness than cast clasp arm, by at least 25%. So it may be used in smaller diameter.

- Greater rigidity with less bulk can be achieved with chromium alloys, as compared to gold.

Reciprocal stabilizing cast clasp arm

- Should be RIGID.
- Average diameter should be more than the average diameter of retentive arm.
- Tapered in OND Dimension only (only length wise); width remains the same.
- **Circumferential clasp arm** = approaches the retentive undercut from an OCCLUSAL DIRECTION.
- **BAR clasp arm** = approaches from CERVICAL DIRECTION.

CLASP ASSEMBLY: Has following components:

- One or more minor connectors.
- Principal rest.
- Retentive arm.
- Non-retentive arm = against horizontal movement, for stabilization and reciprocation.

Basic principle of clasp design

- **More than 180° of greatest circumference** of the crown of the tooth should be included.
- When bar clasp is used = at least 2 areas of tooth contact must embrace more than one half of tooth circumference.
- Occlusal rest should prevent cervical movement of clasp arm.
- Each retentive arm should be opposed by reciprocal arm.
- Retentive clasps should be BILATERALLY OPPOSED.
- Path of removal of retentive clasp end should not be parallel to the path of removal of RPD.
- Should not transmit forces to abutment.
- Reciprocal element should be located at the junction of gingival and middle 3rd of crown.
- Terminal end of retentive arm is placed in gingival 3rd.

- Reciprocal arm stabilizes the RPD against horizontal movement; should be RIGID.
- Reciprocal arm may act as indirect retainer if placed on supra-bulge area anterior to the fulcrum line.
- Retentive and reciprocal arms should be located nearer to the horizontal axis of rotation of abutment (which lies somewhere in its root) to avoid heavy forces on PDL.

BAR CLASP: Parts and functions.

- SUPPORT = by occlusal rest.
- STABILIZATION = by rest, Mesial and Distal minor connectors.
- RETENTION = by buccal I-bar.
- Reciprocation = by location of minor connectors.

CIRCUMFERENTIAL CLASP

- Most logical clasp.
- Approaches from occlusal direction.
- More tooth coverage (so anaesthetic).
- True adjustment is IMPOSSIBLE with cast clasp—it only increases/decreases frictional resistance.
- Better/superior to BAR–CLASP.
- It has one retentive and one stabilizing/non-retentive arm.

RING CLASP

- Encircles nearly all of a tooth from its point of origin.
- Used when a proximal undercut cannot be approached by other means.
- Should always be used with a SUPPORTING STRUT on non-retentive side.
- Covers more tooth surface and is aesthetically objectionable.
- It is used ONLY IF Disto-buccal or Disto-lingual undercut can't be approached from occlusal rest area.

BACK-ACTION CLASP

- Biologically and mechanically unsound.

EMBRASURE CLASP

- Used in unmodified Class II or III RPD.
- Should be used with DOUBLE OCCLUSAL RESTS to avoid food impaction and helps to shunt food.
- It has 2 retentive and 2 reciprocal clasp arms.

MULTIPLE CLASP

- 2 opposing C–clasps joined at terminal ends of 2 reciprocal arms.
- Used when PD replaces entire half of the dental arch.

HALF AND HALF CLASP

- Has a C-clasp retentive arm from one direction and a reciprocal arm from other.
- Used to provide **DUAL retention** only in UNILATERAL denture design.

Reverse action/hair pin clasp

- Engages proximal undercut from occlusal direction (below the point of origin).
- Its lower arm only is FLEXIBLE passing over HOC.

Bar clasp/roach clasp

- Approaches from GINGIVAL DIRECTION.
- RPI system = Rest, proximal plate and I–bar.
- It consists of a mesio-occlusal rest with minor connector placed in Mesiolingual embrasure, but not touching the adjacent tooth.
- I–bar should be located in gingival 3rd of buccal surface, in an 0.01 inch undercut and only 2 mm of its tip only should touch the tooth.

Combination clasp

- Has a WROUGHT wire retentive arm and a cast RECIPROCAL arm.
- Used when **maximum flexibility** is required.
- Being wrought—a **smaller diameter** can be used; so better aesthetic.
- Round in form.
- Most common use = on an abutment adjacent to a distal extension base, where only a Mucogingival undercut exists.
- Advantages = flexibility/adjustability/esthetics/less fatigue failures/line contact with tooth/less tooth area covered.

INDIRECT RETAINERS

- Placed as far as possible from distal extension base, giving best possible leverage advantage against lifting of the distal extension base.
- Placed **on the opposite side** of the fulcrum line, in a REST SEAT.
- Most effective location of IR is incisors, but it is a weak tooth, so canine or 1st PM (mesio-occlusal) may be used.
- Most frequently used is an AUXILIARY OCCLUSAL REST, e.g. in Mandibular Class I arch = MMR of 1st PM is used.
- In Class II PD = MR of first PM on the opposite side of arch from the distal extension base.

DENTURE BASE

- Broader coverage helps in wider distribution of forces.
- Resin is attached to PD framework by MINOR CONNECTOR.
- Space (at least 20 gauge thick) should be there between metal and residual ridge for flow of resin.
- 1.5 mm thick RESIN must be there s.t. RELIEVING may be done if required.
- More ***open ladder like framework*** is preferred over a MESH-LIKE framework.

- Should be located both buccally and lingually.
- Ladder like pattern also prevent warping of resin after processing due to release of inherent strains.
- Metal is preferred as denture base than resin, because it provides stimulation to underlying tissues; intimate contact and good retention; accuracy of fit.
- Distortion of resin base in maxillary denture is manifested as a distortion away from palate in midline and towards the tuberosities.
- Temperature changes get transmitted through the metal bases to basal tissues and help to maintain the health of tissues.
- Metal being more rigid, is used in less BULK and so does not encroach the tongue space.
- Resin may be required if due to extreme tissue resorption, the fullness of tissues is to be achieved by bulk of resin and for contours of functional check and tongue and for aesthetic reasons.

Acrylic teeth can be attached by

1. With acrylic resin.
2. Cemented.
3. Processed directly to metal.
4. Cast with the framework.

- **Porcelain teeth** = are mechanically retained, as they have a PIN on ridge lap area.
- **Diatoric teeth** = have holes on their ridge lap in which resin flows.
- **Resin teeth** = retained by chemical union with [illegible]n.
- Pressing on a resin tooth = i.e. attaching a ready-made resin tooth to the metal base, with acrylic resin of same shade.
- **Metal tooth** = is cast in framework, where only a small space is present.
- Occlusal adjustment on **gold tooth** is easier than chrome alloy teeth.

RELINING

- Base should be made of material, which can be relined/ribased especially distal extension.
- Loss of support of distal extension bases occur from changes in residual ridge and loss of occlusal contact between artificial teeth.
- To check the occlusion—***Wax strip is better*** than articulating paper. The indentation in wax strip are QUANTITATIVE, But in articulating paper are only QUALITATIVE.
- If IR lifts from their rest seat, it also implies need of relining.

STRESS BREAKER

All parts or RPD are rigid except—Retentive arm of DR wrought wire retentive clasp acts as a STRESS BREAKER between denture base and abutment, because of its flexibility.

They allow some movement b/w denture bases and DR and so prevents transfer of forces to the abutments.

2 types

1. Having a movable joint between Denture Base and Direct Retainer, e.g. hinge; sleeve and cylinder; Ball and socket. It permits both vertical and hinge action of distal extension base.
2. Having a FLEXIBLE connection between DB and DR. It is made by DUAL CASTING technique.

PRINCIPLES OF RPD

Simple machines–are of 6 types, i.e.

- Lever, wedge, pulley, screw, wheel and axle; inclined plane.
- Lever and incline plane design should be AVOIDED in RPD.

If effort arm of a lever is larger than the resistance arm, the mechanical advantage is in favour of effort arm.

$$\text{Mechanical advantage} = \frac{\text{Effort arm}}{\text{Resistance arm}}$$

CANTILEVER

- Beam supported at one end only; acts as a first class lever; it should be avoided.
- A tooth can withstand vertical forces better than oblique/horizontal forces. It is because more PDL fibres are activated to resist the application of vertical forces to teeth than are activated to resist off-vertical forces.
- Flat ridge provide good support but poor stability.

Differences b/w different types of RPDs

Class I **Class II with distal extension**	**Class III**
Support derived from tissues under Denture Base, i.e. tissue supported	All support derived from the abutment teeth, i.e. tooth supported
Impression = Dual impression technique is used; functional impression required.	No functional impression required.
Indirect retainer required in Distal Extension Base	Not required
DB material used should be able to be RELINED/REBASED to compensate for tissue changes.	No relieving required
Made of Acrylic/Resin	Metallic
Retentive arm should lie in mesial undercut and should be able to flex to dissipate stresses. Wrought wire retentive arm can flex in all directions.	DR is a clasp at each abutment/end. Retentive arm should be passive and should flex only while removal.

IMPRESSION MAKING

1. **Anatomic form** = recorded s.t. no pressure is exerted on soft tissues beyond their PHYSIOLOGIC LIMITS, s.t. its retentive and stabilizing components may be properly placed, e.g. by Agar, alginate, rubber base materials.
2. **Supporting form** = of soft tissues under the distal extension of RPD should be recorded s.t. FIRM areas are used as PRIMARY SUPPORT BEARING AREAS and easily displaceable tissues are not overloaded, e.g. by ZOE, rubber base impression materials.
    - ♦ Denture made in functional form is generally less irregular and has great cover area than the denture made to anatomic or resting form.
    - ♦ Denture made on anatomic form exhibits less stability under rotating forces than on functional form and fails to maintain occlusal relation.
    - ♦ It also fails to distribute occlusal loads and so damages to abutments.

GUIDING PLANES

- ♦ 2 or more parallel vertical surfaces of abutment teeth, which help to direct RPD during placement or removal.
- ♦ Provide one path of placement or removal of RPD.
- ♦ It should be 2/3rd as wide as the distance between buccal.
- ♦ 1/3rd the buccolingual width of tooth.
- ♦ 2/3rd the length of crown from Marginal Ridge cervically.
- ♦ Should be located on abutment surface adjacent to an edentulous area.
- ♦ Avoid to create buccolingual line angles on the tooth.

SURVEYING

SURVEYOR is an instrument to determine the relative parallelism of 2 or more surfaces of teeth or other parts of cast of dental Arch.

For a clasp to be retentive, its path of escaping must be other than parallel to the path of removal of RPD, otherwise it will not flex.

Retentive arm tip should engage on undercut of 0.01″ (0.25 mm); but wrought-wire clasp can engage 0.02″ provided arm is long enough (at least 8 mm).

Retentive clasp should be placed at a more disto-gingival area for aesthetic purpose.

BLOCK OUT OF THE CAST

1. ***Shaped block out***
   - Done on buccolingual surfaces to locate clasp patterns.
   - Ledges or shelves are blocked out.
2. ***Parallel block out***
   - Done cervical to guiding plane surfaces and overall undercut areas, which will be crossed by major or minor connectors.
3. ***Arbitrary block out***
   - All gingival crevices.
   - Undercuts distal to cast framework.
   - Labial and buccal tooth and tissue undercuts not involved in denture design.

Relief

- Areas in which major connector will contact the tissues, e.g. mid-palatal raphe.
- Beneath the framework extensions on the ridge areas for attachment of resin bases.
- Relief is not used below palatal major connectors except if TORI are present.

STERILISATION (Ref. to section of microbiology for details.)

- Cleaning = scrub with detergent solution and wiping with I_2/Cl_2 solution (dil. Household bleach).
- O clothes = 140°–160°F wash cycle with normal bleach conc. and machine drying (at 212°F/100°C).
- Disinfection by—, 2% glutraldehyde at 10 min.
- Heat sensitive items by ethylene oxide gas.
- Impressions, relines, face bow forks, etc. should be disinfected with IODOPHORES.

Some important points about bones

- Changes in bone calcification upto 25% can't be seen by R/G..
- Trabecular space size tends to decrease slightly from root apex towards the coronal part.
- **Index areas** = are those areas of alveolar support that disclose the reaction of bone to additional stresses.
  - **Positive bone factor**—means there is an ability of building additional support.
  - **Negative bone factor**—i.e. inability to respond favourably to stresses.

LAMINA DURA—is a **R/G feature:**

- Is the **thin layer of hard cortical bone,** which normally lines the sockets of all teeth.
- Gives **attachment to PDL** fibres.
- Withstands mechanical strain.
- **Cortical** in nature.
- Seen as **Radiopaque** line around the teeth.
- During tipping, C rot. of tooth is in apical 3rd of root.
- Bone resorption occurs in pressure zone and deposition in tension zone.
- DURING TIPPING—LD is seen UNEVEN in the R/G.
- If a tooth tips in edentulous area—the LD on that side becomes HEAVIER, which is nature's reinforcement against abnormal stresses. The TRABECULAE are arranged at right angle to heavier LD.
- Bone is 30% organic and mostly PROTEIN.
- Teeth with multiple and divergent roots resists forces BETTER, as forces are distributed to a LARGER AREA.

ALLOYS (Also refer to dental materials section.)

- Gold alloy (type IV) or chrome-cobalt alloy are used.
- Recontouring of abutments depends on MOE (STIFFNESS) of the alloy being used.

- Cr-Co alloy—low density/wt; high MOE, low cost, tarnish resistant.
- Wrought wire components can be soldered to Au or Cr–Co.
- Cr-Co has low yield strength/YS than Au.
- YS is the greatest STRESS applied within elastic limits.
- MOE—STIFFNESS of Au is 1/2 that of Cr-Co alloy.
  - So it is more RIGID in less bulk.
  - Can be good if undercut is very small.
- A high YS and low MOE—HIGHER flexibility.
- Au is 2 times flexible than Cr-Co.
- Greater flexibility of Au allows placement of retentive arm tips in GINGIVAL 3rd of abutment.
- Grain size of Cr-Co is LARGER and associated with low proportional limit/PL and so it may get fractured.
- Cr-Co gets work HARDENED RAPIDLY and so fracture. So adjustment should be done with extreme caution.
- Cr-Co = has low density than Au and so 1/2 as heavy as Au.
- Attrition of enamel is more with Cr-Co than with Au.
- Au more prone to GALVANIC SHOCK to teeth restored with Ag.
- Many mechanical properties of wrought structure are better than cast structure.
- A min YS of 60,000 psi is required for retentive arm.
- If electric soldering of wrought wire is done, the higher heat evolved may cause RECRYSTALLIZATION of grain growth, by changing FIBROUS microstructure of wrought wire to the crystalline structure. It should be avoided by controlling the TEMPERATURE.
- 650 fine gold solder is used.
- Electric soldering is better than torch soldering, because of the localization of heat.
- Flux prevents OXIDATION of parts being joined.
- **Borax flux** = for Au to Au soldering.
- **F-flux** = Cr-Co alloy soldered to alloys having Cr.

- **F-flux** = Au soldered to Cr-Co.
- Au alloy WROUGHT wires are given HARDENING HEAT Rx to increase PL, tensile strength/TS and hardness. It is done at placing at.
  - 840° F × 5 min and then.
  - Coding to 480° F in 30 min.
  - Then quenching in water.

Hydroxyapatite

- Used for bone augmentation.
- No toxicity; non-inflammatory or foreign body response.
- Not resorbable.
- Stops further bone resorption.

Tissue conditioners—are elasto-polymers, which continue to flow for an extended period of time, permitting distorted tissues to rebound and assume their normal form.

Changes seen in an unopposed tooth:

- Loss of orientation of PDL fibres.
- Loss of supporting bone.
- Narrowing of PDL space.

All abutment surfaces facing edentulous areas should be made parallel to the path of placement.

Proximal surfaces are prepared parallel to the path of placement to create guiding planes.

HOC should be lowered till the junction of middle and gingival 3rd.

Mandibular molars are WEAKEST of posterior abutment.

Impression materials

(A) RIGID	–	POP, ZOE.
(B) Thermoplastic	–	modelling plastic; Impression waxes and natural resins.

(C) Elastic – Reversible HC (Agar, Agar).
– Irreversible hydrocolloids (Alginate).
– Merceptan rubber base (Thiokol).
– Silicone.
– Polyethers.

- Difference between impression wax and modelling plastic—impression wax has the ability to flow as long as they are in mouth and so permit equalization of pressure and prevent displacement.
- Most commonly used modelling plastic is red material in cake form —it softens at 132°F and should never be softened at higher temperature.
- Reversible and irreversible HC impressions cannot be stored for any length of time and should be POURED immediately.
- Used for orthodontic impressions, etc.

  For accuracy, Thiokol impression materials should have uniform thickness of 3 mm. Cast made in thikol is SMOOTHER and harder than in HC.
- Used for RPD impressions.

Silicone impression materials.

- Used for FPD impression.
- Addition reaction type is more dimensionally stable and has excellent detail reproduction.

Polyether impression materials:

- Flow characteristics are very low.
- Flow is lowest of any rubber impression materials.
- Stiffness is high.
- Used in FPD, but less in RPD impression.

♦ Agar changes from sol to gel under heat by ***a physical change*** which is reversible.

♦ Alginate changes to gel by ***an irreversible chemical change***.

♦ Syneresis is associated with release of a mucinous exudate, which has a retarding effect on gypsum, and so chalky surface of the cast occurs. It can be prevented by using chemical accelerators, e.g. K_2SO_4.

- So agar impression is placed in 2% K_2SO_4 for 5–10 min before making the cast.

OCCLUSION

Occlusal harmony between RPD and natural teeth is a major factor in the preservation of health of supporting structures.

Simultaneous Bilateral contacts of posterior teeth must occur in CO.

BO is required if RPD is opposed by Maxillary CD.

Working side contacts should be there for mandibular distal extension denture. These should occur simultaneously with working side contacts of natural teeth to widely distribute the stresses.

Simultaneous balancing and working side contacts should be formulated for maxillary bilateral distal extension RPD.

Only working side contacts required for maxillary or mandibular unilateral distal extension RPD.

In Class IV RPD, opposite anterior teeth should contact in ICP so as to prevent continuous eruption of opposing natural incisors.

Contact of opposing incisors in eccentric positions should not be developed.

Contact of opposite posteriors in protrusion is NOT DESIRABLE in any situation, except when an opposing CD is placed.

SPRUE

- Should be large s.t. molten metal will not solidify until the metal in casting is frozen.
- 8–12 gauge ROUND wax is used as sprue.
- Should induce minimum amount of turbulence.
- Should be attached at the bulkier sections of the patterns.
- Should be lightly curved, i.e. no acute angles should be there which can lead to entrapment of gases and turbulence.
- Point of attachment to the patterns should be FLARED OUT, and so shrinkage porosity will be avoided in casting—due to continuous feeding of molten metal.

- Multiple spruing is done for RPDs.
- Main sprue hole = 3/8″.
- Investment for casting gold alloys = plastics (gypsum) bound silica material.
- Casting shrinkage of gold = 1–1.74%.
- Higher the % age of Au in the alloy, the greater is the casting shrinkage.
- Casting shrinkage of Cr-Co alloy is 2.3%, and so silica-bounded investment is used. (Ethyl silicate or sodium silicate as binder); thermal expansion occurs.
- Occlusal adjustment of distal extension RPD is better done on articulator than intra-orally.

CLEFT LIP AND PALATE

VEAU'S classification:

Class	Features
I	Involves soft palate.
II	Involves soft palate and hard palate but not alveolus.
III	Involves SP + HP + Alveolus; UNILATERAL.
IV	Involves SP + HP + Alveolus of both sides leaving free premaxilla.

- CP III, IV are associated with CL also.
- CL closed surgically at = 6–12 weeks.
- CP closed surgically at = 18 months.
- Gag reflex of CP patient is markedly decreased.
- Sounds like /puh/ and /kuk/ are practically impossible.
- Vowel sounds, e.g. a, e and sibilants 'S' aid in assessing palato pharyngeal competence.
- Palatopharyngeal closure = closing off the nasal cavity by the action of ms attached to soft palate.
- Main problems appear in pronouncing B, D, K, P, T sounds.

Levator veli palatini m

- Origin = petrous part of termporal bone and cartilage of eustachian tube.
- Runs D and F.
- Inserts in palatine aponeurosis.
- Action-pulls soft palate upwards and backwards.
- **Makes a SLING** with other side m.

Tensor veli palatine

- Origin = scaphoid fossa, spheroid spine, eustachian cartilage.
- Runs = D and F to lateral aspects of hamulus (used as pulley).
- Insert = in soft palate.
- Action = effects tension on SP in U and B direction.

Pharynx = comes forward and medially by 3 ms:

1. Pterygo-pharyngeal portion of superior constrictor m = it contracts to pull the posterior pharyngeal wall forward to meet the soft palate.
2. Palatopharyngeus m = seen as posterior pillars of tonsils.

   Pharyngopalatal part produces a ridge or bunching up of posterior pharyngeal m. known as PASAVANT'S PAD, which approximates soft palate and pharynx. This ***compensatory structure is USUALLY seen in patients of CP***.
3. Salpingopharyngeus m. = closes lateral pharyngeal wall with soft palate.
   - Helps in producing PLOSIVE sounds.

These close the nasal cavity from oral cavity and pharynx.

Closure of oral cavity

1. By contraction of thyropalatal portion of palatopharyngeus m.
   - Pulls soft palate down towards the tongue.
2. Tensor m. flattens the dome of soft palate.

3. Tongue is forced U and B.
4. Palatoglossus m helps to complete the closure.

SPEECH—Is a function of:

- Respiration = lungs/exchange of air.
- Phonation = vocal cords/change pitch.
- Resonation = nasal/oral/pharynx cavities.
- Articulation = teeth, tongue, lip, palate.
- Integration = brain.

Obturator = serves not to close the soft palate, but rather to fill the space between palatal remnants.

3 types of obturators, viz.

1. Hinge type.
2. Fixed types = most commonly used; fixed type is at the level of palatopharyngeal m/PP.
3. Meatus type.

5

Periodontics

Important points

- **Mean thickness** of PDL is 0.2 mm (0.15–0.38 mm).
- **2 days** old supragingival plaque has = streptococci.
- **Plaque in** caries is = acidic.
- Plaque in PD diseases = is basic.
- **Keye's technique** = i.e. applying hypertonic salts in an oxidative antiseptic for controlling plaque.
- Subgingival plaque is more tenacious than supragingival plaque.
- **Supragingival** contains = 10^{11} bact./gm wet wt.
- Plaque cannot mineralise in = acid environment.
- LJP is usually severe in patients with = defective neutrophils.
- Alveolar bone/ID septum = 1.5 mm below CEJ.
- In plaque, acid fermentation of carbohydrate occurs in = 2–5 minutes, or few seconds.
- Only oral microbes which produces collagenase = bacteroides melaninogenicus.
- Lactobacilli are prominent in caries, because they are secondary invaders and acid atmosphere is favourable for them.
- Bacteria dominant in root surface caries are—**Actinomyces**.
- Bacteria which decrease the damaging potential of lactic acid by using it as a metabolite are—**Neisseria and Veillonella**. So they are anti–caries bacteria. Veillonella acts as ***symboint of streptococci***.

- PH of normal plaque is 7.1; while pH of plaque in caries prone persons is 5.5, i.e. acidic due to lactic acid.
- Sucrose → glucose + fructose.
- Glucose → dextrans (alpha- 1, 3 linkage).
- Fructose → levans.
- Cyanoacrylate = is an adhesive, which can be used instead of sutures.
- Sounding = is known as transgingival probing.
- Free gingival groove is related to = arrangement of supra alveolar fibres.
- **Tartar controlling agents** used in tooth pastes are—triclosan; zinc citrate pyrophosphate.

Causative microbes

Root surface caries	Actinomyces viscosus
Bacteria which form intracellular apatite crystals	Veillonella
Green stain of plaque	Aspergillus and penicillin
Bacteria to colonise first after tooth surface is cleaned	*Strept. Sanguis* and *S mitis*
Early supragingival plaque	G + cocci and rods
Mature supragingival plaque	Spirochetes/G (–) rods, e.g. bacteroides, which causes gingivitis
Tooth ass. sub-gingival plaque	G + cocci and rods, e.g. actinomyces, which cause root caries
Epith ass. sub-gingival plaque	G (–) bacteria
Caries initiated by	*S mutans*
Bacteria prominent in dentinal caries/deep cavity	Lactobacilli
Bacteria prominent in pits and fissures	Lactobacilli

Causative microbes (*Contd.*)

Bact prominent in smooth surface caries	*S mutans*
Bacteria which decrease damagingpotential of lactic acid by using it as a metabolite	Veillonella and neisseria
Symbiont of streptococci	Veillonella

Bluish line of gingiva in plumbism = known as **Burtonian line.**

Immunoglobulins—are glycoproteins; source for preparation of human gamma globulins is placenta.

Ig for auto-immune reactions	IgM
Ig **maximum in saliva**	Salivary IgA
Ig **maximum in sulcular** fluid	IgG
Smallest Ig, **most abundant**	IgG
Ig that **crosses placenta**	IgG
Warm antibodies	IgG
Blocking antibodies	IgG
Largest immunoglobulins	IgM
Earliest antibody to be synthesised	IgM
Natural antibodies	IgM
Mainly **intravascular** immunoglobulins	IgM
Cold antibodies	IgM
Reaginic antibodies (allergies)	IgE
Heat labile Ig	IgE
Ig with **minimum half life**	IgE
Ig that **protects the surface**	Ig A
Commonest Ig **deficiency**	Ig A
Prevents adhesion of bacteria to mucosa	IgA
Ig present in **milk**	IgA and IgG
By G + bacteria	IgG
By G – bacteria	IgM

IgM	First to be formed after infection, i.e. has a role in early stages of infection. Also activates the complement system.
IgE	Responsible for severe acute allergic response. Attaches to mast cells and basophilic leucocytes.
IgD	Binds with B-cells. Triggers lymphocytic stimulation. Does not activate complements (unlike IgG, M).
IgA	Main Ig of exocrine secretions, i.e. tears, milk, saliva, etc. 2 types—serum IgA is monomer; found in GCF; secretory IgA is dimmer; resistant to digestion. Does not activate complements (unlike IgG, M).
IgG	Most abundant in serum; distributed equally b/w blood and extravascular fluids. Neutralizes the bacterial toxins and helps phagocytosis. Passes through placental barrier. Provides newborns with the humoral immunity of the mother.

Cells maximum in sulcular fluid = PMN.

Lymphocytes predominent in sulcular fluid = B-cells.

Lymphocytes predominent in blood = T-cells.

Stages of Gingivitis

Stages	Lesion	Predominant cells
I	Initial lesion	Neutrophils
II	Early lesion	Lymphocytes
III	Established lesion	Plasma cells
IV	Advanced lesion	—

Brushing:

Technique	Directions of bristles	Comment
Scrub tech	Horizontal	Most common to cause abrasion
Bass/	Pointing apically, at **sulcular**	Most common 45 to long axis of teeth recommended tech
Roll tech	Pointing apically, parallel to long axis of teeth	Least efficient
Mod. Stillman's	Pointing apically, at 45 to long axis of teeth	Recommended if gingival recession and root exposures
Charter's tech	Pointing occlusally, at 45 to long axis of teeth	Recommended after gingival surgeries
Fone's tech	Horizontal	Recommended in children
Stillman's	Pointing apically, at 45 to long axis of teeth	

Tooth brushing techniques

Technique	Bristle position	Motion	Effects
Horizontal scrub	90° to teeth	Horizontal strokes	Supraging cleaning Gingival stimulation
Fones	Do	Large circles over teeth and gingiva	Do
Leonard	Do	Vertical strokes	Do

Tooth brushing techniques (*Contd.*)

Technique	Bristle position	Motion	Effects
Smith-Bell	At occlusal surface	Sweep gingivally	Supragingival cleaning
Rolling strokes	Apically at attached gingiva	Sweep in arc occlusally	Supraging cleaning gingival stimulation
Stillman	45 to apex; part on gingival margin, part on cervix of tooth	Vibratory pulsing	Gingival stimulation
Modified charters	90° to teeth	Sweep occlusally, circular vibratory	Interdental cleaning Gingival stimulation
Modified bass	45 to apex; in sulcus	Sweep occlusally, vibratory, horizontal jiggle	Supraging cleaning Gingival stimulation

Important points about tooth brushing

- Most commonly used method which causes tooth abrasions–scrub technique.
- Most commonly recommended method, bass or sulcular method.
- Least efficient method is—roll technique.
- Method which is recommended in gingival recession and root exposures—modified stillman method.
- Method which is recommended after pd surgeries—charter's method.
- Recommended method in children—fones technique.

- Brushing efficiency depends on 3 factors—technique; frequency and duration; brush design.
- Modified Bass technique = only technique which **cleanses the sulcus** effectively; **best technique.**
- Modified Charters technique = useful for cleaning **fixed orthodontic appliances**.
- Horizontal scrub technique = worst; however it is most commonly used technique.
- Fones technique = for children; easy to learn and mastered by children.
- Powered tooth brushes are superior to manual tooth brushes; esp for removing interdental plaque.
- 3 minutes brushing time is ideal.
- Brush should be usually changed once in 90 days/3 months.
- Most widely used ***disclosing agent*** is **erythrosin.**

Differences between adult and child's tooth brush

Adult	Child
Has 4 rows	Has 3 rows
Has 10–14 vertical tufts	6 tufts
Size of head = larger	Is 2/3rd of that of adult brush

- Nylon bristles—flexible; non absorbent; rounded ends.
- Floss—unitufted–multitufted; waxed-unwaxed; twisted-untwisted.
- **Best floss**—unwaxed; multitufted; twisted.
- Each tuft of brush—has 18–20 bristles.
- Tooth pick is made of—**orange wood.**
- Tooth paste—its abrasive content should specify less than or equal to 100 rad, i.e. radioactive dentinal abrasion value.

Important points

- Instruments = best for root planing = curet.
- Most harmful premature occlusal contacts exist on—non-working side; facial incline of max lingual cusps and lingual inclines of mand facial cusps.
- Most frequent osseus lesion in periodontitis = crater.
- Gingival clefts may be caused by = faulty tooth brushing.
- Main result of TFO = mobility.
- First fibre group destroyed to allow JE migration = dentogingival, i.e. G1 fibres.
- In gingivitis:
  - Earliest lesion = neutrophils collect.
  - Established lesions = lymphocytes.
  - Advanced lesions = plasma cells.
- Plaque irritates gingival tissue = **biochemically.**
- Gingivitis in a child is frequently related to each of the following except = SPIROCHETES.
- Treatment of hypersensitivity = in anterior teeth = $SrCl_2$ or $CaCl_2$, as they cause no staining; in posterior teeth = by $AgNO_3$.
- Treatment of hypersensitivity = pot. oxalate is most commonly used agent.
- Treatment of hypersensitivity = apply NaF paste (from NDB).
- Histoplasma = a fungus having both capabilities, i.e. dimorphism and produces gingivitis also.
- Histoplamosis microbes are also found in RE system.

Gingival index by Loe and Silness

- 0 = clinically healthy gingiva.
- 1 = no bleeding upon palpation.
- 2 = bleeding.
- 3 = spontaneous bleeding.

Plaque index by Silness and Loe

Functions of following

1. I_2 = iodine = antimicrobial, astringent.
2. H_2O_2 = kills anaerobes, removes debris by nascent oxygen, RC irrigant.
3. 0.2% chlorhexidine = antiseptic.
4. KNO_3 = desensitizer in tooth paste, cariostatic.
5. 0.2% NaF = remineralisation, antibacterial.

Types of embrasures

1. Type I = floss.
2. Type II = proxa brush.
3. Type III = unitufted brush.

- In periodontitis = an increased IgA would suggest the possibility of an increased response to oral Ag—stimulation.
- First stage of LJP = destruction of principal fibers of PDL; degeneration.
- First step in pathogenesis of PD pocket formation = is breakdown of sulcular epithelium.
- For epithelium to migrate apically = group A, i.e. (G1) fibers must be destroyed, as these are the fibers attached immediately apical to the epithelium attachment.
- Plasma cell gingivitis = is ass. with use of chewing gums.
- Sterile necrosis by TFO.
- Natural Abs = IgM.
- Hemiseptum = one walled bony defect.
- Intra-bony pockets = 3 walled defect.
- After PD surgery—epitheium attachment takes 8 weeks for healing and so floss is not recommended.
- Estrogen and progesterone act as growth factors for bacteroides by substituting for vitamin K, i.e. menadione.
- Epithelium of epithelium—attachment does not contain = rete-pegs, but which are acquired during apical migration.

HYPERSENSITIVITY

Type I, Anaphylaxis or immediate	IgG, i.e. blocking Ab, IgE, i.e. reaginic Ab	IgG + mast cell complex reacts with Ag	Histamine, SRS-A are released
Type II, Cytotoxic	IgG, IgM	(Cell with Ag) r.w. Ab	Cell lysis, e.g. RBCs, as in autoimmune diseases, e.g. pemphigus, pemphigoid, SLE, rheumatoid arthritis, mickulicz's dis
Type III, Arthus' reaction	Local tissue damage, vascular endothelium	Ag rw Ab	Lysosomal enzymes
Type IV, Delayed hypersen-sitivity	No Abs involved here	T-cells r.w. Ag	Lymphokines, OAF, etc. released

Schwartzman's reaction = is not an immune reaction, but an alteration in factors affecting intravascular coagulation. So first dose is intradermal; and second dose is I/V, which then causes necrotic lesion at the site of first dose.

e.g. in Waterhouse = Friderichsen syndrome, acute adrenal deficiency, here, endotoxins play a role in Schwartzman's reaction.

Systemic form of Arthus reaction = is serum sickness.

DISTANCES

1. Mean thickness of PDL is 0.2 mm (0.15–0.38 mm).
2. Marginal gingiva 1 mm.

3. Gingival sulcus 2–3 mm.
4. Attached gingiva max CI = 3.5–4.5 mm, maximum.

   M and CI 3.3–3.9 mm.

   Max First PM 1.9 mm.

   M and first PM 1.8 mm, minimum.
5. Junctional epithelium 0.25–1.35 mm.
6. JE-epithelium bone crest 1.07 mm (in young) 2.81 mm (in olds).
7. Physiologic mesial migration 1.0 cm on each side,
8. Radius of action of plaque 1.5–2.5 mm.
9. Bone loss/year in periodontitis.
10. Bone loss/year after full mouth extractions.
11. Cementum is thickest at apex, its thickness is 150–200 microns.
12. Cementum is thinnest at apex, its thickness is 20–50 microns.
13. Specific gravity of saliva 1.003.
14. Amount of GCF secreted per day by normal gingival 0.5–2.4 ml.
15. Concentration of tetracycline in GCF is 2–10 times that of plasma.
16. Probing depth of normal gingival sulcus is 2–3 mm.
17. Histologic depth of normal gingival sulcus is 1.5–1.8 mm.
18. Oxygen coefficient of normal gingival is 1.6 ± 0.37.
19. Diameter of standard probe tip is 0.35–0.55 mm.
20. Recommended probing force is 0.25 N or 2.5 gm, w.
21. Total no. of intra-oral films recommended for complete full mouth survey is = 18; (IOPA–14; bitewings–4).
22. Plaque contains bacteria as 1.7×10^{11} per gm wt (i.e. 1.7×10^{8} per mg wt).
23. Average daily increment in calculus former is 0.1–0.15%.
24. Minimum levels of cyclosporine in plasma above, which gingival hyperplasia occurs is 150 nanogm/ml.
25. Duration of each masticatory cycle is 0.6–1.0 sec.

26. Number of swallows per day in an individual is 600 times/24 hrs.
27. Total occlusal points in dentition are 138.
28. Normal Ca and P precipitate concentration is 35–40%.
29. Tooth brush abrasion of dentin is more than enamel by 15–25 times.
30. Cementum is abraded more than enamel by 35 times.
31. Conc. of chlorhexidine used in mouthwashes is 0.12–0.2%.

Furcation lesions can be graded as

Grade	Features
I	Incipient early lesion; pocket is suprabony; bone loss is minimal; cannot be detected.
II	Bone destroyed on one aspect of the furcation; a part of PDL and alveolar bone end is intact; partial penetration of probe possible.
III	Interradicular bone is completely absent; probe can be passed through and through; but furcation not visible as it is covered by gingival tissue.
IV	Same as grade III, but furcation is visible and denuded.

1. Grade 1 = bone loss upto 1/3rd of the tooth width, i.e. about 3 mm of horizontal attachment loss.
2. Grade 2 = bone loss b/w 1/3rd and 2/3rd of the tooth width.
3. Grade 3 = a through and through lesion.
    - Extent of furcation is measured by Naber's probe.

Tooth mobility = according to Miller's index is:

1. Score 1 = mobility upto 1 mm.
2. Score 2 = mobility of 1–2 mm.
3. Score 3 = mobility over 2 mm and or rotation or depression in the socket.

Recession: According to Miller's classification.

Class I; prognosis is good to excellent	Marginal gingival recession does not extend to mucogingival line. No soft tissue and bone loss seen in I/D area.
Class II; prognosis is good to excellent	Marginal gingival recession extends to MGL or beyond; no soft tissue and bone loss seen in I/D area.
Class III; partial coverage can be seen	Marginal gingival recession extends to MGL or beyond; soft tissue and bone loss seen in I/D expected area and malpositioning of teeth.
Class IV; hopeless prognosis	Marginal gingival recession extends to MGL or beyond; severe soft tissue and bone loss seen in I/D area and severe malpositioning of teeth.

Periodontal indices

DEBRIS INDEX = by Green and Vermillion 1960.

0 no plaque.

1 plaque covering 1/3rd tooth.

2 plaque covering 2/3rd tooth.

3 plaque totally covering tooth.

Plaque index, Silness and Loe 1964.

0 no plaque detected.

1 looks clean but material can be removed from gingival 1/3rd with probe.

2 visible plaque.

3 tooth covered with abundant plaque.

Modified gingival index, Loe 1967.

0 healthy gingiva.

1 gingiva looks inflammed, but do not bleed on probing.

2 gingiva looks inflammed, and bleeds on probing.

3 ulceration and spontaneous bleeding.

Community periodontal index of Rx needs: CPITN.

CPITN probe = has a ball end of 0.5 mm in diameter; colour coded area extends from 3.5–5.5 mm; probing force of 20–25 gm is recommended.

Code 0	Healthy gingival tissues with no bleeding after probing.
Code 1	Bleeding on probing, plaque present, but no calculus or defective restoration margins, pockets < 3.5 mm.
Code 2	Bleeding on probing, calculus detected or defective restoration margins, but pockets < 3.5 mm.
Code 3	Pockets within colour coded area, i.e. pocket > 3.5 mm to < 5.5 mm.
Code 4	Colour coded area disappears indicating pocket > 5.5 mm.

False pocket = where increased probing depth is due to gingival enlargement without loss of attachment of the PDL.

True pocket = where increased probing depth results from destruction of PDL.

Recession = where the gingival margin lies apical to the CEJ.

ORAL HYGIENE AIDS

Tooth brushes	The mimp features are the size of head, texture of filaments, rounded ends of the bristles.
Electric tooth brush	Beneficial in patients with reduced manual dexterity.
Single tufted brushes	Cleans around lone-standing teeth; partially erupted M3, proximal spaces adj to saddle areas in partially dentate patients.
Floss **Tape**	 Broader than floss; used in i/d areas.

ORAL HYGIENE AIDS (*Contd.*)

Superfloss	Used for cleaning under the bridges.
Floss threader	Used to pass floss below the FPD.
Interproximal/ bottle brushes	Method of choice for i/d cleansing when space permits.
Wooden sticks	Not so effective than interproximal brushes.

Root planning involves removal of subgingival plaque, calculus and infected cementum.

Scaling instruments

Instrument	**Description**	**Area of use**
Chisel/push scaler	Chisel head angled at 45.	Applied from labial to remove gross supragingival deposits from approximal surfaces of mand ant teeth.
Point scaler/ + sickle scalers and jacquettes	Are triangular in cross section and have 2 cutting edges, which converge to a sharp point.	All buccal and lingual embreasures, supragingival and 2–3 mm subgingival. Manipulated with wrist movements.
Hoes	Have a blade set at 100 angle to shank and cutting edge is bevelled at 45. A set of 4 is required to give access to all tooth surfaces.	Access to deep pockets; used in a series of pull strokes. Subgingival depostits.
Curettes	Curved spoon shaped blade with 2 cutting edges, which meet to form a rounded hoe.	Supra, and esp subgingivally throughout the mouth. Used after hoes in root planning.
Ultrasonic scalers		Avoid in patients fitted with a cardiac pacemaker.

Differences between periodontal abscess and periapical abscess

C/F	PD abscess	PA abscess
Pain	Acute onset	H/O tooth ache
Swelling	Usually localised, extra-oral swelling unlikely	Over tooth apex; more likely to be extensive
Pocket	Always present; more likely in p.o. PD disease	Pocket may/may not be present
Sinus	Frequently on attached gingiva	Tracks to the apex
Percussion	Tender to percussion; worse laterally	Tender to percussion; esp axially
Restoration status	More likely if tooth caries free/ unrestored	More likely in heavily filled tooth
Vitality	Tooth is vital	Non-vital
Radiograph	Little evidence in early stages; bone loss	Loss of lamina dura in PA areas; after 10 days or so.

Endo-perio lesions = when infection involves both pulp chamber and PDL space simultaneously.

Splint = a means of increasing tooth support by joining to an adjacent tooth or teeth.

A primary function of the PD tissues is to support the tooth when a load is applied.

Trauma from occlusion cannot induce periodontal tissue breakdown, but in p.o. pre-existing PD disease, excessive occlusal loading may increase the PD breakdown.

- Temporary splint for 2–6 mos.
- Provisional splint for 6–12 mos.
- Permanent splint for > 12 mos.

Important procedures

Procedure	Indications
Currettage	• Supra bony pockets. • New attachment attempts. • Maintenance Rx. • In patients with systemic conditions where surgery is C/I.
Gingivectomy	• Supra bony pockets. • Gingival hyperplasia. • Supra bony PD abscess.
Full thickness flaps	Osseous surgery.
Partial thickness flap	For apical repositioning of flap.
Osseous surgery	Infra bony pockets.
Flaps	• Furcation. • Infra bony pockets. • Osseous defects and gingival enlargement.
Mucogingival surgery	• Widening the zone of the attached gingiva. • Coverage of denuded roots. • Shallow vestibules.

Most common Pathogens causing various PD diseases

Disease	Pathogens
Early gingivitis	Actinomyces.
Long standing gingivitis	Fusobacterium and veillonella.
Adult periodontitis	B gingivalis.
Pregnancy gingivitis	Bacteroides intermedius; it can substitute progesterone/estradiole for vitamin K as growth factor.

Most common Pathogens causing various PD diseases (*Contd.*)

Disease	**Pathogens**
Rapidly progressing periodontitis	B gingivalis; B intermedius; small spirochetes, etc. Functional defects in neutrophils or monocytes.
Refractory periodontitis	B gingivalis, etc.
LJP	A. actinomyecetamcomitans (AA); capnocytophaga; Neutrophil chemotactic defect and decreased phagocytosis. Concentration of AA is 6 times greater than the normal sites; Increased Ab levels to AA esp IgG. Serotype B is the commonest.
GJP	B gingivalis is most common. C high IgG titers esp to serotype C.
Periodontitis in juvenile diabetes	Actinomyces and streptococci.
ANUG	• Principal bacteria = B intermedius; unnamed intermediate sized spirochetes; • Superficial bacteria = **Borrelia vincenti; fusiform bacilli.** • **Increased Ab titers IgG; IgM.**
AIDS	• Bacteroides melaninogenicus. • G + bacilli. • G – wet spreaders.
In IDDM; gingivitis	• Actinomyces. • Streptococci. • Veillonella. • Fusobacterium.

Most common Pathogens causing various PD diseases (*Contd.*)

Disease	Pathogens
In IDDM, periodontitis	• Capnocytophaga. • Anaerobes. • It is different than adult periodontitis in which B gingivalis is predominant.
PD abscess	• B gingivalis.
Prepubertal	• Decreased chemotaxis of PMN and periodontitis monocytes. • Main bacteria are fusobacterium, selemonas, etc.

Important values

- Force applied during brushing = < 500 gm.
- Dentin abraded = 25 times faster than enamel.
- Cementum abraded = 35 times faster than enamel.
- Dentrifrices contain F = 1100 ppm.
- Distance b/w apical edge of calculus and bottom of pocket = 0.2–1.0 mm.
- In gingivitis, ratio of T4–T8 cells = 2:1.
- In periodontitis, ratio of T4–T8 cells = 1:1.
- In AIDS, ratio of T4–T8 cells is << 1.
- In sulcular fluid, ratio of T cell : B cells = 1:3.
- In PBF, the ratio of T cell : B cells = 3:1.
- Zone of J E = 500 microns or 0.25–1035 mm.
- Rate of bone loss = 0.2 mm/yr on facial surfaces, 0.3 mm/yr on proximal surfaces.
- Radius of action required = 1.5–2.5 mm.
- Loss of attachment occurs 6–8 mos before the bone loss.

Tooth whitening systems

- It is the Rx of choice if the patient has realistic expectations; teeth are only moderately stained.

- Power bleaching = is an in office procedure; it uses 30–35% of H_2O_2 with heat or light.
- At home tray based system = has 10% H_2O_2 or 22% urea carbamide peroxide solution; used for more than 2 hrs daily.
- Paint on liquid gel = 6.5% H_2O_2.
- Whitening strips = 6.5% H_2O_2.
- Oral irritation is largely associated with tray whitening systems.
- Potassium nitrate is used to overcome dentinal hypersensitivity.

PERI-IMPLANTITIS

- It is an inflammatory process affecting tissues surrounding the osseo-integrated dental implant.
- In healthy peri-implant tissues = aerobic bacteria; high no. of coccoid cells; low no. of G +ve bacteria.
- In unhealthy peri-implant tissues = G –ve anaerobes; spirochetes; motile organisms.
- Pocket depth of more than 3 mm requires investigation.
- Cleaning of implants is done with = carbon fiber curettes; rubber cups and polishing paste.
- Daily rinsing with chlorhexidine digluconate 0.12–0.2%.
- Antibiotic given if pockets are more than 6 mm; amoxycillin + metronidazole is given.
- If pocket depth is more than 5 mm = surgical intervention is done.

FOR MEDICINE PART

- There is an association between low grade infections and cardiovascular diseases.
- CRP lipoprotein LPa; RAS activation, etc. are the non-traditional risk indicators for heart diseases.
- Viral and bacterial infections, e.g. CMV and chlamydia pneumoniae are associated with atherosclerosis.
- LDL is also known as **bad cholesterol**.

- LPS is a toxic component of G –ve cell wall bacteria, which initiates inflammatory responses and monocytic adhesion to walls of blood vessels.
- Activated monocytes also known as **macrophages**.
- Macrophages filled with LDL are known as **foam cells**.
- Plasma level of CRP, i.e. C–reactive protein indicates systemic inflammation.
- High levels of CRP are predictive of increased risk of heart attack years before they occur.
- NIMIT'S NOTES:

GINGIVA

NORMAL PERIODONTIUM

- It contains 2 hard tissues, i.e. cementum and alveolar bone; and 2 soft tissues, i.e. gingival and PDL.
- Origin of periodontium is dental follicle.
- Gingival has 3 parts, i.e. free gingiva (FG); attached gingiva (AG) and interdental papilla.
- FG demarcated from AG by free gingival groove (FGG).
- AG separated from alveolar mucosa by mucogingival junction (MGJ).
- **Colour** of the normal gingiva = coral pink; it depends on the vascularity; degreee of keratinization and pigmentation.
- Under absolute normal or ideal conditions, the depth of gingival sulcus is or about zero.
- Keratinized gingiva = includes marginal and attached gingival.
- Hard tissues of dento-gingival apparatus are cementum and bone; soft tissue are PDL and gingiva.

Width of attached gingiva

- Is greatest in the incisor region = 3.5 to 4.5 in maxilla; 3.3 to 3.9 mm in mandible.
- Less in posterior segment.

- Least width in the first premolar area = 1.9 mm in maxilla and 1.8 mm in mandible.
- It increases with age and in supra-erupted teeth, although the position of MGJ remains stationary throughout life.

- ♦ Histology of gingival.
- ♦ Gingival epithelium may be orthokeratinized; parakeratinized and non-keratinized.
- ♦ **Orthokeratinized epithelium** has a well defined stratum granulosum with no nuclei in stratum corneum. It has 4 layers, i.e. basale; spinosum; granulosum and corneum.
- ♦ **Parakeratinized epithelia**, stratum corneum retains **pyknotic nuclei** and ***keratohyalin granules*** are dispersed, not giving rise to a stratum granulosum. It has basale; spinosum and corneum layers.
- ♦ **Non-keratinized epithelia** has neither stratum granulosum nor stratum corneum layers. It has only basale and spinosum.
- ♦ **Other cells** = e.g. Langhans cells are antigen presenting cells; Merkel cells are tactile preceptors.
- ♦ Interdental papilla = is pyramidal in shape in anterior segment and col-shaped in posterior segment.
- ♦ Col = facial and lingual papilla joined by a valley like depression.
- ♦ Col is covered by thin, stratified squamous non-keratinized epithelium.
- ♦ **Basal lamina** is seen under an electron microscope. It is 300–400 A thick. It has **2 layers,** viz. *lamina lucida (glycoprotein laminin) and lamina densa* (type IV collagen).
- ♦ **Basement membrane** is seen under light microscope. It consists of ***basal lamina and connective tissue elements***.
- ♦ ***Sulcular epithelium*** and ***non-keratinized stratified squamous*** epithelium are ***without rete pegs*** and extends from the coronal limit of the junctional epithelium JE to the crest of the gingival margins.
- ♦ JE is stratified squamous non-keratinizing epithelium formed by confluence of oral epithelium and reduced enamel epithelium/ REE during tooth eruption.

- JE and the gingival fibers form a functional unit known as **dento-gingival unit**.
- Gingival connective tissue is mainly **collagen fibers type–I**.
- **Gingival sulcus and probing depth**:
  - Under absolutely ideal conditions; the depth is zero or about zero.
  - Histologic depth = 0–6 mm.
  - Clinically normal gingival sulcus = 2–3 mm.
- **Collagen**:
  - Most abundant protein in the animal kingdom.
  - Polypeptide of 3 alpha–chains, i.e. alpha–1, 2, 3.
  - Collagen molecule may be a homotrimer or hetertrimers.
  - Characterized by repeating Glycine amino acid sequence.
  - In vertebrate collagen = the amino acid at gamma position are hydroxyproline or hydroxylysine.
  - Size of collagen molecue is 300 A × 15 Å. (Å = angstrom unit)
  - Collagen fibers are characterized by a special banding of pattern at 64 nm interval.
  - Collagen biosynthesis involve hydroxylation of proline and lysine, which require oxygen; ferrous ions and vitamin C as cofactors.
- **Stippling** = it is orange-peel like appearance of the surface; gingival has a textured surface known as stippling. It is due to the elevations. Only attached gingival and centre of inter-dental papilla is stippled. Effect of age not in infants and in edentulous patients.
- **Active eruption** is the actual movement of the tooth towards the occlusal plane. **Passive eruption** is the exposure of the tooth by apical migration of gingival.
- **Theories of eruption Supra-eruption.**

PERIODONTAL LIGAMENT/ DETAILS (Also refer to section of dental histology in Vol. I.)

- PDL fibers are known as principal fibers.

- Fibers are mainly formed ***by fibroblasts***.
- Terminal parts of principal fibers which is embedded in the bone and cementum is known as Sharpey's fibers.
- PDL fibers are composed of amino acids, the most prominent of these being the ***collagen type I***.
- Types of collagen fibers ____ locations ____.
- Terminal ends of PDL fibers are embedded in the cementum and bone, and are known as **Sharpey's fibers.**
- Epithelial rests of Malassez are remnants of Hertwig's epithelial root sheath _____ details _____ depth _____ function.
- It has the ***shape of hourglass***, being narrowest in the region of the axis of rotation.
- **Types of principal fibers**

Trans-septal	• Also known as supracrestal fibers _____. • Extend inter-proximally over the alveolar crests and are inserted in the cementum of adjacent tooth. • These fibers are reconstructed even after the destruction of bone has occurred in PD disease. • Are responsible for relapse of rotations after orthodontic Rx.
Alveolar	Run from cementum to bone in the _____ apical direction _____.
Horizontal oblique	• Are largest group of the fibers, i.e. maximum in no. • Run from cementum in a coronal direction to the bone. • Bear most of the masticatory load.
Apical	Not seen in teeth with incompletely formed roots, run almost in a vertical direction from the apex of tooth to bone.
Inter-radicular	Seen only in multi-rooted teeth.

- Calcified masses in PDL are known as cementicles.
- **Sensory receptors in the PDL**

Free nerve endings	Carry pain sensations.
Ruffini like organs	Mechanoreceptors; located in apical areas.
Meissner's corpuscles	Mechanoreceptors; located in midroot regions.
Spindle like endings	Pressure and irritations sensations.

CEMENTUM (Also refer to section of dental histology in Vol. I.)

- It is formed by the cells known as cementoblasts.
- It is an avascular, mesenchymal tissue.
- 2 sources of collagen fibers in cementum.
  - **Extrinsic fibers** = i.e. **Sharpey's fibers**; are basically PDL fibers embedded in cementum.
  - **Intrinsic fibers** = which belong to cemental matrix. Are formed by cementoblasts.
- It is of 2 types.
- Acellular cementum—is the ***first formed cementum***. It covers the cervical 3rd or half of the root. It does not contain cells. It is formed before the tooth reaches the occlusal plane.
- Cellular cementum = formed after the tooth reaches the occlusal plane; it contains cells and is ***less calcified than acellular*** type. It covers apical part _____ Its thickness _____, etc.
- Junction between cementum and enamel is of 3 types:

Type of junction	**% age**
Cementum overlaps the enamel	60–65%
Edge to edge butt joint	30%
Cementum and enamel fail to meet	5–10%

- Thickness of cementum varies from 16–60 microns in the coronal half to 150–200 microns in the apical areas.
- Cementum is thickest in apical third and in furcation areas of the tooth.
- Both cementum and PDL are thicker on distal surfaces of roots than on the mesial surface.
- Cementum repair is not affected by the vitality of the tooth.
- Cellular and acellular cementum are differentiated under light microscope.

ALVEOLAR BONE

- Alveolar process is that part of the maxilla and mandible that forms and supports the tooth sockets.
- It is formed by intramembranous ossification.
- **Basal bone** = that part of the jaw located apically to teeth.
- **Alveolar bone proper** is the inner wall of the tooth socket; it is seen as **lamina dura** in R/G; on H/E, it contains small holes through, which neurovascular bundles link PDL with cancellous bone, i.e. ***cribriform plate***.
- **Lamina dura** = the cribriform plate of socket is seen in R/G as thin radiopaque line.
- **Bundle bone** = i.e. bone adjacent to PDL which contains a large no. of Sharpey's fibers. It is localized within alveolar bone proper.
- **Woven bone** = is the first formed bone/immature bone.
- **Lamellar bone**—mature bone made up of layers or lamellae.
- **Cancellous bone/spongy bone/trabecular bone**—it is structurally similar to compact bone, except for the presence of trabecular spaces. More cancellous bone is found in maxilla than the mandible.
- **Bone marrow**—in the embryo and newborns, all bone cavities are occupied by red marrow; in adults, the red marrow changes to yellow/fatty marrow. But red marrow may still be found in ribs, sternum, vertebrae, skull and humerus.

- **Even in jaws,** the foci of red bone marrow may be seen in maxillary tuberosity; maxillary and mandibular molar and premolar areas; and the mandibular symphysis and ramus angle.
- **Periosteum** has 2 layers:
  - Inner layer is composed of osteoblasts surrounded by osteoprogenitor cells.
  - Outer layer is composed of collagen fibers and fibroblasts.
- **Endosteum** is single layered—it is composed of osteoblasts and a small amount of connective tissues.
- Osteoblasts originate from pluripotent stem cells of bone marrow while osteroclasts originate form hematopoietic system.
- Osteoclasts are characterized by their size (50–100 microns); multiple nuclei (2–10); and its presence within resorption lamina at the calcified matrixbone marrow interface.
- Parathormone/PTH acts on bone to produce resorption, thereby increasing the serum calcium levels; but the receptors of PTH in bone are located on osteoblasts (AIPG–99) and not on the osteoclasts.
- Osteoblasts are characterized by the presence of enzyme alkaline phosphatase, while osteoclasts have enzyme acid phosphatase.
- The mesio-distal angulation of the crest of the interdental septum usually parallels a line drawn between the CEJ of the approximating teeth.
- **Fenestrations** are isolated areas, in which the root is denuded of the bone, but the marginal bone is intact. Root is covered only by the periosteum and overlying gingiva.
- **Dehiscence,** i.e. when the denuded areas extend through the marginal bone, it is known as dehiscence.
- Typical feature which distinguishes the gingivitis from periodontitis is the presence of clinically detectable attachment loss.
- Incidence = probability that a person will become a case. It is the ratio of no. of new cases to the no. of persons at risk.
- Prevalence = proportions of persons in a population, who have the disease at a given period of time. It is the ratio of no. of persons with the disease to the no. of persons in the population.

- Sensitivity of a test = is the proportion of subjects with the disease who test positive. It is the ratio of no. of subjects who test positive to the no. of subjects with the disease.
- Specificity of the test = proportion of subjects without the disease who test negative. It is the ratio of subjects who test negative to the no. of subjects without disease.

PLAQUE

- It is a host–associated biofilm. It is defined as soft deposits that form the biofilm adhering to tooth surface or other hard surfaces in the oral cavity.
- Acquired pellicle _____.
- Most common sites are near the orifices of salivary glands.
- More than 500 distinct bacterial species are found in plaque.
- Inorganic component is mainly Ca and P.
- Initial bacteria colonizing the pellicle coated tooth surface are predominantly gram positive facultative microbes, e.g. actinomyces viscosus and streptococcus sanguis.
- Pregnancy associated gingivitis is associated with dramatic increase in the level of P. intermedia/which uses steroids as their growth factors.
- Scurvy diabetes mellitus _____.
- Bismuth pigmentation/Burtonian line is linear, steel grey in colour _____. Other lines of pigmentations lead arsenic, etc. silver, etc. _____.
- Main Ig in saliva = IgA.
- Main Ig in GCF = IgG.

PERIODONTAL MICROBIOLOGY

Plaque = soft deposits that form the biofilm adhering to the tooth surface or other hard surfaces in the oral cavity including removable and fixed restorations.

Materia alba = soft accumulations of bacteria and tissue cells that lack the organized structure of dental plaque and are easily displaced by water spray.

Calculus = is the mineralized plaque.

Plaque = 3 types, i.e. supragingival; marginal; subgingival.

Supragingival plaque causes root caries; calculus formation.

Marginal plaque causes gingivitis.

Subgingival plaque is of 2 types = tooth associated (which causes root caries and calculus) and tissue associated (which causes periodontitis).

More than 500 distinct microbial species are found in dental plaque.

During plaque formation, the initial bacteria colonizing the pellicle coated tooth surface are gram-positive facultative micro-organisms, e.g. actinomyces viscosus and streptococcus sanguis.

The composition of plaque formed on all types of restorative materials is similar with the exception of that formed on silicate.

Pregnancy gingivitis is associated with increases levels of Provetella intermedia, which uses steroids as growth factors in place of vitamin K.

Viruses associated with chronic periodontitis are EBV–1; HCMV.

Localized aggressive periodontitis = actinobacillus actinomycetamcomitans serotype–B (gram negative rods).

Necrotizing periodontal diseases = by P. intermedia and spirochetes.

Calculus = 2 types, i.e. supragingival and subgingival.

Supragingival calculus—most common locations are buccal surfaces of maxillary molars and the lingual surfaces of mandibular anterior teeth. It is because of the presence of the openings of major salivary glands in these vicinity.

Location and extent of subgingival calculus may be evaluated by careful tactile perception with an explorer.

Saliva is the source of mineralization for supragingival calculus, while GCF provides the minerals for subgingival calculus.

Differences between supragingival and subgingival calculus:

Properties	supragingival	subgingival calculus
Colour	Yellow	Black
Consistency	Soft	Hard
Source	Saliva	GCF

Inorganic component of calculus is crystalline in nature. The four main crystal forms are:

1. Hydroxyapatite = 58%.
2. Magnesium whitlockite = 21%.
3. Octacalcium phosphate = 12%.
4. Brushite = 9%.
5. Brushite is more common in ***mandibular anterior region***.
6. Hydroxyapatite and octacalcium phosphate are detected most frequently.
7. Magnesium whitlockite is common in the posterior region.

BACTERIOLOGY

Bacteria	Features	Importance
Neisseria	G negative cocci, anaerobe	
Veillonella	G negative cocci, anaerobe	
Peptostreptococcus	G positive cocci, anaerobe	
Bacteroides	G negative bacilli	
Eubacterium	G positive bacilli	
Actinobacillus actinomycetam comitans	Gram negative rods	
Provetella	G negative bacilli	
Campylobacter	Gram negative vibrio	
Porphyromonas	G negative bacilli	
Fusobacterium	G negative bacilli	

- Interproximal attachment loss is generally a consequence of bacteria induced periodontitis. While buccal and lingual attachment loss is frequently the result of tooth brush abrasion.

DIABETES

- There is an alteration of oral flora with greater preponderance of Candida albicans; hemolytic strept; staphylococci.
- There is an increased collagenase activity and decreased collagen synthesis render the periodontal tissues more susceptible to destruction.

PREGNANCY

- Pregnancy itself does not cause gingivitis.
- Gingival disease during pregnancy is caused by bacterial plaque, but hormonal change during pregnancy accentuates the gingival response to plaque and modifies the resultant clinical picture.
- Bacteria which increase significantly during pregnancy is = Prevotella intermedia.
- Gingival has "rasp-berry like" appearance.

GINGIVAL ENLARGEMENT

- Hyperplasia vs hypertrophy—No. of cells increase in former.
- Drugs causing gingival enlargement are phenytoin; cyclosporin; nifedipine.
- Idiopathic gingival enlargement involves/affects gingival margin; attached gingival and interdental papillae.
- Capnocytophaga species is implicated in the initiation of pubertal gingivitis.
- Epulis are inflammatory (non-neoplastic) masses of the gingiva.

ACUTE GINGIVAL INFECTIONS

- ANUG; primary herpetic gingivo-stomatitis and pericoronitis are acute gingival infections.

- ANUG is caused by spirochetes Treponema intermedia and fusiform bacilli.
- ANUG is also known as trench mouth.
- Primary infection of AHG is asymptomatic.

PERIODONTAL POCKETS

- It is the pathologically deepened gingival sulcus.
- The only reliable method of locating pocket and determining their extent is CAREFUL PROBING.
- ***Pseudopocket/gingival/false/relative pocket***: Are caused by gingival enlargement without destruction of the underlying periodontal tissues.
- ***True pockets/periodontal/absolute pockets***: It is formed by the destruction of supporting periodontal tissues. It is of suprabony and infrabony types.
- ***Suprabony pockets***: Also known as supracrestal or supraalveolar pocket; bottom of the pocket is coronal to the underlying alveolar bone.
- ***Infrabony pocket:*** Also known as infrabony, subcrestal or intra-alveolar pocket; bottom of the pocket is apical to the level of the adjacent alveolar bone.

Difference between suprabony and infrabony pockets

Suprabony	Infrabony
Base of pocket is cornonal to alveolar crest.	Apical to crest of alveolar bone.
Pattern of destruction of underlying bone is horizontal.	Vertical/angular.
Interproximally, the transseptal fibers restored during PD disease are arranged horizontally.	Obliquely arranged.
PDL fibers below the PD pocket follow normal horizontal-oblique course.	Follow angular pattern.

- ***Simple pocket*** = involves one-tooth surface.
- ***Compound pocket*** involves 2 or more tooth surfaces.
- ***Complex pocket*** = it originates from one tooth surface and twisting around the tooth to involve one or more additional surfaces. Involves more than 2 tooth surfaces. These are spiral type of pockets. These are most common in furcation areas.
- The only reliable method of locating the periodontal pocket is by probing of the gingival margin along each tooth surface.
- Periodontitis is always preceded by gingivitis, but not all gingivitis proceed to periodontitis. Most important cause of gingivitis is plaque.
- The distance b/w the apical extent of calculus and the alveolar crest in human periodontal pockets is most constant, having a mean length of 1.97 mm ± 33.16%.
- The distance b/w JE and alveolar bone is relatively constant.
- Distance b/w attached plaque and bone is 0.5 mm–2.7 mm.
- Intrabony pockets most often occur interproximally, but may be located on facial and lingual tooth surfaces.
- Horizontal bone loss vs vertical bone loss.
- ***Angular bony defects/vertical bony defects*** are classified on the basis of the no. of osseous wall remaining, i.e. 1-walled, 2-walled; 3-walled defects, combined, 1½ walled, circumferential defects.
- 3-walled defects are also known as ***intrabony defects***; they mostly occur on mesial aspect of 2nd and 3rd molars.
- 1–walled defects is also known as ***hemiseptum***.
- Prognosis of 3 walled defects is better than the 2-walled defects; worst prognosis is of 1-walled defects.
- ***Combined osseous defect*** = i.e. the number of walls in the apical portion of the defect are greater than its occlusal part.
- **Other angular defects** can be shallow and narrow; shallow and wide; deep and narrow; deep and wide. Surgical exposure is the only sure way to determine the presence and configuration of vertical osseous defect.
- **Most common** location of vertical defects is on distal surfaces of molars.

- **Most common bony lesion** = crater.
- ***Craters*** = concavities in the crest of interdental bone confined within the facial and lingual walls.
- ***Reverse architecture*** = bony defects produced by loss of interdental bone including the facial and lingual plates or both, *without concomitant loss of radicular bone* thereby reversing the normal architecture. These are more common in maxilla.
- Radiological evaluation of bone changes in periodontal disease is based mainly on the appearance of the I/D septa, because the relatively dense root structure obscures the facial and lingual bony plates.
- Crest of the I/D septa is parallel to the line b/w the CEJs of the adjacent teeth.
- Healthy gingiva is associated with coccoid cells and straight rods; while diseased gingival is associated with increased numbers of spirochetes and motile rods.
- ***Histopathology*** = pocket formation starts as an inflammatory change in CT wall of gingival sulcus.
- ***Many zones*** are present: junctional epithelium; zone of destroyed collagen; zone of partial destruction; area of normal attachment;
- Collagen destruction may be due to enz collagenase; and increased numbers of **PMN cells**. If volume of PMN cells reaches approx 60% of JE, it detaches from the tooth surface and migrates apically. PMN increase in number, which migrate through the gaps b/w epithelial cells.
- Discoloration is due to circulatory stagnation; bleeding is due to. engorged vessels and pain is due to ulceration of inner aspect of the pocket wall.
- **Plasma cells** increased in CT; JE is reduced to 50–100 microns (normal width of JE is 500 microns); migration of JE along the root requires the presence of healthy epithelial cells. So degeneration of JE retards the pocket formation. Degenerative changes at the base of pocket, i.e. in JE are less severe than those in the epithelium of lateral wall of the pocket.
- Pockets are said to be healing lesions, but the rate of destructive changes are more than the rate of healing/constructive changes.

- **Root caries** = here, proteolysis of Sharpey's fibers occurs and cementum gets softened; this caries tends to progress around rather than into the tooth. Main cause is **Actinomyces viscosus**.
- Main bacteria in PD abscess are G (–) anaerobic rods.

TRAUMA FROM OCCLUSION

It refers to the tissue injury but not the occlusal forces. It is the tissue injury that results when occlusal forces exceed the adaptive capacity of the tissues. It occurs in supporting tissues and does not affect the gingival. It does not cause pockets formation.

- **Traumatic occlusion**—i.e. an occlusion producing such injury. Any occlusion which produces periodontal injury is traumatic.
- **Acute TFO**—i.e. which occurs from an abrupt change in occlusal forces.
- **Chronic TFO**—more common; develops from gradual changes in the occlusion produced by tooth wear, drifting movements; bruxism, etc.
- **Primary TFO**—i.e. if TFO is the main cause of periodontal destruction. More than normal occlusal forces are the cause. It does not alter the level of CT attachment an do not initiate pocket formation, because supracrestal fibers are not affected and so JE does not migrate.
- **Secondary TFO**—i.e. when the adaptive capacity of the tissues to withstand normal occlusal forces is impaired. Alveolar bone loss is the most common cause of secondary TFO. The periodontium becomes vulnerable to injury, e.g. decrease in PD area due to marginal inflammation.
- **Capillary** pulse pressure is 20–26 gm/sq. cm; width of PDL is 0.2–0.25 mm.
- Bifurcation and trifurcation are the areas most susceptible to injury from increased occlusal forces.
- Most common sign of TFO is mobility of teeth and R/G there is widened PDL; thickened lamina dura; vertical bone loss; root resorption, etc.
- **Pathologic migration**—occurs mostly in anterior region; mobility and rotation of the affected teeth occur. It occurs under

conditions that weaken the PD support and/or increase or modify the forces exerted on the teeth.

- **Drifting**—it is different from pathologic migration, in that it does not result from destruction of PD tissues. It usually occurs mesially with tilting or extrusion. Premolars drift distally.

Oral manifestations of AIDS

Manifestations	Clinical features
Oral hairy leukoplakia	• Primarily occurs in persons with HIV infections, esp due to **Epstein Barr** virus. • Found esp on the **lateral borders of tongue**; frequently has a bilateral distribution. • Lesion does not rub-off. • Lesion has hyperparakeratosis and acanthosis and balloon cells, which contain Ebviruses. • Microscopically, it contains some characterisitic koilocytes/**balloon cells,** which contain virus particles of herpes group. • Lesions also reveal surface colonization by candida, but it is a secondary invader.
Candidiasis	• Most common oral lesion in HIV esp on hard and soft palate. • Is due to diminished host resistance. • Seen in approx 90% of AIDS patients. • Diagnosis of candidiasis is made by H/E of a tissue sample or smear of material scraped from the lesion.
Kaposi sarcoma	• Is a rare, vascular neoplasm. • Closely associated with **human herpes virus-8**.

Oral manifestations of AIDS (*Contd.*)

Manifestations	Clinical features
	• In its classical form, it is a localized and slow growing lesion; but in AIDS patient it is a much more aggressive lesion. • Contains mononuclear inflammatory cells esp of **plasma cells**.
Bilateral epithelioid angiomatosis	• Infectious vascular proliferative diseases. • Caused by rickettessia like organism, bartonellaciac henselia; quintana or others.
Atypical ulcers	• Patients have a higher incidence of ***recurrent herpetic lesions and aphthous stomatitis***. • In non-HIV patients, herpes presents on the keratinizing mucosa and aphtae on non-keratinizing surfaces. But in HIV patients, herpes may involve all mucosal surfaces and extend to the skin.
Linear gingival erythema	• It may be limited to marginal tissue or may extend into AG in a punctate or a diffuse erythema or extend into alveolar mucosa. • Candida dubliniensis has been implicated in some cases of LGE.
Atypical periodontal disease	• Severe soft tissue necrosis; like ANUG. • Rapid PD destruction. • Deep interdental craters. • Exposure of alveolar bone and sequestration. • Severe pain .

- Is caused by HIV/HTLV–3 and is characterized by destruction of lymphocytes.
- It affects CD 4 cells, i.e. T–cells.
- Lower ratio of T 4–T 8 cells (reversed helper to suppressor cells ratio).
- AIDS related complex ARC = 2 clinical findings and 2 hematological findings.
- HIV patients are potential candidates for conventional periodontal Rx procedures to include periodontal surgery and implant placement.
- **Clinical diagnosis and radiographic criteria:**
  - The complete R/G survey of mouth requires a minimum of 14 intra-oral films and 4 posterior bitewing films.
  - OPG provides an informative overall R/G picture of distribution and severity of bone destruction in PD disease. But for PD diagnosis, and Rx planning, a complete intra-oral series is required.
  - Halitosis—is primarily caused by volatile sulfur compounds, specifically hydrogen sulfide and methyl mercaptan, which result from the bacterial putrefaction of proteins containing sulfur aminoacids.
  - Proximal contact relations can be checked by clinical observation and by dental floss.
- **Level of attachment**—is the distance from the base of pocket to the CEJ.
- **Pocket depth**—distance from the base of the pocket to the gingival margin.

GINGIVAL DISEASES

- Gingivitis = is the inflammation of gingival with no attachment loss.

Stages	Predominant cells	Important features
Initial lesion/ subclinical	PMN cells	
Early lesion	Lymphocytes	JE and Sulcular Epith show rete peg formation.
Established lesion	Plasma cells	

- Gingival pigmentation from systemically absorbed metals results due to perivascular precipitation of metallic sulfides in the subepithelial CT. Pigmentation occurs only in areas of inflammation, where the increased permeability of irritated blood vessels permits the seepage of the metals in the surrounding tissues.
- Bismuth = bluish black discoloration of the gingival margin in the areas of pre-existent gingival inflammation.
- Lead = Burtonian's line, i.e. linear steel–grey gingival pigmentation.
- Mercury = linear gingival pigmentation.
- Increased melanin pigmentation in the oral cavity is seen in:
    - Addison's disease—caused by adrenal dysfunction.
    - Peutz–Jeghers synd.
    - Albright's syndrome, i.e. polyostotic fibrous dysplasia.
- Gingival abscess—localized collection of pus limited to the marginal gingival or interdental papilla. (AIPG—2004).
- Periodontal abscess involves the supporting periodontal tissues.

Drug induced gingival enlargement

- Seen with **phenytoin** (anti-convulsant); **cyclosporine** (immuno-suppresent); **nifedipine** (calcium channel blocker).
- It occurs in the areas where teeth are present, and **not in the edentulous areas;** the enlargement disappears in the areas from which the teeth are extracted.

- Besides phenytoin, other hydantoins known to induce gingival enlargement are ethotoin and mephenytoins.
- Other anticonvulsants that have the same side effects are succinimides, methsuxinimide and velproic acid.
- Cyclosporine may be substituted by another immuno-suppressant ***Tacrolimus*** that causes much less severe gingival overgrowth.
- Attached gingival is involved in idiopathic gingival enlargement.
- Gingival enlargement is seen in pregnancy—known as pregnancy epulis/angiogranuloma.
- Epulis–inflammatory tumor like gingival enlargement.
- Pyogenic granuloma—gingival enlargement that is considered an exaggerated response to minor trauma.
- Gingival enlargement seen in leukemia patients occurs commonly in acute leukemia, but may also be seen in subacute leukemia. It seldom occurs in chronic leukemia.

ANUG

- Is inflammatory destructive disease of gingival.
- Etiology: **fusiform bacillia** and **spirochetes**.
- Characteristic lesions-punched out crater like depressions at the crest of I/D papilla, covered by a pseudomembrane and demarcated by a pronounced linear erythema.
- Vincent's angina: fusospirochetal infection of the oropharynx and throat.

PERIODONTAL INDICES

Index—defined by Russel in 1961, as a numerical value describing the relative status of a population on a graduated scale, with a definite upper and lower limit, designed to permit and facilitate its comparison with other population, classified by the same criteria and method.

It estimates only the relative prevalence or occurrence of the clinical condition.

Properties of an index

1. Clarity, simplicity and objectivity—the index should be reasonably easy to apply so that there is no undue time lost during field examinations. The criteria for the index should be clear and unambiguous, with mutually exclusive categories.
2. Validity—it should measure what it is intended to measure, so that it correlates with the clinical stage of disease under study.
3. Reliability/Reproducible—ability of an index to measure condition in the same subject repeatedly and obtain the same score each time.
4. Quantifiability—should be amenable to statistical analysis, so that the status of a group can be expressed by a number.
5. Sensitivity—i.e. detect reasonably small shifts.
6. Acceptability—the use of the index should not be painful or unacceptable to the subject.

Types

1. Reversible—measures cumulative changes that can be reversed from diseased to healthy, e.g. Gingivitis index.
2. Irreversible—measures the cumulative conditions that cannot be reversed, e.g. Caries index.

GINGIVAL INDICES

1. PMA index—Given by Schour and Massler in 1948.

The primary impetus which led to the development of the PMA index was the need for some quantitative method of recording readily observable inflammatory conditions of the gingivae to replace the then gross assessment of gingivitis in both children and adults as mild, moderate or severe.

The index was intended to survey gingival changes in relatively large groups for epidemiological purposes and study. The basic philosophy used in the development of PMA index was very similar to the DMF index, i.e. the number of gingival units affected were counted rather than the severity of inflammation.

Facial surface of gingiva around a tooth was divided into 3 scoring units:

1. Mesial dental papilla (P).
2. Marginal gingiva (M).
3. Attached gingiva (A).

Criteria

P	0	Normal; no inflammation.
	1+	Mild papillary engorgement; slight increase in size.
	2+	Obvious increase in size of the papillary gingival; haemorrhage on pressure.
	3+	Excessive increase in size with spontaneous haemorrhage.
	4+	Necrotic papilla.
	5+	Atrophy and loss of papilla.
M	0	Normal; no inflammation visible.
	1+	Engorgement; slight increase in size; no bleeding.
	2+	Obvious engorgement; bleeding upon pressure.
	3+	Swollen collar; spontaneous haemorrhage; beginning infiltration into attached gingivae.
	4+	Necrotic gingivitis.
	5+	Recession of the free marginal gingivae below the CEJ due to the inflammatory changes.
A	0	Normal; pale rose; stippled.
	1+	Slight engorgement with loss of stippling; change in colour may or may not be present.
	2+	Obvious engorgement of attached gingivae with marked increase in redness. Pocket formation present.
	3+	Advanced periodontitis. Deep pockets evident.

P, M and A values for all tooth were totaled separately and then added together to express the PMA score per person.

Advantages

(i) Main usefulness of this index was in the examination of children in whom the early stages of gingivitis were usually seen without obvious changes in the other periodontal tissues.

(ii) Broad application in epidemiological surgery and clinical trials.

(iii) Served as the basis for many other indices.

2. Gingival component of PDI—By Ramfjord in 1959.

Teeth examined $\dfrac{6 \quad 14}{41 \quad 6}$

Criteria

0 Absence of inflammation.

1 Mild to moderate inflammatory changes not extending all the tooth.

2 Mild to moderately severe gingivitis extending all around the tooth.

3 Severe gingivitis characterized by redness, swelling, tendency to bleed and ulceration.

$$\text{PDI Score: } \frac{\text{Sum of score of all six teeth}}{\text{No. of teeth examined}}$$

Importance—used in epidemiologic surveys, longitudinal studies on periodontal disease and clinical trials of therapeutic or preventive procedures.

3. Gingival index—By Loe and Silness in 1963.

Most frequently index of gingivitis nowadays.

Scoring surfaces are:

1. Buccal
2. Mesial
3. Distal
4. Lingual

Criteria

0 Normal gingiva.

1 Mild inflammation, slight change in colour, slight edema, no bleeding on palpation.

2 Moderate inflammation, redness, edema and glazing, bleeding on probing.

3 Severe inflammation, marked redness and edema, ulcerations; tendency to spontaneous bleeding.

Scoring

0.1–1.0 Mild gingivitis.

1.1–2.0 Moderate gingivitis.

2.1–3.0 Severe gingivitis.

Totaling the score around each tooth and dividing by 4 yields the GI score for the tooth. Totaling all the scores and dividing by the number of teeth gives the GI score per person.

Advantages

1. Distinguishes clearly between those with little or no gingivitis.
2. Used to determine prevalence and severity of gingivitis both in epidemiologic surveys and in an individual.

4. Modified gingival index—By Lobene and associates.

Modification of gingival index in which the bleeding criteria is eliminated making the index non-invasive.

Criteria

0 Absence of inflammation.

1 Mild inflammation slight change in colour, little change in texture of any portion of the marginal or papillary gingival unit.

2 Mild inflammation, criteria as above, but involving the entire marginal or papillary gingival unit.

3 Moderate inflammation, glazing, redness, edema and/or hypertrophy of the marginal or papillary gingival unit.

4 Severe inflammation, marked redness, edema and/or hypertrophy of the marginal or papillary gingival unit, spontaneous bleeding congestion or ulceration.

Advantage

The criteria for mild and moderate inflammation is well defined, which increase the index sensitivity in the lower portion of the scoring scale.

5. Periodontal screening examination—By O'Leary and co-workers (1963).

They used a combined gingival periodontal index, in which the mouth is divided into 4 posterior and 2 anterior segments. The gingival scoring for each segment is based upon the gingival unit with the greatest severity in each segment providing the score for that segment.

Criteria

0 Normal gingiva.

1 Slight to moderate inflammation not surrounding any particular tooth.

2 Similar inflammation but completely surrounding one or more teeth.

3 Marked inflammation.

4 Presence of buccal or lingual recession.

Adv- O'Leary gingival evaluations lend themselves mainly to broad surveys.

6. End point method of assessing gingivitis—By Fischman and co-workers (1973).

The rationale of this index was that the time it took for a subject with pre-existing gingivitis to reach an arbitrary level of gingivitis would be a measure of the efficacy of a preventive agent. This arbitrary level of gingivitis could be defined in terms of the Loe index. The authors felt that this system would permit the evaluation of the potential therapeutic agents in groups with pre–existing gingivitis.

One of the criticisms of this system is that it measures deterioration in gingival health and not an improvement, although the criteria could be reversed in terms of the end-point.

Adv: It permits the evaluation of the therapeutic agents without the need to empirically search for an optimum time period to evaluate a drug's effect.

7. Suomi and Barbano (1968), suggested an index based upon a 3 point system of 0, 1 and 2, scoring both facial and lingual units for each of 12 segments of the mouth (molar, premolar and anterior for each quadrant). Although this index separates subjects well on the presence or absence of gingivitis, it is found to be too limited in its description of the severity of gingivitis.

INDICES OF GINGIVAL BLEEDING

1. Sulcus bleeding index—By Muhlemann and Mazor in 1958.

Index used bleeding on probing as an indicative of gingival inflammation.

Criteria

0 No inflammation, no bleeding on probing.

1 Bleeding from gingival sulcus on gentle probing tissue otherwise appears normal.

2 Bleeding on probing, change in colour due to inflammation.

3 Bleeding on probing, change in colour and slight edema.

4 Bleeding on probing, change in colour and obvious edema.

5 Bleeding on probing, change in colour, spontaneous bleeding, marked edema, with or without ulceration.

Sulcus bleeding index is determined by averaging all of the scores for the individual.

2. Bleeding point index—By Lenox and Kppezyk in 1973.

Developed to assess in patient's oral hygiene performance. It determines the presence or absence of bleeding interproximally and on the facial and lingual surfaces of each tooth. A periodontal probe is drawn horizontally through the gingival crevice of a quadrant and the gingiva is examined for bleeding after 30 seconds.

3. Gingival bleeding index—By Carter and Barnes in 1974.

This index also assesses the presence or absence of gingival bleeding, but only at the interproximal sites and using unwaxed dental floss. All interproximal areas having a mesial and distal sulcus are considered to be susceptible to gingival inflammation and these areas are recorded as total areas at risk. Although these involve two sulci, they are scored as one gingival unit. The mouth is divided into six segments and flossed in the following order—upper right, upper anterior, upper left, lower left, lower anterior and lower right. Gingival bleeding score is obtained by noting total units of bleeding and the total susceptible areas at risk.

4. Gingival bleeding index—By Ainamo and Bay in 1975.

Easy and suitable way for the practitioner to assess patient's progress in plaque control. Presence or absence of bleeding is determined by gentle probing of gingival crevice with a periodontal probe. Appearance of bleeding within 10 seconds indicates a positive score, which is expressed as percentage of total number of gingival margins examined.

The authors felt that this index was well suited for epidemiological studies, short term clinical tests and in the daily practice of dentistry.

5. Papillary bleeding index—(PBI) By Muhlemann in 1977.

Criteria

0 No bleeding.

1 Bleeding some seconds after probing

2 Bleeding immediately after probing.

3 Bleeding on probing spreading towards the marginal gingiva.

Barnett and Colleagues (1980), modified the Muhlemann PBI by precisely defining the placement of the probe at the mesial line angle of the tooth and gently sweeping the probe forward into the mesial papilla. They timed the appearance of bleeding and graded it as follows:

0 No bleeding within 30 sec of probing.

1 Bleeding between 3 and 30 sec of probing.

2 Bleeding within 2 sec of probing.

3 Bleeding immediately upon probe placement.

The authors showed modified PBI to be more sensitive than the visual aspects of the GI in assessing changes in gingival health.

6. Interdental bleeding index (Eastman IBI)—By Caton and Palson in 1985.

A triangle shaped toothpick made of soft, pliable wood is inserted interproximally from the facial surface, depressing the interproximal papilla by up to 2 mm. It is inserted and removed 4 times and the presence or absence of bleeding within 15 seconds is noted.

IBI score is determined by dividing no. of bleeding site by no. of sites evaluated.

7. Index used by NIDR

Assesses gingival inflammation by the presence or absence of bleeding.

This index is based on the objective that bleeding is a more objective sign than colour change and provides evidence of recent plaque exposure.

Two sites per tooth (mesial–buccal interproximal and mid buccal on all teeth excluding molars; and mesial buccal interproximal and mid-buccal of the mesial root of molars) on one half of the maxillary arch and the contralateral half of the mandibular arch are examined after excess moisture is dried with air.

Left or right arch selection is randomly decided.

NIDR probe is inserted 2 mm into the gingival sulcus at the mid-point of the buccal and than gently down into the mesial-buccal interproximal area. Total numbers of bleeding site divided by total sites examined and multiplied by 100 gives the percentage of sites with gingival bleeding.

Criteria

0 No bleeding present.

1 Bleeding after NIDR probe is placed in sulcus up to 2 mm and drawn along the inner surface of sulcus.

8. Bleeding Index—By Edwards in 1975.

In this index a dental tape is wrapped around a proximal tooth surface in a bucco-lingual manner and inserted into the base of the crevice. This procedure is repeated twice. If no bleeding occurs after 15 sec, a score of 0 is recorded and 1 if bleeding occurs.

PLAQUE INDICES

Most of these indices utilize a numerical scale to measure the extent of the surface area covered by plaque.

1. Plaque component of PDI—Given by Ramfjord in 1959.

Index teeth examined $\dfrac{6 \quad 14}{41 \quad 6}$

Surfaces examined—interproximal, facial and lingual surfaces.

Criteria and scores

0 Absence of Plaque.

1 Plaque at interproximal surface and not covering more than 1/3 of tooth surface.

2 Plaque covering more than 1/3rd but less than 2/3rd of the tooth surface.

3 Plaque covering more than 2/3 of the tooth surface.

Advantage

Index is suitable for longitudinal studies of periodontal disease.

Shick and Ash modified the original criteria of Ramfjord by excluding consideration of the interproximal areas of teeth and restricting the scoring of plaque to the gingival half of the facial and lingual surfaces of the index teeth.

Score

0 Absence of dental plaque.

1 Dental plaque in the interproximal area at the gingival margin covering less than one third of the gingival half of the facial or lingual surfaces of the tooth.

2 Dental plaque covering more than one-third, but less than two third of the gingival half of the facial or lingual surface of the tooth.

3 Dental plaque covering two thirds or more of the gingival half of the facial or gingival surface of the tooth.

$$\text{Plaque score} = \frac{\text{Total score}}{\text{No. of teeth examined}}$$

2. Quigley Hein Plaque Index—(1962).

It measures plaque on the gingival third of the facial surfaces of the anterior teeth using basic fuchsin as disclosing solution.

0 Absolutely no plaque.

1 Single line of plaque.

2 Clear line of plaque along large extents of the gingival margins.

3 Plaque on only the cervical third of crown.

4 Plaque extending on the middle third of the crown.

5 Plaque extending into the occlusal third of crown.

$$\text{Q.H index} = \frac{\text{Sum of scores}}{\text{No. of surfaces evaluated}}$$

3. Turesky-Gillmore-Glickman modification of the Quigley-Hein Plaque index—(1970).

Plaque is assessed on the facial and lingual surfaces of all the teeth after using a disclosing agent.

0 No plaque.

1 Separate flicks of plaque at the cervical margin of the tooth.

2 A thin continuous band of plaque (up to 1 mm) at the cervical margin.

3 A band of plaque wider than 1 mm, but covering less than one third of the crown.

4 Plaque covering at least one-third but less than two thirds of the crown.

5 Plaque covering two thirds or more of the crown.

$$\text{Plaque score} = \frac{\text{Total score}}{\text{No. of teeth examined}}$$

Advantages

1. Relatively easy to use because of the objective definition of each numerical score.
2. Can be applied to longitudinal studies and clinical trials of preventive and therapeutic agents.

This index is one of the two indices of choice when assessing plaque in clinical trials.

4. Plaque index—By Sillness and Loe in 1967.

Uniqueness of this index is that it ignores the coronal extent of plaque on the teeth surface area and assesses only the thickness of plaque at the gingival area of the tooth.

It does not exclude or substitute for teeth with gingival restoration or crowns.

Tooth scoring units = distofacial, facial, mesiofacial and lingual.

Criteria and Scores

0 No plaque in the gingival area.

1 A film of plaque adhering to the gingival margin and adjacent area of the tooth. The plaque may be recognized only by running a probe across the tooth surface.

2 Moderate accumulation of soft deposits within the gingival pocket and on the gingival margin and/or adjacent tooth surface that can be seen by the naked eye.

3 Abundance of soft matter within the gingival pocket and/or on the gingival margin and adjacent tooth surface.

$$\text{PI} = \frac{\text{Sum of individual scores}}{\text{No. of surfaces examined}}$$

Index can be used for longitudinal studies and clinical trials.

5. Simplified oral hygiene index

Given by Greene and Vermillion in 1960 and later modified by them to include only six tooth surfaces, representative of all the anterior and posterior segments of the mouth.

The imprecise term ‘debris’ was used because it was not practical to distinguish among plaque, debris and materia alba.

It measures the surface area of tooth covered by debris.

Index teeth are facial surfaces of 3, 18, 14 and 24 and lingual surfaces of 19 and 30.

A mouth mirror and a sickle shaped explorer is used.

The explorer is placed on the incisal third of the tooth and moved towards the gingival third.

Criteria and Scores

0 No debris or stain present.

1 Soft debris covering not more than one-third of the tooth surface or the presence of extrinsic stains without other debris, regardless of surface area covered.

2 Soft debris covering more than one-third, but not more than 2/3 of the exposed tooth surface.

3 Soft debris covering more than 2/3 of the exposed tooth surface.

$$\text{Debris index score} = \frac{\text{Total score}}{\text{No. of surfaces examined}}$$

Interpretation of scores:

0.0–0.6 Good

0.7–1.8 Fair

1.9–3.0 Poor

6. **Patient hygiene performance index** (PHP)—Given by Podshadley and Haley in 1968.

First index developed for the sole purpose of assessing an individual's performance in removing debris after toothbrushing instructions.

Same six teeth are used as in OHI-S.

Each tooth surface is divided into five areas–3 longitudinal thirds with the middle third subdivided horizontally into thirds.

Presence or absence of debris is recorded as 1 or 0 using the six surfaces.

Index is easy to use and can be quickly performed.

Index can be applied to individual patient education.

7. **Navy-plaque index**—Given by Elliott in 1972.

Index teeth are $\dfrac{6 \quad 14}{41 \quad 6}$

Each tooth surface is divided into 9 scoring units.

Criteria

0 Absence of plaque.

1 Plaque present.

$$\text{Navy plaque index} = \frac{\text{Totalling all 9 subdivision scores for 6 teeth}}{\text{No. of tooth surfaces examined}}$$

8. **DMPI system**—by Cancro (1983).

This index places more emphasis on the gingival or cervical portion of the tooth as well as the interproximal areas. These areas are frequently missed by the toothbrush and may be used to study the effects chemical agents brought to the tooth by such vehicles as toothpaste or mouthrinse without interference by the mechanical action of toothbrushing.

Each area is scored as

0 Absence of plaque

1 Plaque covering 1/3rd of the area.

2 Plaque covering 2/3rd of the area.

3 Plaque covering the entire area.

The remaining area is scored as 1 or 0 depending on the presence or absence of plaque.

Plaque score can be represented as sums per tooth, per quadrant, or per area of all teeth.

Recent studies have shown that this index is easily learned by hygienists and is reproducible in clinical trials.

9. Bonded bracket index—By Ciancio, et. al. in 1984.

This index assesses plaque in orthodontic patients.

It scores bracket associated plaque as follows.

0 No plaque on bracket or tooth surface.

1 Plaque on brackets only.

2 Plaque on brackets, tooth, no extension to gingiva.

3 Plaque on bracket, tooth, extension to papilla.

4 Plaque on bracket, tooth, partial coverage to gingiva.

5 Plaque on bracket, tooth, full coverage to gingiva.

CALCULUS INDICES

1. Calculus component of simplified oral hygiene index

Calculus is assessed by gently placing an explorer into the distal gingival crevice and drawing it subgingivally from the distal contact area to the mesial contact area.

Criteria and Scores

0 No calculus present.

1 Supragingival calculus covering not more than one-third of the exposed tooth surface.

2 Supragingival calculus covering more than one-third, but not more than 2/3rd of the exposed tooth surface or the presence of individual flicks of subgingival calculus around the cervical portion of the tooth or both.

3 Supragingival calculus covering more than two-thirds of the exposed tooth surface or a continuous heavy band of subgingival calculus around the cervical portion of the tooth or both.

$$\text{CI} = \frac{\text{Total score}}{\text{No. of surfaces examined}}$$

2. Calculus component of periodontal disease index

Teeth recorded $\dfrac{6 \quad 14}{41 \quad 6}$ (facial and lingual surfaces)

Criteria and Scores

0 Absence of calculus.

1 Supragingival calculus extending only slightly below the free gingival margin (not more than 1 mm).

2 Moderate amount of supragingival and subgingival calculus or subgingival calculus alone.

3 An abundance of supragingival and subgingival calculus.

$$\text{Calculus score per person} = \frac{\text{Total score}}{\text{No. of teeth examined}}$$

Advantages

1. Has a higher degree of examiner reproducibility.
2. Can be quickly performed.
3. Best application in epidemiologic surveys and longitudinal studies.

3. **Probe method of calculus assessment** (Volpe and Manhold Index, 1961).

- Index was developed for longitudinal studies of the quantity of supragingival calculus formed.
- A periodontal probe graduated in mm is used to measure the vertical extent of calculus deposits on the lingual surfaces to mandibular incisors and canines.
- This index has a high degree of inter- and intra-examiner reproducibility.

4. **Calculus surface index**—By Ennever in 1961.

Index teeth—Mandibular incisors.

Surfaces examined—All four surfaces.

Criteria

0 Absence of calculus.

1 Presence of supra/sub-gingival calculus.

Maximum score can be 4 × 4 = 16.

Adv: Used in short-term (< 6 weeks) clinical trials of calculus inhibiting agents.

5. **Marginal line calculus index**—By Muhlcmann and Villa in 1967.

- This index was developed to assess the accumulation of supragingival calculus on the gingival third of the tooth or more specifically, supragingival calculus along the margin of gingival.
- Used in short-term clinical trials of anti-calculus agents.
- Calculus content is observed along the previously cleaned lingual gingival margin of the mandibular incisors.
- Scoring is given in percentage.

6. **Calculus index used by NIDR**

Unlike gingival assessment, calculus under assigns only one score per tooth, after examining both the mid-buccal and mesial-buccal inter proximal sites, on one half of the maxillary arch and contralateral mandibular arch.

Criteria

0 Calculus absent.

1 Supragingival calculus, but no sub gingival calculus is present.

2 Supra calculus, or sub gingival calculus only, is present.

Indices to measure periodontal destruction.

1. Gingival sulcus measurement component of PDI—By Ramfjord in 1967.

A university of Michigan probe # 0 probe is used for the purpose. The probe should be held with a light grasp such that the angle formed by the working end of the probe and the long axis of the crown of the tooth is approximately 45°.

Only buccal and mesial measurements are undertaken since it was found by Jamison and Ash in separate extensive analysis, that there is no significant loss of accuracy in the PDI index from omitting the distal and lingual scores. Also omitting lingual and distal scores enhances reproducibility in buccal and mesial scoring. The crevicular measurements are made in the following manner: The distance from the free gingival margin to the cemento-enamel junction and the distance from the free gingival margin to the bottom of the gingival crevice or pocket is measured for the buccal and mesial aspect of each tooth examined. The buccal measurements should be made at the middle of the buccal surfaces. The mesial measurement should be made at the buccal aspect of the interproximal contact area with the probe touching both teeth if there is a neighbor tooth present.

If the gingival margin is on enamel, measure from gum margin to CEJ and record the measurement. If the epithelial attachment is on the crown and the CEJ cannot be felt by the probe, record the depth of the gingival crevice on the crown. Then record the distance from the gingival margin to the bottom of the pocket if the probe can be moved apically to the CEJ without pain or resistance. The distance from the CEJ to the bottom of the pocket can then be found by subtracting the first from the second measurement.

If the gingival margin is on the cementum, record the distance from the CEJ to the bottom of the gingival crevice as a plus value. Both loss of attachment and actual crevice depth can be assessed from these scores.

2. **Periodontal index**—By Russel in 1956.

- This index considers periodontal diseases as a slowly progressing, continuous disease process extending from gingivitis to advanced periodontal disease.
- This index was intended to estimate the intent of deeper periodontal disease by determining the presence or absence of gingival inflammation and it's severity, pocket formation and masticatory function.
- It is an epidemiologic index with a true biologic gradient since it measures both the reversible and irreversible aspects of periodontal disease.

Criteria and Scores		**Add. radiographic criteria**
0	Negative. There is neither overt inflammation in the investing tissues or loss of function owing to destruction of supporting tissues.	Normal radiographic appearance.
1	Mild gingivitis. There is an overt area of inflammation in free gingival, but this area does not circumscribe the tooth.	
2	Gingivitis. Inflammation completely circumscribes the tooth, but there is no apparent break in epithelial attachment.	
4	(Used when radiographs are available.)	Early notch like resorption of the alveolar crest.

Criteria and Scores	Add. radiographic criteria
5 Gingivitis with pocket formation. Epithelial attachment is broken and there is pocket formation. No interference with normal masticatory function. The tooth is firm and has not drifted.	Horizontal bone loss involving the entire alveolar crest up to the length of tooth root.
6 Advanced destruction with loss of masticatory function. The tooth may be loose, may have drifted, may sound dull on percussion with a metallic instrument or may be depressible in the socket.	Advanced bone loss involving more than half of the tooth root or a definite infra bony pocket with widening of the periodontal ligament. There may be root resorption or rarefaction at the apex.

$$\text{PI score} = \frac{\text{Sum of individual scores}}{\text{No. of teeth present}}$$

Interpretation of score:

0–0.2	Clinically normal tissues.
0.3–0.9	Simple gingivitis.
0.7–1.9	Beginning destructive periodontal disease.
1.6–5.0	Established destructive periodontal disease.
3.8–8.0	Terminal disease.

Disadvantages

It tends to underestimate the true level of periodontal disease, since only a mouth mirror is used.

Importance. 1. It was used in Ten-state Nutrition survey (1968–70), National Health Survey (1960–62), National Health and Nutrition

Examination Survey (1971–74), and Hispanic Health and Nutrition Examination Survey (1982–83).

3. **Extent and severity index:** Given by JP Carlos, MD Wolfe, and Kingman in 1986.

- This index considers periodontal disease a chronic process with intermittent periods of activity and remission that affects individual teeth and site around teeth at different rates within the same mouth.
- Unlike periodontal index which uses only a mouth mirror, this index uses periodontal probe to determine the attachment levels.
- It expresses the percentage of site that exhibits disease (E for Extent) and at the same time measures mean attachment loss in mm (S for Severity). (Disease is any site with more than 1mm of attachment loss).
- Attachment loss is measured at the mesio-buccal interproximal and mid-buccal location on all teeth excluding molars and at the mesio-buccal interproximal and mid-buccal of the mesial root of molars, in one half of the maxillary arch and the contralateral half of mandibular arch.

4. **Radiographic approaches to measure bone loss**

(a) **Gingival-Bone Count Index**—Developed by Dunning and Leach in1960.

It records the gingival condition and the level of the crest of the alveolar bone. The bone level is assessed by clinical examination, but radiographs are recommended for greater accuracy. The gingival is assessed on a scale of 0 to 3, and the bone involvement is scored on a scale of 0 to 5.

The Gingival-Bone Count Index is the average gingival score per person plus the average bone score.

(b) **Periodontitis Severity Index**—Developed by Adams and Nystrom.

It consists of two components. The presence or absence of clinical inflammation is scored 0 or 1 respectively. The presence or absence of interproximal bone loss is determined radiographically using a modified Schei ruler. Each 10% increment in bone loss corresponds to a bone loss score of 1, to a maximum score of 10. The periodontitis severity index is a product of clinical inflammation score and bone loss score.

The index has promise in longitudinal studies, but is limited in epidemiologic surveys because of the need of the periapical radiographs.

INDICES TO ASSESS TREATMENT NEEDS

1. **GPI index** by O'Leary in 1967.

   G–Gingival status.

   P–Periodontal status.

   I–Irritation index (triad of materia alba, calculus and overhanging restorations).

- Modification of Ramfjord's PDI and is used for the purpose of screening person to determine the need for periodontal treatment.
- Maxillary and mandibular arch is divided into 3 segments, anterior, left posterior and right posterior.
- Each segment is assesses for the 3 components of the index.
- The objective is to determine the tooth or surrounding tissues with the severest conditions within each of the six segments.

Criteria

0 Tissue tightly adapted to teeth; firm consistency with physiologic architecture.

1 Slight to moderate inflammation, indicated by changes in colour and consistency, involving one or more teeth in the same segment, but not completely surrounding any one tooth.

2 Above changes either singly or combined completely encircling one or more teeth in a segment.

3 Marked inflammation, as indicated by loss of surface continuity (ulcerations), spontaneous haemorrhage, loss of faciolingual continuity, as any interdental papilla, marked deviation from normal contour, recession and clefts.

- Area with highest score determines the gingival score for the entire segment.

$$\text{Gingival status of mouth} = \frac{\text{Sum of gingival score of segments}}{\text{No. of segments}}$$

1. **Periodontal treatment need system** (PTNS)—By H.T. Bellini in 1973).

- This index assesses plaque, calculus, and gingival inflammation and pockets more than 5 mm, in each quadrant of mouth, and place individuals into 4 groups.

PTNS	Unit	Plaque	Calculus and /or Overhangs	Inflammation	Pocket Depth
Class O	Mouth	No	No	No	Not considered
Class A	Mouth	Yes	No	No	d ≤ 5 mm
Class B	Quadrant	Yes	Yes	Yes	< 5 mm
Class C	Quadrant	Yes	Yes	Yes	> 5 mm

2. **CPITN**—621 method according to WHO technical series publication.

- By WHO in 1997.
- Combines GPI and PTNS.
- Periodontal status is assessed by 3 indicatiors:
  (a) Presence or absence of gingival bleeding.
  (b) Supra/sub gingival calculus.
  (c) Periodontal pocket-shallow (4–5mm) or deep (6 mm or more).

CPITN probes

Epidemiological probe—Probe has markings from 3.5–5.5 mm with a 0.5 mm diameter ball at the tip.

Clinical probe—Probe has markings from 3.5–5.5 mm and from 8.5–11.5 mm with a 0.5 mm ball at the tip.

The ball prevents the probe from being pushed through inflammatory tissues at the base of pocket. Probing force is 20 gm.

Index teeth

17 16 11 26 27	For 20 years and above
47 46 31 36 37	

16 11 26	For upto 19 years
46 31 36	

This avoids classifying deepened crevices associated with eruption as periodontal pockets. For same reason periodontal pockets are not covered for children under 15 years of age.

Principles

1. Mouth is divided into sextants.
2. Last molar is not included.
3. It second molar is extracted and 3rd molar has shifted in its position, it can be included.
4. Tooth indicated for extraction is not included.
5. Tooth with vertical mobility due to periodontal diseases should not be included.
6. If only one tooth is present in one segment, it should be included in the adjoining segment.
7. Two or more teeth should be present in a segment for study.

Criteria

0 Healthy periodontium.

1 Bleeding observed, directly or by using mirror.

2 Calculus felt during probing, but the entire black area of probe (3.5–5.5 mm) is visible.

3 Pocket 4 to 5 mm (gingival margin on black area of probe).

4 Pocket > 6 mm (black area not visible).

Treatment needs

0 No treatment needed.

1 Oral hygiene needs improvement.

2 1+ professional scaling.

3 1+ professional scaling.

4 1+ professional scaling + complex treatment.

Advantages

1. Permits rapid examination of a population to determine periodontal treatment needs.
2. American Academy of Periodontology has proposed that the index may be used for periodontal screening and recording tool for general practioner.

Periodontitis as a manifestation of systemic diseases

Disease	Features
Papillon-Lefevre syndrome	• Characterized by hyperkeratotic skin lesions, severe destruction of periodontium and in some cases, ***calcification of dura***. • Cutaneous and periodontal changes appear together before the 4 yrs age. • It follows an autosomal recessive pattern. Parents are not affected and both must carry the autosomal gene for the syndrom to appear in child. Males and females are equally affected.
Down synd; trisomy 21	• Prevalence of periodontal disease in it is higher, i.e. almost 100% in patients younger than 30 yrs.
Chediak-Higashi	• Decreased neutrophil chemotaxis and secretion. • Neutrophil granules fuse to form large granules known as megabodies.

Periodontitis as a manifestation of systemic diseases (*Contd.*)

Disease	Features
Hypophosphatasia	• Rare; familial; skeletal disease. • C/F: rickets; poor cranial bone formation; premature loss of primary teeth; esp the incisors. • Low levels of serum alk Pase enz. • Phosphoethanolamine is present in serum and urine. • Teeth are lost with no clinical evidence of gingival inflammation and show reduced cementum formation. • In adolescent, the disease resembles localized juvenile periodontitis.
Localized aggressive periodontitis	• Age of onset is around puberty. • Involvement of first molars and incisors • A ***striking feature*** of this form is **lack of clinical inflammation** despite the p.o. deep pockets. • Amount of plaque on affected teeth is minimal. • Plaque contains elevated levels of **Actinobacillus actinomycetamcomitans** and in some patients, Porphyromonas gingivalis. • **Other C/F: distolabial migration** of max incisors with concomitant diastema formation. Increased mobility of first molars; sensitivity of denuded root surfaces to thermal and tactile stimuli and deep, dull radiating pain during mastication. • **R/G: arc-shaped loss** of alveolar bone extending from the distal surface of 2nd premolar to mesial surface of the 2nd molars **Immunological defects**.

Periodontitis as a manifestation of systemic diseases (*Contd.*)

Disease	Features
	• Functional defects of PMNs, monocytes or both; these defects can impair either the chemotactic ability or their ability to phagocytose. • Hyperresponsive monocytes producing large quantity of PGE-2 on lipopoly-saccharide stimulation. • Poorly functional form of monocyte receptor, Fc-gamma-RII, the receptor for IgG 2 antibodies.

Skeletal disturbances manifested in the jaws (Also refer to the section of oral pathology in volume I for details.)

Osteitis fibrosa cystica	• Also known as **Recklinghausen's dis of bones.** • Develops in advanced primary or sec. hyper-parathyroidism and causes osteoclastic resorption of bone with fibrous replacement and haemorrhage with **hemosiderin deposition** creating a mass known as **brown tumor.** • It results in scattered cyst like radiolucent areas throughout the jaws and a **generalized disappearance of the lamina dura**.
Paget's disease	• **Lamina dura is absent**. • Normal trabecular pattern is replaced by hazy, fine trabecular markings or scattered radiolucent areas may contain irregularly shaped radiopaque zones.
Fibrous dysplasia	• May appear as a small radiolucent area at a root apex or as an extensive radiolucent area with irregularly arranged trabecular markings.

	• **Ground glass appearance.** • **Obliteration of lamina dura.**
Langerhans cell histiocytes	• Appear as single or **multiple radiolucent areas** which may be unrelated to the teeth or entail destruction of tooth supporting bone.
Osteopetrosis	• The **outlines of the roots may be obscured** by diffuse radiopacity of the jaws.
Scleroderma	• The **PDL is uniformly widened** at the expense of surrounding alveolar bone.

EPIDEMIOLOGY

Incidence = i.e. number of new cases occurring in a defined population during specific period of time.

I = no. of new cases of specific dis. During a given time period × 1000/population at risk.

Prevalence = all current cases, i.e. old and new. Existing at a given point of time (point prevalence) (AIPG–2004) or over a period of time in a given population (period prevalence).

P = no. of all current cases of specified dis existing at a given point or period time × 1000/estimated population.

Relationship = prevalence = incidence × mean duration.

Cross-sectional study = single examination of a cross section of population at one point in time.

Longitudinal study = observations are repeated in the same population over a prolonged period of time by follow up examinations.

Case control study, i.e. retrospective study

- Both exposure and outcome/disease have occurred before the start of the study.
- Study proceeds backwards from effect to cause.

- Study uses a control or comparison group to support or refute an inference.

Cohort study, i.e. prospective study

- Cohort—A group of persons exposed to the same sort of environment.
- Proceeds forward from cause to effect.
- A study began in 1970 with a group of 5000 adults who were asked about their Gutka consumption; the occurrence of cancer was studied in this b/w 1990–1995. This is an example of cross-sectional study/retrospective cohort study/concurrent cohort study/case–control study.
- **Epidemic** = the unusual occurrence in a community or region of disease clearly in excess of expected occurrence.
- **Endemic** = constant p.o. of a disease or infectious agent within a given geographic area or population group.
- **Sporadic** = sporadic means scattered; cases occur irregularly from time to time.
- **Pandemic** = an epidemic affecting a larger proportion of population and occurring over a wide geographical area such as section of a nation, a continent or the world.
- **Sensitivity** = proportion of subjects with the disease **who test positive.**

  Se = no. of subjects who test positive/no. of subjects with disease.
- **Specificity** = proportion of subjects without the disease **who test negative.**

  Sp = no. of subjects who test negative/no. of subjects without disease.

Question

The usefulness of a screening test in a community depends on (AIPG-2004).

Sensitivity/specificity/reliability/prediction values _____.

Normal development of a child

Prenatal:Embryofetus	End of 2nd week to 1 month From 1 mo till birth
Postnatal	
Neonate	2 wk to 1 mo
Infant	1 mo to 1 yr
Preschool	1 yr to 3 yrs
Primary school	4 yrs to 8 yrs
Middle school	8 yrs to 12 yrs
Pubertal	13 yrs to 15 yrs

Self notes:

GINGIVAL INFLAMMATION

Stage	Lesion
I	Initial
II	Early
III	Established
IV	Advanced

Main features of different stages of gingivitis

Stage I	Stage II	Stage III
Also known as initial lesion	Also known as early lesion	Also known as established lesion
Of 2–4 days duration	Of 4–10 days duration	Of 2–3 wks duration
Acute inflammation		Chronic inflammation
Main cells are PMNs	Lymphocytes antibodies	Plasma cells which produce

Main features of different stages of gingivitis (*Contd.*)

Stage I	Stage II	Stage III
Vascular changes, i..e. dilatation of capillaries is the first response	Erythema, i.e. colour change is seen; Bleeding on probing.	Colour modified due to congested blood vessels, Hb breakdown, etc.
Loss of perivascular collagen	Collagen destruction esp of circular and dento-gingival fibers	Increased collagenolysis due to enz collagenase
Most coronal portion of JE is altered	JE shows rete pegs formation	Increased rete pegs
Esp Fibrin present		Increased levels of enz alk and acid Pases.

Important points

- Gingivitis is the **most common** type of gingival disease.
- **Chronic marginal gingivitis/simple gingivitis** is the most common type of gingival disease.
- **Contained gingivitis** = the stage in which T-lymphocytes are preponderant. As the severity increases, the no. of B-cells increase.
- Initial response of gingival to plaque is = **subclinical**.
- First clinical **symptom**—bleeding.
- In stage II, the first clinical **sign** of gingivitis is = colour change.
- Cells of acute inflammation are—PMN and lymphocytes.
- PMNs = also cause phagocytosis in gingival.
- Intercellular spaces in JE widen through which the PMN cells migrate in the gingival sulcus.
- Bacterial composition in gingivitis is cocci and rods, which changes to spirochetes and motile organisms in periodontitis.
- Cells of chronic inflammation are—macrophages, lymphoid cells
- Collagen destruction occurs especially of circular and dento-gingival fibers are affected.
- Main fibers affected are circular and dento-gingival fibers.

- Extension of lesion into alveolar bone is the fourth stage known as advanced lesion or the stage of **periodontal breakdown.**
- 2 earliest s/s of gingivitis are—increased GCF formation and bleeding on probing.
- **Bleeding** on probing appears earlier than change in the colour, etc. It is an objective sign. Mostly, the sites which bleed are predominantly lymphocytic, i.e. stage II.
- Most common cause of abnormal gingival bleeding is chronic gingival inflammation.
- Bleeding is due to dilatation and engorgement of the capillaries, which come closer to the surface of the epithelium. And thinning /ulceration of SE.
- Bleeding sites are collagen poor and inflamed CT have cellular infiltrate rich in lymphocytes.
- Bleeding in ANUG = is due to ulceration of necrotic surface epithelium and the engorged blood vessels are exposed in the CT.
- Systemic causes of bleeding—purpura; hypoprothrombinemai, i.e. vitamin K deficiency; hemophilia; leukemia; Christmas disease; multiple myeloma; anticoagulants, e.g. dicumarol and heparin; salicylates, etc.

Surface texture

Condition	**Surface**
Gingivitis	Loss of stippling
Chronic inflammation; exudative	Surface is smooth and shiny
Chronic inflammation; fibrotic	Surface is firm and nodular
Senile atrophic gingivitis	Smooth
Chronic desquamative gingivitis	Peeling of the surface
Hyperkeratosis	Leathery
Non-inflammatory gingival hyperplasia	Minutely nodular surface

Colour change: Normal colour is coral pink.

- Black line = due to Bi, As, Hg.
- **Burtonian line** = i.e. bluish red/deep blue linear; due to Pb.
- Violet marginal line = due to Ag argyria.

Types of gingivitis

Type	Features
Acute	Painful; comes suddenly; short duration.
Subacute	Less severe phase of acute condition.
Recurrent	Reappears after treatment or spontaneously disappears and reappears.
Chronic	Slow; of long duration; painless.
Localized	Confined to gingival irt a single or a group of teeth.
Generalized	Involves entire mouth.
Marginal	Involves gingival margins.
Papillary	Involves I/D papillae but may involve margins also; earliest signs of gingivitis most often occur in papillae.
Diffuse	Affects gingival margins + AG + I/D papillae.
Localized marginal	Confined to one or more areas of marginal gingival MG.
Localized diffuse	Extends from the margin to mucobuccal fold but limited in areas.
Localized papillary	Confined to one or more interdental spaces in a limited areas.
Generalized marginal	i.e. GM irt all the teeth are involved.
Generalized diffuse	Involves entire gingival; the **alveolar mucosa/ AM is also affected**; so the demarcation b/w AM and AG is lost.

SULCULAR FLUID

- Also known as gingival crevicular fluid, i.e. GCF.
- Is an inflammatory exudates, not a continuous transudate.
- Very little or no fluid found in strictly normal gingival.
- Collected by microcapillary pipette or absorbing strips.
- **Brill technique** = strip is placed inside the sulcus or pocket.
- **Loe and Holm Pederson technique** = strip is placed at the entrance of the pocket.
- Measurements are done by periotron.
- JE and SE are permeable to substances of M wt upto 1 million.
- Glucose conc is 3–4 times greater than in serum.
- Total protein conc is very less as cp to serum.
- Main Ig present are = G, M, A.
- C3 and C4 also present.
- **Protective role** = as cleansing agent; antibacterial agent; due to WBCs, Abs and adhesive actions.
- **Circadian rhythm** = GCF increases from 6 AM to 10 PM; and then decreases.
- Female sex hormones increase GCF as they increase vascular permeability, e.g. in pregnancy; oral contraceptives; ovulation, etc.
- Vigorous gingival brushing increases GCF.
- GCF increases during healing after the PD surgery.
- Tetracycline/doxycycline excreted in GCF; and so it is preferred in gingival diseases.
- **Main WBCs** found in GCF are **neutrophils,** i.e. PMN cells approx 92%, these are phagocytic and protective; these are also present in saliva, where their main source is gingival sulcus.
- Ratio of T-cells to B-cells is 1:3, which is the reverse of serum, i.e. 3:1.

Saliva (Also refer to section of physiology and dental histology in vol 1 and 2.)

- Antibacterial factors: lysozymes, Lactoperoxidase–thiocynate system/i.e. LPT; antibodies.
- LPT system is bactericidal to certain strains of Lactobacillus and Strept. By preventing accumulation of lysine and glutamic acid.
- Main antibodies in saliva = secretory IgA.
- **Main antibodies in GCF** = IgG.
- IgA of parotid saliva can inhibit attachment of oral mucosal and dental surfaces.
- Major enz in saliva is **parotid amylase**.
- Certain glycoproteins bind to many plaque–forming bacteria which aids in formation of plaque.
- Certain glycoproteins having BLOOD GROUP REACTIVITY inhibit sorption of bacteria to tooth surface and mucosa.
- Most important **salivary buffer**—is bicarbonate–carbonic acid system.
- **Coagulation factors** present in saliva are 8–12 factors.
- **Principal cells** are PMN cells; WBCs reach saliva by passing through gingival sulcus lining.
- **Xerostomia** = it is seen in Sjogren's syndrome; Mikulicz disease; sarcoidosis; irradiation, etc. it causes increases dental caries; gingival diseases, etc.

Normal clinical features of gingiva

Colour	• Normal colour is coral pink; esp of AG and MG. • AG is demarcated from adjacent alveolar mucosa by mucogingival line MGL. • Alveolar mucosa is red; shiny and smooth. • H/E = epithelium of alveolar mucosa is thin/non-keratinized; no rete pegs present. • CT of alveolar mucosa = loosely arranged; more numerous blood vessels.

Normal clinical features of gingiva (*Contd.*)

Contour	• MG—collar like fashion and follows scalloped outline on facio-lingual surfaces. • Gingival margin is knife-edged.
Consistency	• Firm and resilient, tightly bound to underlying bone except free margin. • Collagenous lamina propria/CT and gingival fibers cause firmness.
Surface texture/ stippling	• Orange peel appearance of surface due to stippling. • AG is stippled; MG is not. • Central part of I/D papilla is stippled; but its margins are smooth. • Less on lingual surface than the facial surface. • Varies with age; absent in infancy; begins to disappear in old age. • Is produced due to papillary layer projecting into elevations on the epithelial surface. • Is a form of adaptive specialization or reinforcement for function and is a feature of healthy gingiva. • Degree of keratinization and prominence of stippling are related. • It disappears in gingival disease due to oedema.
Keratinisation	• It is also a protective adaptation to function. • There is a CT based genetic determination of the type of epithelial surface.
Position	• Is the level at which gingival margin is attached to the tooth. • Varies with eruption of tooth but depth of gingival sulcus is maintained by remodeling of OE, JE, REE.

Continuous tooth eruption

- Eruption continues throughout life.
- It has active and passive phases.
- **Active eruption** is the movement of tooth towards OP; it is coordinated with attrition.
- **Passive eruption** is exposure of tooth by apical migration of gingival; is a **pathological process**.
- **Anatomic crown** = part of the tooth covered by enamel.
- **Anatomic root** = part of the tooth covered by cementum.
- **Clinical crown** = part of the tooth projecting in oral cavity.
- **Clinical root** = part of the tooth covered by PD tissues.
- When tooth reaches the OP at its functional antagonist, the clinical crown is approx 2/3rd of the anatomic crown.
- **Passive eruption** is divided in 4 stages:

Stage	JE position	Base of gingival sulcus
I	On enamel	On enamel
II	Partly of enamel partly on cementum	On enamel
III	On cementum	At CEJ
IV	On cementum	At cementum; a part of cementum is exposed.

- Proliferation/migration of JE on root is due to degeneration of gingival and PDL fibers and their detachment from the tooth.
- Distance b/w apical end of JE and alveolar crest remains same throughout continuous tooth eruption, i.e. 1.07 mm.
- Exposure of tooth by apical migration of gingival is known as gingival recession/atrophy.

DENTIFRICES

Components	% age	Functions
Detergent, e.g. sodium lauryl sulfate;	1–2	• Lowers the surface tension. • Loosens the debris/stains for easy removal. • Foaming action.
Abrasive	25–60	• Abrasive action on deposits.
Binder, e.g. alginate; cellulose, etc.	1–2	• Prevents separation of solid and liquid ingredients. during storage.
Humectant, e.g. glycol; sorbitol, etc.	20–40	• Retains moisture and prevents hardening on exposure to air.
Flavoring agent, e.g. peppermint oil; cinnamon oil, menthol, etc.	1–1.5	• Helps to mask the less pleasant flavors of other ingredients.
Water	15–50	• To create gel or paste consistency.
Preservative, sweetener and colouring agents	2–3	• Preservative to prevent the bacterial growth, e.g. alcohol, benzoates, formaldehyde, etc. • Sweeteners give pleasant taste, e.g. sorbitol, glycerine, etc. • Colours give attractiveness, e.g. vegetable dyes.
Therapeutic agents	0–2	• Fluorides = anticaries, e.g. NaF, etc. • Plaqueinhibitors, e.g. chlorhexidine, triclosan, etc.

DENTIFRICES (*Contd.*)

Components	% age	Functions
		• Desensitizing agents = occlude the open dentinal tubules, e.g. stannous fluoride; potassium nitrate; strontium chloride, etc. • Tartar controlling agents = inhibit the formation of calculus supragingivally, e.g. disodium pyrophosphate; zinc citrate, etc.
Recently incorporated therapeutic agents		• Anti-plaque = triclosan; chlorhexidine; stannous fluoride; vitamin P factor; sanguinarine. • Anti-tartar = enz pyrophosphatase. • Anti-calculus = 0.3% triclosan; 2% gentrez.
PM tooth brush, i.e. proton magnesium brush		• No tooth paste required. • Electrically operated. • It uses saliva to conduct an electric shock to remove plaque.

GINGIVAL ENLARGEMENT

Localized	Limited to the gingival adj to a single tooth or group of teeth.
Generalized	Involves the gingival throughout the mouth.
Marginal	Confined to MG only.
Papillary	Confined to I/D papillae.
Diffuse	Involves MG, AG and I/D papillae.

GINGIVAL ENLARGEMENT (*Contd.*)

Discrete	An isolated tumor like growth.
Drug induced	Esp by phenytoin; cyclosporine and nifedipine; it is generally gingival hyperplasia, i.e. increased no. of cells; lesion is mulberry shaped; firm pale; minutely lobulated; does not occur in edentulous area; fibroblast to collagen ratio is normal; elongated rete pegs and hyperplasia of CT occurs; only GM and I/D papillae are involved, (as cp to idiopathic gingival hyperplasia, in which MG, AG and I/D papillae are involved).
Leukemic enlargement	Is due to dense infiltration of immature and proliferating leukocytes; it is mainly found in acute or subacute leukemia but seldom in chronic leukemia. Gingival is bluish red and moderately firm.

- Systemic administration of phenytoin accelerates the healing of gingival wounds in non-epileptics by decreasing collagen degradation due to production of an inactive fibroblastic collagenase. But may cause megaloblastic anemia and a folic acid deficiency (AIPG—95).
- Cyclosporine is immuno-suppresent drug to prevent organ transplant. It reversibly inhibits helper T-cells;

ANUG

- Also known as trench mouth; **Vincent's infection,** etc.
- **Vincent's angina** = i.e. with involvement of the throat and larynx also.
- Punched out; crater like depressions at the crest of the I/D papillae extending to the marginal gingival; surface covered by gray pseuodmembranous slough.
- Metallic taste; thick pasty saliva; constant radiating gnawing pain; foul smell.

- It **does not lead to formation of PD pockets,** because the necrotic changes involve the JE; and a viable JE is required for formation of the pockets.
- Caused by **spirochetes (borrelia vincenti) and fusiform bacilli (treponema)**. Specific cause of ANUG has not been established.
- **4 zones** of the lesion are seen as:
  - zone 1 **bacterial zone** = most superficial.
  - zone 2 **neutrophil rich** zone.
  - zone 3 **necrotic** zone.
  - zone 4 zone of **spirochetal infiltration.**
- Mostly, intermediate sized spirochetes are found.
- There is increased levels of IgG and IgM antibodies to intermediate sized spirochetes and B. melaninogenicus subsp intermedius.
- Depression of host defense mechanism—Depressed PMN chemotaxis and phagocytosis.
- **Role of cortisol** = stress causes increased secretion of cortisol, which is associated with **depression of lymphocytes and PMN functions,** which may predispose to ANUG.
- ANUG is non-contagious but transmissible.
- It is more common in children with Down syndrome than in other retarded children.
- In agranulocytosis–inflammation is very less than ANUG, which is due to decreased host resistance and decreased number of PMN cells.
- Streptococcal gingivostamatitis is caused by strept. Viridans.
- Gonococcal stomatitis is caused by Neisseria gonorrhoeae.
- Acute herpetic gingivostomatitis is caused by herpes simplex virus HSV. It most frequently occurs in children younger than 6 yrs of age. Inclusion bodies are found in nucleus of the cells, which may be colony of virus particles. It is contagious and may be present as subclinical infection.
- Vesicles of Acute herpetic gingivostomatitis; H. zoster; varicella/ chicken pox reveal eosinophilic intranuclear inclusion bodies in the peripheral cells.

Differences b/w slow progressing and rapidly progressing periodontitis

Slow progressing periodontitis	**Rapidly progressing**
In 50–60 yrs age	In 20–35 esp in young adults
Associated with abundant plaque	Scantier plaque
Slow pace of development	Rapid bone destruction
No defects in neutrophils functions	Defective neutrophils and monocytes chemotaxis

Types of marginal periodontitis according to severity and degree of tissue destruction:

- Mild if 2–4 mm loss of attachment.
- Moderate if 4–6 mm loss of attachment.
- Severe if more than 7 mm loss of attachment.

♦ Juvenile periodontitis occurs in children and adolescents.

♦ Post juvenile periodontitis occurs in adults, i.e. 18–30 yrs age.

♦ Refractory periodontitis = cases not responding to treatment or recurring after treatment.

♦ Generalized juvenile periodontitis = e.g. in Papillon-Lefevre syndrome; hypophosphatasia; agranulocytosis and Down's syndrome, etc.

Extension of gingival inflammation

♦ It extends along collagen fibers and follows the course of blood vessels and loose tissues. Interproximally, it spreads in the loose CT and transseptal fibers and then in the bone at the crest of interdental septum. It leads to **horizontal bone loss**. The site at which it enters the bone depends on the location of vascular channels; facially and lingually, it may spread along outer periosteal surface.

- In TFO, the inflammation spreads b/w transseptal fibers directly into the PDL. It leads to **vertical bone loss** in TFO.
- Rate of bone loss—0.2 mm/yr on facial surfaces; and 0.3 mm/yr on proximal surfaces. Loss of attachment precedes the loss of alveolar bone by 6–8 mos.
- Osteoclast remove the inorganic part of the bone, while mononuclear cells remove organic part of the bone. During bone resorption, fatty marrow is replaced by fibrous marrow. Periodontal destruction is **episodic**. During destructive activity, T-cells change to B-cells and plasma cells. During healing, bone is formed adj to sites of bone resorption to buttress weakened bony trabeculae, which is known as **Buttressing bone formation**. The shelf like thickening of alveolar margin is known as **lipping**.
- The newly formed osteoid is more resistant to resorption as it is non-calcified, than the mature bone.
- Radius of action of bone resorption factors is 1.5–2.5 mm. Beyond 2.5 mm, they do not have any effect. Interdentally, the angular defects can only occur in spaces wider than 2.5 mm. On facial surfaces of anterior teeth, the bone thickness is lesser and so only horizontal bone loss occurs.

Furcation involvement

- Mandibular first molars are most common sites and the maxillary premolars are the least common.
- Diagnosis is done by Naber's probe which is a blunt probe.

Different gradings

Grade I	Incipient bone loss
Grade II	Partial bone loss
Grade III	Total bone loss
Grade IV	Total bone loss with gingival recession. It is also known as visible furcation.

- Furcation areas are most sensitive to injury from excessive occlusal forces.

JUVENILE PERIODONTITIS

- 2 types, i.e. localized and generalized.
- Causes of generalized JP—Papillon-Lefevre syndrome; Downs syndrome; nerutopenia; leukemia; hypophosphatasia; prepubertal periodontitis.
- Papillon-Lefevre syndrome = hyperkeratotic and ichthyosis skin lesion; severe loss of periodontium; calcification of dura; the cutaneous and periodontal lesions appear before the age of 4 yrs; primary teeth are lost by 5–6 yrs of age; and permanent teeth by 15 yrs of age; there is no osteoblastic activity; autosomal recessive.
- Downs syndrome = is trisomy 21; mental and growth retardation; high incidence of PD dis and gingivitis esp in lower anterior regions; decreased resistance to infection; defective T-cell maturation and chemotaxis; increased no. of B. melaninogenicus.
- Hypophosphatasia = abnormal alk Pase activity; early loss of primary teeth esp incisors.
- **Prepubertal periodontitis** = occur during or after eruption of primary teeth; neutrophil and monocytic defects; extreme acute inflammation of gingival tissues and rapid bone loss.

LOCALISED JP; LJP = is a disease of periodontium occurring in an otherwise healthy adolescent, which is characterised by a rapid loss of alveolar bone about more than one tooth of the permanent teeth; the amount to destruction manifested is not commensurate with the amounts of local irritants.

- **Main bacteria** involved = Actinobacillus, actinomycetemcomitans and capnocytophaga.
- Site = esp the first molars and incisors area which are the first erupted teeth, with least destruction of canine-premolar area; bone loss is bilaterally symmetrical.
- Rapid bone loss; 3–4 times than in the typical periodontitis.
- Bone loss is vertical and arc shaped.
- Absence of clinical inflammation in p.o. deep PD pockets.
- Plaque does not tend to mineralize.
- Mobility and migration (esp distolabial migration of max incisors) of involved teeth.

Histopathology

- Bacteria invade the CT reaching the bone surface.
- Mainly plasma and blast cells accumulate.
- More **unattached plaque** is present; plaque is non-mineralized.
- Epithelial attached subgingival plaque is responsible for LJP.
- There is **functional chemotactic defect of PMN** as the main cause.

Destructive mechanisms are:

- **Inhibition of PMN chemotaxis**; and hence pahgocytosis is reduced.
- Due to endotoxins and leucotoxins produced by the microbes.
- Due to production of fibroblast inhibitory factors.
- Collagen destruction by proteolytic enzymes.
- By direct lytic action.

Treatment options

- LJP has better prognosis than GJP.
- Surgery and antibodies are required, because microbes remain in the tissues even after scaling and root planning.
- Scaling, root planning, curettage, bone grafts, etc.
- Antibiotics = tetracycline 250 mg qid for 14 days every 8 weeks; bone loss was stopped.
- Transportation of 3rd molar to 1st molar site
- Extraction of teeth is the last resort.

Host response: **the basic concepts**

- Difference b/w tissue/host collagenase and bacterial collagenase is that former destroys the collagen completely, while latter just splits the collagen, which have the tendency to reunite when bacteria are removed.
- Monocytes form macrophages, which give cell mediated immunity.

- T-cells provide cell mediated immunity.
- B-cells provide humoral immunity.
- B-cells/B-lymphocytes form plasma cells in spleen and lymph nodes.
- Plasma cells form Ig, which give **systemic humoral immunity**.
- Plasma cells form Abs, which give **local humoral immunity**.
- Ig has 2 parts, i.e. Fc and Fab. Fc is heavy chain and is complement binding site, while Fab is light chain and is Ab binding site.
- **Secretory IgA** is more resistant to digestion by proteolytic enzymes than other Igs.
- IgA is in salive.
- IgM is first formed after infection.
- IgE appears in allergies; is reaginic Ab.
- IgG is most abundant; known as blocking antibody.

Tissue responses

- Type I/anaphylaxis = (mast cells + IgE complex) reacts with Antigen/Ag—and then histamine, etc. are released which lead to tissue damage.
- Type II/cytotoxic = cell's Ag reacts with Ab, e.g. RBC, autoimmune disease and produce hemolysis of cells.
- Type III/Arthus' reaction = Ag reacts with Ab and lead to local tissue damage due to lysosomal enzymes.
- Type IV/delayed hypersensitivity—CMI = lymphocytes react with Ag and so lymphokines are released. Here, no Abs are involved.

PLAQUE: Also known as **microcosm**

- It is a thin, transparent film on the tooth surfaces which are not properly cleaned, consisting of bacteria; leucocytes; desquamated epithelial cells; etc.
- It is complex, metabolically interconnected highly organized system.

- It appears as a thin tenacious gelatinous film on the tooth surface, which accumulates within 24–48 hrs after removal to its normal thickness.
- An important component of plaque is **acquired pellicle,** which is a glycoprotein derived from saliva and adsorbed on tooth surface and it covers the whole tooth and facilitates plaque formation. It does not have any bacteria; but may serve as a nutrient for bacteria; it is formed within 30 min after removal and within 24 hrs to its normal thickness (0.1–0.8 microns). It is acellular.
- ***Materia–alba*** can be removed with water jet but plaque cannot be.
- In plaque; most numerous organisms were aciduric streptococci in caries process.
- PH of plaque in caries active person is approx 5.5.
- ***3 main organism in plaque*** are strept mutans; veillonella and actinomyces.
- *S mutans* synthesise **Glucan** from dietary sucrose. This glucan/dextran is insoluble, sticky gel, inert and resistant to attack by bacterial hydrolytic enzymes, which causes plaque to adhere to the tooth surface and acts as a barrier against the diffusion of salivary buffers which tend to neutralize the acid produced by the bacteria.
- **Sucrose** gives rise to glucose and fructose. Glucose forms dextrans and fructose forms levans.
- Dextrans are maximum carbohydrate in plaque.
- Plaque is mainly bacteria, i.e.70–80%.
- 1 cu.mm = 1 mg plaque = contains 10^8 bacteria.
- Types of plaque—supragingival and subgingival.
- Supragingival is—coronal and marginal types.
- Subgingival is—tooth associated, i.e. attached; epithelium associated; and unattached.

Bacterial adherence

In gingival sulcus	On enamel	On tongue
Bacteroides	Str mutans	Str salivarius
Spirochetes	Str sanguis	A. naeslundii
	Lactobacilli	
	Actinomyces viscosus	

Composition of plaque according to its age—with accumulation of plaque and development of gingivitis, there is both qualitative and quantative change in plaque.

1 day	Cocci
3 days	Rods
5–7 days	Filaments
7–10 days	Spirochetes
3 wks	Corn cob appearance
2 mos	Bristle brush appearance
Early gingivitis	Actinomyces filaments
Long standing gingivitis	Fusobacterium and veillonella
On active sites	B gingivalis; B intermedius; A actinomycetamcomitans
On Treated sites	Esp str. sanguis
Adult periodontitis	B gingivalis

- Salivary IgA—prevents bacterial attachment.
- Most nutrients for the formation of supragingival plaque are provided by saliva. Strept and actinomyces are initial colonizers, they use salivary carbohydrates as nutrients.

Attached plaque/tooth associated subgingival plaque	1. Mainly G + bacteria predominate. 2. G(–) rods in apical part 3. Cocci and filaments are perpendicular to tooth surface. 4. They cause: calculus formation; **root caries** and resorption and alveolar bone loss (**slow** progressing PD diseases). 5. Apical border of plaque is **some distance from JE** and that gap is filled up with WBCs.
Epithelial associated subgingival plaque	1. **Extends upto JE** 2. Mainly consist of G (–) rods; cocci and spirochetes. 3. Causes **rapid alveolar bone destruction.** 4. **No root caries.** 5. Extremely periodontopathic. 6. Has higher virulency. 7. May penetrate epithelium and CT.
Unattached plaque	1. Has G(–) rods; cocci. 2. Extends to JE. 3. Is associated with gingivitis.
In LJP and rapidly	1. Tooth associated plaque is minimal; progressing periodontitis but epithelial associated plaque is extensive. 2. Plaque is very virulent. 3. Epithelial associated plaque is more dangerous.

- Microbes are 43 millions to 5.5 billions/ml; average is 750 millions.
- Most of the salivary bacteria are derived from dorsum of the tongue.

- Str sanguis and other G + cocci are the major bacteria which initiate supragingival plaque.
- At healthy sites, especially G + cocci, e.g. str. sanguis mainly and A. viscosus facultative bacteria are present.
- In patients with PD diseases, influence of supragingival microbes and plaque–control procedures appear to be limited to approx 4 mm into the pocket.
- Subgingivally, main source of Ig and C is GCF.
- Athymic rats show increased bone loss.
- Progressive PD dis are associated with B-cells dominated lesions.
- After scaling and root planning, increased Abs levels occur esp to Bacteroides.

Major bacteria which initiate supragingival plaque	Str sanguis and other G + cocci.
In healthy sites	G + cocci, e.g. str sanguis mainly and facultative A. viscosus
Initial gingivitis	By A viscosus and A israelii, G + rods. Bacterial succession is required to produce disease, i.e. from G + cocci to G + rods to G(–) rods.
Pregnancy gingivitis	Bacteroides intermedius and capnocytophaga; are anaerobes. It is associated with increased levels of estrogen and progesterone, because these hormones serve as nutrients for these species.
ANUG	Borrelia vincenti; Bacillus fusiforme.
Slow progressing periodontitis	By A israelii; and A naeslundii; by tooth attached plaque.
In subgingival plaque	Increased G(–) capnophilic and anaerobes.

Rapidly progressing PD	By B gingivalis; B intermedius; Wollinella recta; Eikenella corrodnes; Actinobacillus actinomycetamcomitans;
Refractory periodontitis	By B gingivalis; B intermedius; Actinobacillus actinomycetamcomitans;
LJP	Main microbes are sacchrolytic, capnophilic, anaerobic G(–) rods; e.g. **Actinobacillus actinomycetamcomitans** is the most common microbes; which can penetrate into **connective/ gingival tissues**; they produce leucotoxins; epitheliotoxins; collagenase, etc. for its spread into the CT; so antibiotics are must for the Rx. Other microbe is capnocytophaga. There is altered chemotactic effect.
Prepubertal PD	Occurs during or after eruption of primary teeth; most common microbe is Actinobacillus actinomycetamcomitans; also capnocytophaga and B intermedius. Severe defect of PMN and macrophages.
Mainly G(–) facultative anaerobes are main bacteria associated with PD disease	e.g. bacteroides species, i.e. B gingivalis; B intermedius; Wollinella recta; Eikenella corrodnes; Actinobacillus actinomycetamcomitans.

Pathogenic mechanism of bacteria in PD diseases

Invasion

Production of exotoxins

Role of cell constituents, i.e. endotoxins; surface components; capsule, etc.

Production of enzymes.

Evasion of immunologic host responses.

Host-bacteria interaction

Endotoxins	1. Penetrate gingival epithelium. 2. Alternate path of complement system is activated—occurs at C3 but C1, 4, 2 is byepassed. 3. Cause localised Schwartzman reaction. 4. Activate factor 12 causing intravascular clotting. 5. Is cytotoxic. 6. Cause bone resorptin.
Hyaluronidases	1. Influence gingival permeability by allowing apical proliferation of JE along the root surface and increases intracellular gaps. 2. Bacteroides and A actinomycetamcomitans produce collagenases. 3. Phopholipase A may initiate alveolar bone resorption as a precursor of prostaglandins.
Ig	Are deactivated or destroyed by proteases.

Immune findings in periodontal diseases

ANUG	1. Periodontal chemotactic defects. 2. Increased Ab titers to B intermedius.
Adult periodontitis	1. Increased Ab titers to B gingivalis, etc. 2. Immune complex present in tissues. 3. CMI to gingival bacteria. 4. Immediate hypersensitivity to gingival bacteria.
LJP	PMN chemotactic defect and depressed phagocytosis increased Ab titers to A actinomycetamcomitans
GJP	PMN chemotactic defect and depressed phagocytosis increased Ab titers to B gingivalis
Prepubertal	PMN and monocytic chemotactic defect.
Refractory periodontitis	Reduced PMN chemotaxis.

Facts about immunoglobulins

Reaction	Ig	Cells, etc.
Anaphylactic/regain dependant reaction	IgE	From mast cells, basophils
Cytotoxic	IgM, IgG	
Immune complex/ Arthus reaction	IgM, IgG– lysozymes	Complexes occur in tissues and blood vessels
Cell mediated/ delayed hypersensitivity	Lymphokines, Osteoclast activating factors	T-cells

Neutrophil associated PD diseases

Neurophil disorders associated with PD disease	1. Diabetes mellitus. 2. Papillon-Lefevre syndrome. 3. Down syndrome. 4. Chediak-higashi syndrome. 5. Drug induced agranulocytosis. 6. Cyclic neutropenia.
PD diseases with neutrophil disorders	1. ANUG. 2. LJP. 3. Prepubertal periodontitis. 4. Rapidly progressing periodontitis. 5. Refractory periodontitis.

Cellular predominance

In healthy sites	G + cocci
In early gingivitis	T-cells predominate
In advanced gingivitis	Plasma cells predominate
In periodontitis	B-cells predominate
T4:T8 ratio	2:1 in gingivitis 1:1 in periodontitis < 1 in AIDS (reversed ratio due to destruction of T4-cells)

CALCULUS

- Calculus is mineralized plaque.
- It helps to keep plaque in close contact with the gingiva.
- 2 types: supragingival; subgingival.
- **Supragingival calculus** = coronal to the gingival margin; whitish yellow in colour; hard clay-like consistency; easily detached from tooth; esp present on the lingual surface of lower incisors opposite Whaton's duct; buccal surface of maxillary molars opposite Stensen's duct; also called **salivary,** because it is derived from saliva.

- **Subgingival calculus** = below the crest of the marginal gingival; is not visible in oral cavity; dense dark brown colour; hard in consistency; firmly attached to tooth; also called **serumal,** because it is derived from GCF and blood serum.
- **Supragingival calculus** has 70–90% inorganic component; mainly consisting of calcium phosphate.
- **The ratio of** Ca to P is higher subgingivally, and the Na content increases with the depth of PD pocket.
- Calculus is mineralized plaque, which starts b/w 1–14 days of plaque formation. At 2 days, it is 50% mineralized, and at 12 days, it is 60–90% mineralized. Microbes are not required for calculus formation.
- Plaque cannot mineralize in acidic atmosphere. Calcification starts in the inner surface of supragingival plaque and in the attached component of subgingival plaque; **filamentous bacteria increase** with the calcification.
- Average daily formation of calculus is 0.10–0.15% of dry wt.
- Material-alba = is an acquired bacterial coating; is clearly visible without the use of disclosing agents. It can be flushed away with a water spray. It lacks a regular internal pattern which is seen in plaque.

Dental stains

Brown	Fe; pigmented pellicle. Tobacco stains are dark brown; tenacious.
Black	Fe; Ag; chromogenic bacteria, e.g. Actinomyces (main cause); B melaninigenicus. Black stains which occur on human primary teeth is typically associated with low incidence of caries.
Green	Cu; Ni. Penicillium and Aspergillus. Usually occur on the facial surface of the maxillary anteriors.

Dental stains (*Contd.*)

Orange	Serratia marcescens and Flavobacterium lutescens.
Metallic	**Mn-black stains.** **Hg-greenish black.**
Chlorhexidine stains	Retention is due to its affinity to sulfate and acidic groups yellowish to brownish colour appears.

Old bacteria with new terminology

Bacteroides gingivalis	Porphyromonas gingivalis
Bacteroides intermedius	Prevotella intermedius
Bacteroides	Prevotella melaninogenicus
Wolinella recta	Campyobacter recta

Classification of mobility of the teeth

Grade I	0.5–1.0 mm facially or lingually.
Grade II	1–2.0 mm facially or lingually.
Grade III	> 2 mm in horizontal or vertical/apical direction.
Physiologic mobility	Shows circadian rhythm, i.e. highest in morning, lowest in evening greater in females; increases in pregnancy; decreases in lactation; most mobile are upper incisors.

Gingival grafting procedure

Condition	Procedure
Long narrow gingival defect on a single tooth.	Best is laterally positioned flap.
Pockets extending to MGJ; thick manageable pocket wall.	Apically positioned flap.
Soft friable pocket wall.	Gingival extension procedures with free gingival graft
Absence of AG with no pockets only recession is present with non pathologic dehiscence.	Free gingival graft.

Interdental embrasures

Type I	No gingival recession	Dental floss is indicated.
Type II	Moderate papillary recession	I/D brush like proxa brush, miniature bottle brush indicated.
Type III	Complete loss of papilla	Unitufted brush indicated

Differences b/w gracey and universal currets

Area of use	Area specific	Universal; anywhere
Cutting edge	Only outer edge; used with pull stroke	Both edges are used
Curvature	2 planed; curvature is upwards and sidewards	One plane instrument
Blade angle	Offset of 60 degrees	90 degrees
Side specificity	For left and right side separate	No specificity

Suturing techniques

Technique	Indications
Direct or loop sutures	Need for coverage of I/D bone with I/D papilla. When bone graft is used.
Figure of eight	When flaps are not in close adaptation due to apical flap displacement of non-scalloped incisions.
Sling ligation	When flap involving 2 I/D spaces and opposite flap not reflected.
Horizontal mattress suture	Used in wide I/D spaces to adapt the I/D papilla against the bone.
Anchor suture	Closing of flap mesial or distal to tooth as in mesial or distal wedge procedure.
Periosteal suture	Used to hold apically displaced partial thickness flap.

Special days

2003	International year of fresh water.
11th April	National safe motherhood day.
11th July	World population day.
14th Nov	World's diabetes day.
16th Sept	International ozone day.
1st July	Doctor's day.
1st Oct	Senior citizen day.
1st Oct	International blood donation day.
21st May	Anti-terrorism day; Rajiv Gandhi's death day.
22nd March	World water day.
22nd May	World biodiversity day.

Special days (*Contd.*)

24th March	World TB day.
26th June	International day vs drug abuse.
26th Sept	World's heart day.
27th Sept	World tourism day.
2nd Sunday of May	International mother day.
31st May	World no-tobacco day.
4th May	World asthma day.
5th June	World environment day.
7th April	World health day.
7th April	WHO day.
8th March	International women's day.
Road safety	Theme of world health day 2004.

- White ribbon alliance for safe motherhood/India: WRAI.
- National nutrition week—1–7th sept 2004.

Common occlusal interferences

Position	**Maxillary cusps**	**Mandibular cusps**
RCP	Mesial inclines of lingual cusps (CR); these are to be removed first	Distal inclines of lower cusps and MR of PM and molars
Protrusive prematurities	Distofacial inclines	Mesiofacial inclines
Mediotrusive or balancing contact	Inner inclines of lingual cusps or non-working (not a pathologic interference)	Inner inclines of buccal cusps
Laterotrusive or working	Inner inclines of buccal cusps	Inner inclines of lingual cusps

VARIOUS DENTAL MEDICAMENTS

Component	Function
EDTA	Chemical reaming of root canals;
Disodium edetate	Chelating agent for reaming RCs
Parachlorophenol + thymol + camphor	Antiseptics for RC disinfection
Dexamethasone	Decreases inflammation of RCs
Chlorohexidine digluconate 20% and ethyl alcohol	For RC decontamination by acting on anaerobes
Iodoform paste	Acute and chronic infections of RC Esp in deciduous teeth Does not interfere with permanent teeth
Calcium hydroxide	RC decontamination; due to its high pH Helps sec dentin formatin Has a chemical neutralizing effect on acids from cements/mouth
Endomethasone	RC sealer; has ZnO + eugenol; Antiseptic; thymol iodide + para-formaldehyde Anti-inflammatory; corticosteroids Radiopaque; barium sulfate
Tetrachloroethylene	RC filling remover
Pulp sedative for pulpitis	Lidocaine HCl as anesthetic Creosote as sedative Phenol/eugenol as antiseptic and disinfectant
Pulp vitality testing	Tetrafluororethane and ethyl alcohol
KNO_3; HEMA; sodium fluoride	For Rx of dentinal hypersensitivity
Fluoride Rx	Knutson's tech; at 3, 7, 10, 13 yrs age

VARIOUS DENTAL MEDICAMENTS (*Contd.*)

Antiseptic for hands	By chlorohexidine gluconate + methyl parahyeroxybenzoate + propyl parahyeroxy-benzoate
Disinfection of instruments	Aldehyde + quaternary ammonium compounds + corrosion inhibitors
Disinfection of impression material	By ampholytic surfactants + isopropyl alcohol (bactericidal, fungicidal, viricidal) also 2% glutraldehyde solution for 10 min.

Nutritional deficiencies

Vitamin C deficiency = known as scurvy; retardation of wound healing; increased susceptibility to infections; haemorrhagic lesions into ms of extremities and joints; defective formation and maintenance of collagen; retarded osteoid formation.

Relation of vitamin C deficiency and PD diseases.

- Low levels of vitamin C influence the metabolism of collagen in periodontium, and so affect the ability of tissues to regenerate and repair.
- It interferes with bone formation leading to loss of periodontal bone.
- It increases the permeability of oral mucosa and of crevicular epithelium.
- Vit C is required to maintain the integrity of the PD vasculature.
- Vit C deficiency interferes with the ecologic equilibrium of bacteria in plaque and so increases the pathogenicity of plaque.
- PD fibers least affected by vitamin C deficiency are those below the JE and above the alveolar crest.

Vitamin D deficiency = it may lead to rickets in infants and osteomalacia in adults.

Osteoporosis of alveolar bone; reduction in the width of PDL; defective mineralization of osteoid and cementoid; generalized partial to complete disappearance of lamina dura; increased radiolucencies of trabecular interstices, etc.

Hypervitaminosis D = increased osteoblastic activity; osteoscelerosis; dystrophic calcification in PDL; hypercementosis and ankylosis of many teeth.

Calciphylaxis = is a condition of induced systemic hypersensitivity, in which tissues respond to appropriate changing agent with local calcification.

Hormonal influences on periodontium

Hypothyroidism	Causes cretinism in infants and myxodema in adults. Delayed physical and mental development occurs. Increased weight; feeling of cold; non-pitting edema of subcutaneous tissues; low BP and BMR. Chronic PD dis with severe bone loss.
Hyperthyroidism/ thyrotoxicosis	High BP; cardiac enlargement; loss of wt; high BMR; heat intolerance; exophthalmos; increased growth and development; early eruption of teeth. Osteroporosis of alv bone; increased size of marrow spaces and increased width of PDL.
Hypopituitarism	Due to deficiency of hormone by anterior pituitary. Retardation of growth of all tissues; dwarfism; delayed eruption of teeth; skeletal Class II relation of jaws; underdeveloped sinuses esp frontal sinus.
Hyperpituitarism	Due to increased secretion of hormone by anterior pituitary. Acromegaly or gigantism occurs; disproportionate growth of facial and body

Hormonal influences on periodontium (*Contd.*)

	bones; skeletal Class III jaw relation esp increased size of mandible. Marked overgrowth of alveolar process; increased size of dental arches; spacing b/w teeth; hypercementosis.
Hypoparathyroidism	Due to accidental removal of parathyroid gland. Hypocalcemia and tetany occurs; if it occurs in infancy, it causes enamel hypoplasia.
Hyperparathyroidism	Generalized demineralization; bone cysts; giant cells tumor; serum Ca conc. increased; serum P level decreases. Tooth mobility; malocclusion; alveolar osteoporosis; widening of PDL; absence of lamina dura.
Diabetes mellitus	Hypofunction of beta cells of islets of Langerhans; glucose levels of blood and GCF high; a decreased camp levels in GCF; (camp reduces inflammation, so in diabetics, there is more inflammation). Altered response of PD tissues to local irritants; Altered flora of oral cavity; decreased salivary flow. Reduction in defense mechanism, increased susceptibility to infections; increased bone loss. Tendency of abscess formation; diabetic periodontoclasia; greater loss of attachment; increased tooth mobility.

Hormonal influences on periodontium (*Contd.*)

	H/E: thickened walls and narrowed lumen of arterioles; increased thickness of basement membrane of capillaries. Main bacteria: S epidermidis; staphylococci. Immunology—infections are due to PMN deficiencies resulting in impaired chemotaxis; defective phagocytosis, etc.
Gonads	Progesterone produces dilatation of gingival microvasculature, which increases susceptibility to injury and exudation; Estrogen-counteract tendencies of hyperkeratosis of epithelium and fibrosis of vessel walls; also stimulates bone formation and fibroplasia. Testosterone—retards downgrowth of sulcular epithelium over the cementum; restores osteoblastic activity; increases cellularity in PDL.
Pregnancy	Gingivitis increases during 2nd or 3rd month and decreases during 9th month depending on the levels of hormones; gingival is edematous; pitting; bright red to bluish red in colour; raspberry appearance. Main microbe is B intermedius, it can substitute progesterone or estradiole for vit K as growth factor. Progesterone produces dilatation of gingival microvasculature and stasis, which increases susceptibility to injury and exudation.

Hormonal influences on periodontium (*Contd.*)

	Destruction of gingival mast cells by increased sex hormones and release of histamines may lead to increased inflammatory response.
HEMATOLOGIC EFFECTS ON PERIODONTIUM	
Leukemia	Immature leukocytes infiltrate the gingival corium leading to enlargement esp of I/D papilla. Highest incidence is in cases of acute monocytic leukemia; then acute myelo-monocytic leukemia. Not found in edentulous patients. Gingival colour is bluish red and cyanotic. Gingival bleeding is due to thrombo-cytopenia, which is due to replacement of bone marrow by leukemic cells; it also decreases the tissue resistance to in-fections and leads to ulceration.

Reader's Notes

Reader's Notes

Reader's Notes

Reader's Notes

Reader's Notes

Reader's Notes

READER'S RESPONSE FORM

Readers are requested to fill the following form and mail it to us giving their invaluable suggestions about the strength and weaknesses of this book for further improvement of the future editions and volumes of this book. The successful students are also requested to contribute generously their ideas and notes for inclusion in further editions of this series for the benefit of their younger friends preparing for the PG entrance examinations. The criticism from the fellow readers and students will be highly appreciated.

1. **Name and address of the student:**
2. **Qualification:**
3. **Phone No. and E-mail i.d:**
4. **Good points about the book:**
5. ______________________________

____

____

____

____

____

____

6. **Problems faced while studying this book:**

____

____

____

____

____

____

____

____

____

7. **Experience of successful candidates while preparing:**

8. **Missing points / topics in this book:**

9. **Contributions from the students in the form of tables, MCQs, latest patterns of exams in different states etc:**

Thanking all of you in anticipation.

Dr. Sandeep Goyal